Acclaim for The Concussion Crisis

"Thoughtfully passionate and comprehensive. . . . Quite a devastating testament. It lays it all out and forces us to ponder how a civilized people can blithely accept an entertainment that does such damage to young men's minds. . . . One lays *The Concussion Crisis* down wondering where future American gridiron gladiators will come from; surely not from families who read this book."

—Frank Deford, *The Washington Post*

"In *The Concussion Crisis*, health writer Carroll and sportswriter Rosner team up to offer a jolt on the head—intellectual only—to those who've tended to dismiss blows to the noggin as innocuous. . . . The book is a clarion call to take full measure of the broken brains and bodies among us."

—*The Globe and Mail* of Canada

"Important. . . . A book everyone involved with football or concerned about the sport must read."

—Gregg Easterbrook, ESPN.com

"*The Concussion Crisis* should be required reading for parents, teachers, amateur and professional athletes, coaches, trainers, and anyone interested in the health of children and young people. . . . Linda Carroll and David Rosner have crafted a riveting look at a health crisis that is finally coming to light after decades of denial. They make a convincing case. . . . People who read this fascinating and eye-opening book will never think about concussions and head injuries in the same old way."

—Connie Goldsmith, R.N., *New York Journal of Books*

"A very hot topic. . . . This noteworthy book issues a challenge to the 'macho play-through-the-pain' sports culture and urges a rethinking of safety versus spectacle."

—*Publishers Weekly*

"A cautionary wake-up call about addressing a seemingly innocuous hit to the head with critical care. . . . A comprehensive, anecdote-laden analysis of concussive head traumas."

—*Kirkus Reviews*

"A powerful call for action on the part of parents, coaches, and older athletes. . . . A good primer for parents whose kids play contact sports such as football."

—*Booklist*

"This valuable book brings an important public health issue to light. Highly recommended."

—*Library Journal*

"This book makes a convincing case for a radical shift away from [macho] attitudes, towards an understanding of concussion as a mild traumatic brain injury with potential for long-term, permanent changes in brain functioning and behaviour. . . . Anyone involved in contact sports, and many who aren't, will find *The Concussion Crisis* accessible and educational. It could help prevent a lot of needless and preventable suffering."

—**Ursula Fuchs, R.N.**, *Winnipeg Free Press*

"*The Concussion Crisis* puts a human face on traumatic brain injury through real-life stories of athletes and soldiers. The authors define the problem, explain the science, and accentuate the need for prevention. This informative book sounds a much-needed alarm for medical intervention, continued research, and a reassessment of how we play sports."

—**Michael J. Stuart, M.D.**, co-director of the Mayo Clinic's
Sports Medicine Center and chief medical officer of USA Hockey

"There is no injury I worry about as a coach more than concussions, and this book shows why. It's a must-read for athletes and their parents."

—**Anson Dorrance, coach of the USA's first World Cup women's soccer champions and of UNC's twenty-time NCAA champions**

"Carroll and Rosner tell some utterly heartbreaking stories, but their book, ultimately, offers hope by giving readers the information and resources they need to confront a public health crisis. They show us that a concussion does not have to be a life-altering event, but it can be if it is not properly recognized, respected, and treated."

—**Michael Sokolove, author of *Warrior Girls: Protecting Our Daughters Against the Injury Epidemic in Women's Sports***

"Linda Carroll and David Rosner convincingly maintain that lots of people regard concussions as a nuisance rather than as potentially life-altering brain injuries. If their book educates some of those people—particularly those of them coaching and/or parenting young athletes—then they will have performed a worthwhile service."

—**Bill Littlefield, host of NPR's *Only a Game***

THE
CONCUSSION
CRISIS

Anatomy of
a Silent
Epidemic

**Linda Carroll
and David Rosner**

Simon & Schuster Paperbacks

New York   London   Toronto   Sydney   New Delhi

Simon & Schuster
1230 Avenue of the Americas
New York, NY 10020

First Simon & Schuster trade paperback edition February 2012

SIMON & SCHUSTER and colophon are registered trademarks
of Simon & Schuster, Inc.

For information about special discounts for bulk purchases,
please contact Simon & Schuster Special Sales at
1-866-506-1949 or business@simonandschuster.com.

The Simon & Schuster Speakers Bureau can bring authors
to your live event. For more information or to book an event,
contact the Simon & Schuster Speakers Bureau at
1-866-248-3049 or visit our website at www.simonspeakers.com.

Designed by Nancy Singer

Manufactured in the United States of America

10 9 8 7 6 5 4 3 2 1

The Library of Congress has cataloged the hardcover edition as follows:

Carroll, Linda, 1956–
    The concussion crisis : anatomy of a silent epidemic / Linda Carroll, David Rosner.
        p. cm.
    1. Brain—Concussion. 2. Brain—Phisiology. 3. Cognitive neuroscience. 4. Sports
injuries—Treatment. I. Rosner, David, 1956–. II. Title.
    RC394.C7C37 2011
    617.4'81044—dc22
      2011010457

ISBN 978-1-4516-2722-0
ISBN 978-1-4516-2745-9 (pbk)
ISBN 978-1-4516-2746-6 (ebook)

For all those whose lives have been changed by the invisible injury

Contents

Contents

Introduction

For more than a decade, a small cadre of scientists had been raising the alarm. Their message was simple and scary: concussions were on the rise and research was showing that these jolts to the brain were a lot more dangerous than any of us thought. While the impact of one jolt to the head tended to be transient, researchers were learning that the brain damage from concussions could not only add up, but also become permanent. And that was especially true if these "mild" traumatic brain injuries occurred in rapid succession.

Since most of us had been brought up with the assumption that a head injury that didn't result in a trip to the hospital could be ignored, no one was keeping count of our own—or our children's—concussions. Moreover, since we'd been raised in a culture that celebrated hard knocks as a rite of passage, we didn't think twice when our kids got banged around on the ballfield.

But as it turned out, some of the most frightening research was in children—especially those playing contact sports. Kids' brains, scientists learned, were exquisitely sensitive to repeated jolting. Concussions, if they weren't managed properly, could derail a kid's life. Thinking could be slowed, attention dulled, judgment impaired, memory muddled. Those changes could make school impossible and send a kid on a downward spiral.

Unfortunately, studies had also shown that many parents were unaware of the dangers facing their children. A 2010 survey found that just 8 percent of parents felt they had a good background on the dangers of repeat concussions. More than a third said they knew virtually nothing about concussion risks, while fully half said they didn't even know whether their children's school had a policy detailing when a student-athlete could return to play after a concussion.

Other studies showed that this was a particularly bad time for parents to be ignorant about the dangers of concussions. A silent epidemic of these unseen brain injuries among kids had been exploding right under our noses. And nowhere was that more true than on the nation's playing fields. In just ten years, visits to the emergency room for concussions among eight- to thirteen-year-olds had doubled, while visits among fourteen- to nineteen-year-olds had more than tripled, a 2010 study showed. And that was just the tip of the iceberg, experts warned, since it didn't include all the kids who were seen by their family doctors or had never even told anyone about their symptoms. It was clear that the public had to be warned and educated about the danger of injuries that had long been dismissed as "dings" and "bumps on the head."

The Concussion Crisis lays out the history of how we came to underestimate the damage resulting from jolts to the head and how scientists, over the last couple of decades, began to recognize that there was an emerging silent epidemic of brain injuries, especially in sports. While nobody knows exactly how many concussions occur, estimates by the Centers for Disease Control and Prevention range anywhere from 1.6 million to 3.8 million sports-related brain injuries in the United States annually. Those CDC estimates don't include concussions from accidents such as playground falls and bicycle collisions. Whatever the actual number of concussions is, one thing researchers do know is that nearly a quarter of a million new patients turn up each year with long-term deficits resulting from these so-called mild traumatic brain injures.

In the following pages, you will see how the epidemic was able to explode unseen into a major public health crisis. It was partly because of the invisible nature of the injury: we didn't understand how people could develop life-altering deficits as the result of something that didn't even show up on a brain scan. Making matters worse was the macho attitude threading throughout our culture: we figured that anyone who complained about issues related to simple bumps on the head was either a sissy or a malingerer.

Nothing can convey the menace of concussions more clearly than the heartrending stories of people whose lives have been irrevocably changed by these seemingly minor injuries. In the pages that follow, you'll read about individuals like the twelve-year-old boy who was so disoriented after a concussion that he couldn't even recognize familiar faces for almost a year, the college football player who had to drop out after a series of concussions made schoolwork impossible, the Ph.D. economist whose career was ended after her thinking was muddled by a jolt in a fender bender.

Until very recently, many people, including doctors, thought of concussions as "a different animal" from severe traumatic brain injuries. But as you read the stories of people who survived horrific car wrecks and wartime bomb blasts, you'll be struck by how similar their symptoms are to those experienced by people whose lives have been derailed by repeated concussions.

Only in the past few years has science begun to explain why that is so. This book will take you into the labs where cutting-edge research is showing why concussions are such serious injuries. You'll meet the scientists who discovered how multiple concussions could add up and leave the same kind of damage as a single severe brain injury.

While all this new science is scary, even more frightening is emerging evidence that concussion damage can remain hidden for years only to show up later as early-onset dementia. You'll learn how scientists discovered that repeated blows absorbed by boxers set many of them up for neurodegenerative disease and how a small band of researchers recognized that the boxing paradigm could also be applied to football. What drove these researchers was a need to explain the haunting stories of National Football League players who slipped into early-onset dementia before they even hit middle age. The latest research shows that a single moderate to severe brain injury can result in changes that increase a person's risk of dementia, while multiple jolts to the head can have the same impact.

Although better testing and treatments may someday help reduce the scourge of concussion damage, what is needed today is for Americans to learn about the true nature of this invisible injury—and to understand its severity and potential to upend a life.

Chapter 1

Just a Bump on the Head

Concussions caught up with Dave Showalter before he could play a single down of college football.

A big, burly kid whose passion for the sport seemed wound as tightly through his DNA as his large brown eyes and fine chestnut hair, Showalter was playing tackle football almost from the time he could walk. While he impatiently waited to grow old enough to join a team, he made do roughhousing at home with his two big brothers. The three would shove the furniture against the walls and position the couch as a goalpost, turning the living room into a playing field for games of "knee football." Their objective wasn't so much to score touchdowns as to rough each other up in the process; casualties of the games often included their mother's bric-a-brac as well as their own heads.

When he reached fourth grade, Showalter finally got his chance to strap on the shoulder pads, pull on a helmet, and play for real. He was grateful that his parents had chosen to send him to a Catholic school that, unlike the neighboring public schools in central Pennsylvania, allowed kids as young as nine to play tackle football.

Already weighing well over a hundred pounds, he was so big that by league rules his helmet had to be marked with a black X and he wasn't allowed to carry the ball or to play glamour positions such as quarterback and running back. An offensive lineman by default, he quickly learned to make the most of his size. At the center of all the crashing and crunching on the line of scrimmage, he would often thrust headfirst into opposing linemen with reckless abandon.

By the time he reached high school, Showalter seemed an indestructible force at six foot four and 260 pounds, his imposing size amplifying the sense of invincibility that naturally comes with youth. All of that allowed him to shake off his concussions as if they were common colds. He played through headaches and nausea and a strange metallic taste that exploded in his mouth after hard helmet-to-helmet hits. He kept quiet about the scary symptoms for fear that telling anyone—his coaches, his trainers, even his parents—might cost him playing time; and besides, having been weaned on football's just-rub-dirt-on-it ethos since fourth grade, he could shrug off each jarring hit as "just getting my bell rung."

It wasn't until the summer before his junior year that a concussion symptom finally brought Showalter up short. He'd be walking around the house and suddenly his vision would fade to black. The blackouts would last several seconds, and though he never lost consciousness, he'd have to grab on to something solid to steady himself. He didn't understand what was happening, and he was frightened that it meant something had gone seriously wrong with his brain. He suspected that the blackouts were related to a concussion he had sustained during summer football camp when he was kneed in the head and briefly knocked unconscious. As much as he loved the game, he decided to give it up and concentrate on other sports.

That resolve lasted barely a season. One afternoon before basketball practice, his old football coach strode into the locker room looking for Showalter. The coach dropped a plastic shopping bag full of recruiting letters on the bench where Showalter was suiting up and said, "I was going to throw these away, but it's a federal offense to mess with your mail. This is something you need to think about, something you could be missing out on." Showalter pulled out a handful of unopened envelopes and saw return addresses from some of college football's powerhouses— Notre Dame, Nebraska, Penn State. As he ripped open the envelopes and started reading, Showalter for the first time realized that he might be able to parlay one more season of high school football into a college scholarship. The more he mulled it over, the less he could think of any reason not to return to the gridiron, especially since his concussion symptoms had completely disappeared.

His comeback seemed perfect. Showalter was playing better than ever, his team was rolling through the season undefeated, and his head felt fine. Even when he took a hard helmet-to-helmet hit late in the season, he just shook it off and kept playing until his team scored a touchdown. Only after he returned to the sideline did anyone notice something was wrong. The trainer glanced down the bench and saw that Showalter seemed dazed, just staring up at the stars beyond the Friday night lights. After taking a closer look, the trainer determined that Showalter was dizzy and disoriented enough to be pulled from the game. During halftime, Showalter tried to argue his way back onto the field, uncharacteristically crying, yelling, and even cursing at the trainer. This time the concussion was so bad that the trainer sidelined Showalter not only for the rest of that game, but also for most of the next week's practices. By the following Friday night's game, Showalter had convinced the trainer that he'd recovered enough to return to action.

As his team moved through the state playoffs, racking up two victories before losing in the quarterfinals, Showalter came more into focus for college recruiters. Now they could see firsthand that not only was he big, at six foot five and 280 pounds, but he was also quick and agile. They recognized raw potential that could be shaped by weightlifting and the right coaching. They could see that this kid had the brawn to excel in major-college football, the brains to shine in the classroom, and the determination to make all those dreams come true. By the time Showalter chose which athletic scholarship would be his ticket out of the depressed railroad town of Altoona, his concussion symptoms were a distant memory and his prospects seemingly boundless.

At Rutgers University, the coaches had big plans for their rough, uncut gem. They would "redshirt" him as a freshman, sitting him out of games through the 1998 season so he'd start his playing career as a sophomore with all four years of eligibility remaining. That gave them a year to sculpt his maturing body through long, grueling hours in the weight room and to teach him blocking techniques that relied more on using his hands than his helmet. He began his sophomore year, an inch taller and forty pounds stronger, as the backup offensive tackle to a senior bound for National Football League stardom.

Then, just a month into his first season on the Scarlet Knights roster, while Showalter was warming up for a game he wasn't even scheduled to play in, his life was upended in a split, and stunning, second. Since it was just pregame warm-ups, he hadn't bothered to buckle his chinstrap or to put in his mouthpiece, and he certainly wasn't expecting his own teammate to crash into him with enough force to knock him to his knees. He knew he was in trouble right after the helmet-to-helmet hit flooded his mouth with that familiar and frightening metallic taste. Although teammates later told him he spent the game on the sideline charting plays as usual, he remembers nothing until halftime, when he asked for Advil to quiet a searing headache. After that, he doesn't remember anything—not the second half of the loss to Wake Forest, not the plane ride home to New Jersey from North Carolina, not even a minute of practice the next day.

Despite amnesia, insomnia, headaches, and dizziness, Showalter soldiered on all week as if nothing had happened. He continued banging helmets every day at practice, then ratcheted up the intensity on Saturday when he finally got into a game. At the next day's film session, as he watched replays of the game with his teammates, Showalter couldn't remember a single play he'd made, not even the block he threw to clear the way for his roommate's touchdown run. As if by pure instinct, he kept right on practicing each weekday and then playing on Saturdays as a late-game substitute. Every time he made contact, his symptoms worsened—the headaches growing into migraines, the dizziness escalating into vertigo. Within a few weeks, just a hundred-yard sprint down the field was enough to send his head spinning.

Still, it wasn't any of the symptoms he experienced on the gridiron that finally persuaded Showalter to seek help—it was something that happened in the classroom. A month after the Wake Forest game, he dug out his spiral notebooks to prepare for midterms. As he leafed through the pages filled with meticulous notes, he started to get scared. Nothing looked familiar. He tried to recall the lectures that went with the notes and realized he couldn't remember even being in the classes that the handwriting proved he'd attended.

Showalter had always had the kind of memory that allowed him to read through a page of notes and immediately conjure up an image of the professor actually speaking the words. He was prouder of that detailed and dependable memory—and the academic achievements it helped garner—than any of his athletic accolades. He had graduated near the top of his high school class, earning membership in the National Honor Society with a 3.75 grade point average. He had chosen to attend Rutgers, over universities with stronger football programs, because of the academic opportunities it promised. Once there, despite the full-time commitment of playing big-time college football, he continued to shine in the classroom, making dean's list with a 3.5 grade point average and securing a spot on the Big East Conference All-Academic Team.

Now suddenly, before he could complete his first season playing for Rutgers, the athletic prowess that had earned him this academic opportunity was threatening to take it away. Worried he was on the verge of losing everything he'd worked so hard to achieve, Showalter finally was able to push past football's macho code and admit to the team physician, "Listen, I think something has happened to me." Exactly what that was would remain a mystery until Showalter went to see the team neuropsychologist.

Jill Brooks looked up from the medical charts spread out on her desk as Dave Showalter stepped into her office for his initial consultation. She was struck by his soft, rounded features and his kind brown eyes. The face didn't seem to fit the powerful, sculpted form towering over her; and his soft-spoken, easygoing manner didn't match the intense and fierce temperament usually associated with the position he played. Brooks could see this was not your typical jock.

When Showalter started to describe what had happened to him, though, it became clear that his story was all too typical. It was a story Brooks had heard countless times in nearly a decade of treating college and high school athletes for concussions at Robert Wood Johnson University Hospital in New Brunswick, New Jersey.

She started to prod Showalter for more details about the helmet-to-helmet collision in the warm-ups at Wake Forest.

"Do you remember getting a strange taste in your mouth after you got hit?" she asked.

Showalter's large eyes widened. "Yes," he said slowly. "How did you know that?"

"Was it a kind of metallic taste?" Brooks asked.

His eyes widened further. He was surprised that this specialist seemed to know all the details of a bizarre symptom he thought he alone had experienced. "Yes. It's happened every time I got hit hard. Nobody's ever been able to tell me what it was."

Brooks explained that the taste was a sign he'd suffered an "impact seizure" and that it was not uncommon for badly concussed athletes to experience one. "What it means is that the force of the hit was so hard and so directed that you had a seizure on impact. The electrical activity in your brain was disrupted because of the force. We call it an impact seizure because you might think you had epilepsy if we simply called it a seizure and typically impact seizures are just one-shot events."

Showalter was silent, the word "seizure" leaving him too stunned to respond.

"The other symptoms—how long did it take for them to go away?" Brooks asked.

Showalter hesitated. He was getting more nervous. "They haven't gone away," he said. "They've just gotten worse."

Showalter told Brooks about his amnesia, the dizziness, and the headaches. He told her that his brain felt foggy and that he'd been having trouble concentrating. He admitted that the symptoms worsened with even the slightest bump by another player.

Brooks wrote it all down, and then, after a brief pause, told him what it meant.

A concussion, she explained, was a serious injury. It wasn't just a "ding" or just "getting your bell rung."

"You can't look at it any other way, because this is an injury to your brain," she said, "and your brain controls everything that you do—from breathing to moving your extremities to your thinking to your emotions. Your brain controls it all. And if you get repeated injuries and repeated impact seizures, you start having difficulties with thinking in class and with follow-through and with sadness and with all that other stuff."

A concussion, she went on, needed to be taken as seriously as any visible injury—more seriously, in fact. She told Showalter he needed to give his brain time to heal. He would have to take time off from all physical activities. There would be no football, no weightlifting, no running, no stationary bike. What Brooks couldn't tell him was exactly when he'd be better. "If you broke your ankle, I could tell you it would take six weeks to heal," she said, "but with a brain injury, it's not like that and there's no way of telling how long it's going to take."

Showalter took a few moments to process all the new information. Finally, he said, "I'll be back by next season, right?"

"Dave, you should not be playing football," Brooks said, drawing a deep breath. "You should *never* think of playing football again."

Showalter stiffened. A swarm of thoughts spun through his mind: "This can't be right. She's just being overprotective. I'm young; I'll heal; I'll be fine by next season."

As Brooks watched him mulling over the unwelcome advice, she worried that she had not driven her point home. The silence was going on too long.

"Dave, this could be permanent," she said finally. "You've had multiple concussions—there's no way of knowing how many—and the effects can be cumulative. Your brain might not heal one hundred percent. Your memory might never come all the way back."

The short walk back to campus from the hospital was all a blur as Showalter desperately tried to get his mind around everything Brooks had just told him. As he passed the school's colonial buildings and the site where Rutgers had hosted the nation's first intercollegiate football game in 1869, Showalter pondered the doctor's orders to give up the sport that had defined his identity for as long as he could remember. He had walked into Brooks's office still harboring dreams of playing in the NFL, and now he suddenly had to resign himself to this new reality that didn't include football at all.

Over the next few months, Showalter followed her prescription for allowing his brain to heal. By the end of the school year, all the concussion symptoms seemed to have resolved. His memory was back, his brain clear. He felt so much better that he figured he could ignore Brooks's recommendation to give up football.

He played the next season for Rutgers without being sidelined by concussions—but his transcript was starting to reflect their impact. That semester, he failed a course for the first time ever as his grades spiraled downward. He couldn't understand why schoolwork, which had always come so easily, was now impossible. He was embarrassed by his grades, and depressed.

To make matters worse, when Showalter's injured ankle failed to rebound the following spring from a third surgery, his coach pulled him aside and said, "You're done." Cut from the team, Showalter tried to concentrate full-time on academics. But by then, not even all the extra study time could help. He would read the same paragraph over and over and over again, and still not remember a word. That semester, he failed three of his four courses. When fall rolled around, Showalter felt even more depressed, and alone. Unable to count on his brain anymore, he decided to drop out of school.

He moved into a tiny one-room apartment above a corner store, just a short walk from the classrooms where he once felt at home. He traded the semester's scholarship check for a $3,000 car so he could support himself making daily deliveries for a local bagel shop. When Rutgers officials noticed that he had cashed his check but not shown up for classes, they demanded the money back. He immediately started paying down the debt in $25 weekly installments.

In 2007, six years after dropping out of college, Showalter was still living in the same ten-by-ten apartment with a futon for a bed and a hot plate instead of a stove. He still had the delivery job and had begun working with autistic children in the afternoons and evenings at a New Brunswick community center. Some days, he'd sit back and survey his sparsely decorated room and reflect on how his life had turned out. He'd think about the careers he once considered pursuing—teaching, public relations, medicine. This certainly wasn't where he thought he'd be at age twenty-eight. When he left the modest two-story brick house that his parents bought with money scraped together from their jobs at the phone company, he thought his possibilities were boundless. Of the six Showalter children, Dave had been the one everybody knew would make it big. Now he could only dream of someday going back to Rutgers and resuming his studies.

Trying to make some sense of it all, Showalter started giving occasional lectures on the dangers of concussions to coaches and trainers. "I feel like I got lost in the shuffle," he'd tell them, "so it's important to me to raise awareness about brain injuries. They can make a huge impact on a person's life. I mean, I can't even remember much of what happened my last two years in college."

The cautionary tale would always amaze his listeners. Who would ever think that seemingly innocuous bumps on the head could erase entire years from a memory and derail a life?

Chapter 2

The Emerging Epidemic

In the classic image of a concussion, a player is lying motionless on the turf with teammates hovering over him and a trainer racing across the field. Smelling salts are waved under his nose, and the player shakes his head as he comes to. The trainer asks him, "How many fingers am I holding up?" The player's answer is the same as always: two. That's because the trainer makes it easy by always holding up the same number of fingers and then rewarding the correct answer by sending the player right back into the game.

That inside joke among players and trainers depends on the belief that concussions are as harmless and transient as the cartoon stars floating around Sylvester the Cat's head every time he gets bonked. Even the words used to characterize a hit to the head—from merely getting "dinged" to just getting your "bell rung"—make light of any possible consequences. It's hard to take seriously an invisible injury with subtle symptoms that often seem to pass quickly.

Since even before the first recorded wrestling matches five thousand years ago in Mesopotamia, concussions have been an unavoidable part of sports. Nevertheless, they have remained at once the most common and most confusing of head injuries. Only in the past decade have brain injury specialists finally come to a consensus on what constitutes a concussion: any change in mental status such as confusion, disorientation, headache, or dizziness following a hit or jolt. And they all agree that a concussion, contrary to popular belief, does not require loss of consciousness or even a bump on the head.

This definition, however, has yet to permeate the sports world. Many athletes don't even realize when they've sustained a concussion. Unless they're knocked senseless or seeing stars, they'll dismiss symptoms as no more worrisome than a scratch and cover them up for fear of appearing weak. For their part, coaches, trainers, and even team physicians don't understand concussions much better than athletes do.

Because people take them so lightly, concussions often go undiagnosed and undocumented. That's why nobody really knows how many athletes actually sustain concussions each year, let alone how many Dave Showalters are living with permanent brain damage from them. Estimates by the Centers for Disease Control and Prevention (CDC) range anywhere from 1.6 million to 3.8 million sports-related concussions in the United States annually. Whatever the actual number in a nation with more than forty-four million kids playing sports from youth leagues through high school, there's one thing experts agree on: the problem has reached epidemic proportions.

It's remarkable how poorly understood concussion remains today considering that the condition was formally identified over a millennium ago. In the year A.D. 900, the renowned Persian physician and alchemist Rhazes introduced the concept of concussion to the medical world, defining it as a transient impairment of mental status following a jolt to the head. After that, the misconception of concussions as mild, short-lived phenomena would stick stubbornly in the public consciousness. They were the butt of jokes in popular culture everywhere from the Three Stooges to Wile E. Coyote.

But all the concussion jokes stopped being funny when stories started to circulate about kids dying after seemingly innocuous hits on the football field. These weren't highly paid pro football players being knocked out in a profession predicated on violence; they were kids playing a kids' game. Suddenly, the symptoms weren't subtle anymore. They were dramatic and deadly.

• • •

On a brisk fall New England morning in 1984, Dr. Robert Cantu could be found hiking up and down the sidelines of the local high school football field, eyes scrunched in concentration and hands stuffed deep inside his jacket pockets for warmth. Each time one of the teams moved the ball downfield, Cantu would stride after the players and reposition himself on the line of scrimmage. As the sideline physician for high school games in and around Concord, Massachusetts, he wanted to stay as close to the players as possible so he wouldn't miss any potentially serious spine or head injuries.

With a young son already playing Pop Warner football, Cantu had stepped up when town officials came looking for a volunteer to fulfill the state's mandate that a doctor be present at every high school game. He figured that a neurosurgeon, like himself, would be best prepared to spot and to handle the types of injuries inherent in football. So each Saturday morning, the slim, redheaded physician would pull on his jeans, running shoes, and, depending on how bitingly cold the weather was, a windbreaker or parka and then drive over to monitor that week's game. Although Cantu always felt a little nervous as he looked out for injuries, he enjoyed watching football, especially from a vantage point so close to the action.

But on this particular Saturday, Cantu was more worried than usual. As he strode up and down the field, he couldn't get his mind off an article he'd recently read in a medical journal. That article described the death of an unnamed nineteen-year-old college football player three years earlier following a seemingly minor jolt to the head.

In late October of 1981, Enzo Montemurro, a compact five-foot-eight, 190-pound fullback on Cornell University's freshman team, took the field at Dartmouth College eager to show the moves that had made him Toronto's high school MVP. Right from the opening kickoff, Montemurro looked like he was going to have the best game of his young college career, gaining a total of thirty-two yards the first six times he carried the ball. Then, on a routine play where his assignment was to block would-be tacklers from getting to a ball-carrying teammate, Montemurro bumped an opposing player. The contact hadn't been particularly solid, so everyone was shocked when the college freshman suddenly collapsed on the sideline after walking off the field with no apparent problem. The team physician and trainer immediately raced over to help, but within seconds Montemurro lost consciousness and became completely unresponsive. He was loaded into an ambulance and rushed the quarter of a mile to the Dartmouth hospital.

The instant Montemurro was wheeled through the emergency room door, Dr. Robert Harbaugh, the neurologist on call that day, recognized that the situation was dire. Montemurro was in a deep coma, and his breathing was so irregular that he had to be put on a ventilator. A quick test suggested that the pressure in his head was dangerously high. Harbaugh promptly paged the hospital's chief of neurosurgery, Dr. Richard Saunders, who was in the midst of morning rounds. Saunders ordered a CAT scan, which confirmed that there was extensive swelling on the right side of Montemurro's brain.

As the two doctors conferred over what would be the best course of action, Harbaugh looked down at the young Ivy League athlete lying motionless on the hospital bed and thought, "This is a person who has his whole life ahead of him—we've got to do something." Saunders told him that the only hope was to remove a section of Montemurro's skull to relieve the pressure on the brain. Saunders wasn't optimistic about Montemurro's chances, but he agreed that they should do everything possible to try to save the teen's life. Although the operation successfully relieved the pressure on Montemurro's brain, it didn't improve his condition. Four days later his family decided it was time to disconnect the ventilator, and Enzo Montemurro died.

Saunders and Harbaugh were haunted by the heartbreaking tragedy of an athlete inexplicably dying young. At the very least, they needed to be able to explain how such a minor jolt on the playing field could have killed a fit, healthy teen so quickly. While waiting for the autopsy report, they began to ask Montemurro's family, teammates, and coaches about the weeks leading up to the fateful game.

Teammates told Saunders and Harbaugh that Montemurro had been punched in the head during a fistfight four days before the game. He had briefly lost consciousness and went to the Cornell infirmary the next morning complaining of headaches and nausea. Doctors there told him that he had sustained a concussion and should avoid any contact sports until his symptoms resolved. The day before the Dartmouth game, Montemurro asked for medical clearance to play, insisting that his headaches had all but disappeared.

These new details brought to mind a report Saunders had read a few years earlier describing the case of a college football player who died suddenly after a minor hit during a game. The eminent neurosurgeon who wrote the report suggested that that death might have been related to a concussion the player had sustained in an earlier game.

When Montemurro's autopsy results came in, it was clear there had been microscopic damage to his brain that predated the Dartmouth game by several days. That got Saunders thinking about an animal study he'd read years earlier. The study showed that once a certain pressure in the brain was reached, an irreversible sequence of events was triggered that eventually killed the animal. Saunders reasoned that the fistfight had raised the pressure in Montemurro's brain to a dangerous but not fatal level and that the minor jolt during the game had pushed the pressure beyond the point of no return.

The more Saunders and Harbaugh thought about the case, the more they realized its grave implications for all the young athletes playing America's most popular sport. You didn't need a big hit to kill a kid—a series of minor jolts could add up to a catastrophe. Saunders and Harbaugh wrote up their findings to warn doctors across the nation about this unrecognized threat. Wanting to reach the broadest possible audience, they submitted their paper to one of America's most prestigious medical journals. The two-page article, published in the *Journal of the American Medical Association* in 1984, introduced a syndrome that Saunders and Harbaugh dubbed "second impact."

The warning was clear: second-impact syndrome could occur any time an athlete suffered a jolt to the head too close on the heels of an earlier concussion. If the brain didn't have enough time to recover from the initial concussion, a second one could have a much more devastating impact—even when the second resulted from nothing more than a light tap. That second hit could cause the brain to swell catastrophically. But it was the first hit, Saunders and Harbaugh discovered, that had made the player into a walking time bomb.

Saunders and Harbaugh's little paper had a big impact on doctors like Robert Cantu. As he walked the sidelines, Cantu realized that if he missed a concussion today, some kid might get bumped next week and die.

Cantu wasn't worried just about the kids playing right in front of him.

He was thinking about all the kids playing across the nation. He knew that precious few states required sideline physicians as Massachusetts did; few required even an athletic trainer at games. Cantu figured the best way to protect kids from second-impact syndrome was to draw up a set of guidelines that could help coaches and medical personnel figure out when and for how long a concussed player should be sidelined.

At the time, there was no real science to guide him. There weren't studies to show how long it took concussed athletes to recover; there wasn't even a consensus among experts on the definition of a concussion. Cantu could only draw on his more than twenty years of clinical experience diagnosing and treating concussions, not just in athletes injured on the playing field but also in patients who came to his office after falls, car crashes, and other accidents. What he came up with was a set of guidelines linking the severity of concussions to the length of time a player should be sidelined. An athlete with a "moderate concussion," for example, could return to play one week after symptoms had completely dissipated, whereas a "severe concussion" would sideline a player for at least a month.

When Cantu's guidelines were published in the October 1986 issue of *The Physician and Sports Medicine*, there was finally a reference for people trying to manage concussions. While Cantu was the first to admit that his choice of suggested recovery periods was "pure seat of the pants," he figured that they would at least make the point that concussions were serious business and that players often needed to be sidelined.

Moreover, the very existence of a published set of guidelines would send the message that doctors might be able to prevent deaths from second-impact syndrome. Just in case his fellow physicians weren't as scared as he was by the specter of a second-impact death occurring on their watch, Cantu reminded them that lawyers also read journal articles like his. The clear implication was that malpractice lawsuits over poor concussion management were now possible because there was proof that letting a kid come back before his brain had healed could lead to his death. As Cantu traveled the country explaining his guidelines and preaching his gospel that everyone should err on the side of caution, he would drive his point home with his favorite mantra: "When in doubt, sit them out."

The guidelines had far less impact on the medical community than

Cantu had hoped. Kids with significant concussions were still being sent back into the same game in which they'd been injured. Kids who'd been sidelined were returning to play while still symptomatic from concussions suffered weeks earlier. And every parent's worst nightmare was still occurring: kids were still being killed by concussions.

Parents would be reminded of the danger whenever the tragic story of a schoolboy dying after a minor hit cropped up in the local newspaper. On Long Island, seventeen-year-old Billy Rideout played through a concussion sustained in a 1986 high school game, collapsed two weeks later on the sideline right after another hit, and died three weeks afterward without ever regaining consciousness. In West Texas, seventeen-year-old Gabriel Sanchez suddenly collapsed and died after suffering his second concussion of the 1988 season. In Southern California, seventeen-year-old Freddy Mendoza shrugged off headaches from a concussion that knocked him out of a 1991 game, collapsed after a hit in the following week's game, and died two days later.

Though it grabbed headlines and hearts whenever it struck, second-impact syndrome was nevertheless a relatively rare phenomenon. The CDC documented seventeen deaths from the syndrome between 1992 and 1995, though its report cautioned that this could be an underestimate. All the deaths were in young athletes, mostly teens. That didn't surprise brain injury experts because immature brains were known to be more vulnerable to concussions in general.

Although second-impact syndrome didn't always kill, it was always devastating. The aftereffects would plague survivors like Brandon Schultz for their entire lives.

Schultz was a high school sophomore in 1993 when a jarring collision in a junior varsity game briefly knocked him unconscious and sent him to the sideline with a headache so bad that he was grimacing and screaming in pain. Although he continued to complain of headaches all week, none of his coaches ever suggested that he see a doctor or get medical clearance before returning to play—a standard practice in his Anacortes, Washington, school district for even the most minor orthopedic injuries, but not for head injuries. Back in action on the defensive line just a week after the concussion, Schultz made a routine tackle on the last play of the first half. Ten minutes later in the team's halftime huddle, he dropped to the ground convulsing in seizures and lapsed into a coma. He was rushed to the hospital, where doctors discovered that his brain was swelling rapidly and performed the first of four emergency surgeries to reduce pressure on it.

Schultz survived, but with severe brain damage that left the onetime A-student cognitively impaired, partially blind, and physically disabled. With no hope of ever living independently, he was transferred to a long-term-care facility in California. Schultz's family sued the school district on his behalf for neglecting to institute a concussion policy. In a landmark settlement in 1998, five years almost to the day after his life-altering concussion, the school district agreed to pay for the medical care and rehab services Schultz would need for the rest of his life—an estimated $12.6 million.

Despite its catastrophic consequences, second-impact syndrome was easy for athletes to rationalize away: they figured it was so rare that they were more likely to be run over by a car than struck by second-impact syndrome. A far more prevalent problem would be harder to dismiss. It was becoming increasingly clear that repeated hits to the head could lead to lasting symptoms even when concussions came months or years apart. And if you were among the millions watching America's most popular spectator sport on any given Sunday, it was impossible to miss this phenomenon.

With a berth in the 1994 Super Bowl on the line, Troy Aikman wasn't about to let a little thing like being kneed in the helmet by a 290-pound lineman deter him. So the Dallas Cowboys quarterback picked himself off the ground after the crushing tackle and played out the series of downs as if nothing had happened. When he returned to the sideline and started talking gibberish, the team trainer asked if he was OK. "Fine," Aikman shot back. But twenty seconds later, it was clear he wasn't fine. "Give me some smelling salts," he told the trainer. "I'm a little fuzzy. Something's not right." After Aikman began asking what day it was and who the Cowboys were playing, the team doctor diagnosed a concussion and sidelined the superstar quarterback for the rest of the afternoon. When the game was over, Aikman was sent to the hospital for overnight observation as a precaution.

Later that night, his agent, Leigh Steinberg, drove over to Baylor University Medical Center to visit Aikman. As Steinberg made his way through the streets of Dallas, he was struck by the intensity of the city's impromptu celebration: fireworks were booming, horns were honking, fans everywhere were shouting and screaming. The revelry outside contrasted sharply with what he found in the hospital room. It was dark and silent, and Aikman was sitting alone, looking confused and oblivious. As Steinberg made his way over to the hospital bed, his twenty-seven-year-old client's boyish face brightened.

"Where am I?" Aikman asked.

"You're at Baylor," Steinberg replied.

"Was there a game today?" Aikman wondered.

"Yes," Steinberg nodded.

"Did I play?"

"Yes."

"How'd I play?"

"You played well."

"Did we win?"

"Yes."

"Where does that put us?"

"You're gonna go to the Super Bowl."

Aikman's blue eyes lit up and a big smile spread across his face, and then the conversation moved on to other topics. Five minutes later, Aikman paused and asked, "Where am I?"

"You're at Baylor," Steinberg answered hesitantly.

"Was there a game today?" Aikman queried.

"Yes."

"Did I play?"

"Yes."

"How'd I play?"

"Well."

"Did we win?"

"Yes."

"Where does that put us?"

"In the Super Bowl."

Aikman's face brightened into a big smile, and he moved on to another subject. A few minutes later, he again asked Steinberg, "Where am I?" That touched off an instant replay of the exact conversation they'd already had twice. Steinberg was shaken. He had never seen anything like this, and he was worried about what would happen when he left the hospital and was no longer around to answer Aikman's questions. Finally, Steinberg decided to write all his answers down on a sheet of paper so he could leave it on the bedside table when visiting hours ended.

The next day, Aikman flew with his teammates to Atlanta for the Super Bowl. During the week leading up to Super Sunday, he was plagued by headaches and nausea. When Steinberg called to check up on him, Aikman again sounded confused and seemed to think he was still playing for the Henryetta Fighting Hens, his old high school team back in Oklahoma.

Even though Aikman led the Cowboys to their second straight National Football League title that Sunday, he wasn't the same quarterback who had dominated the previous Super Bowl with the clockwork precision of a field general. Afterward, while watching Aikman struggling to recall any plays from the game, Steinberg couldn't shake a feeling of foreboding. Though his marquee client had managed thus far to come back from his concussions, other players hadn't been quite so resilient.

In the fall of 1992, one of football's most electrifying stars, Al Toon, had been forced to retire prematurely by a host of debilitating post-concussion symptoms that wouldn't ease off. Initially, the concussion that knocked Toon out of the NFL didn't faze him any more than the previous eight. A wiry All-Pro wide receiver who'd awed New York Jets fans for eight seasons by making acrobatic catches and withstanding brutal hits, Toon expected to bounce right back from a tackle he didn't think was particularly hard. He shrugged off the usual headaches, dizziness, and mental fog, figuring the symptoms would disappear after a couple of days just as they had after all his previous concussions. But this time, the symptoms tenaciously hung on and then got even worse. He was experiencing memory loss, vertigo so bad he couldn't stand up in the shower, headaches so intense he needed to spend whole days bedridden in a darkened room. Toon went from specialist to specialist in search of relief and answers. None of those doctors could tell him how long it would take for his symptoms to abate or if he'd ever fully recover, but they all agreed that he shouldn't risk another blow to the head. Three weeks after his last concussion, Toon tearfully announced his retirement at the age of twenty-nine.

With that retirement, a new concept entered the sports lexicon: post-concussion syndrome. Toon's story provided a textbook case to illustrate how repeated concussions could lead to a syndrome in which symptoms take longer and longer to ease. It also provided a frightening example of how long the syndrome's classic symptoms—headaches, dizziness, fatigue, mental fogginess, memory loss, irritability, depression—might dog a player.

By the night in 1994 when Steinberg visited Aikman in the hospital, Toon had already been battling his crippling concussion symptoms for more than a year. Steinberg couldn't help but think of the retired player's plight as he spoke with his own bewildered client. He started to wonder how many concussions Aikman's brain could withstand before he wound up in the same situation as Toon. He worried about all the other players on his deep, star-studded client roster—especially the quarterbacks. As the superagent who represented half the starting quarterbacks in the NFL, he knew they were the most vulnerable to the kind of hits that led to severe concussions.

Over the years, Steinberg had become increasingly troubled that the defensive linemen and linebackers who targeted his quarterbacks on every play were growing bigger, stronger, and quicker. Aikman, the prototypical drop-back passer at six foot four and 219 pounds, was easy prey for linemen a hundred pounds heavier than he was.

More worrisome was the situation with Steinberg's other superstar quarterback, Steve Young. As if it wasn't enough that he had already played five seasons longer than Aikman had, Young was even more vulnerable to hard tackles because of his bold scrambling style. A peerless all-around athlete at six foot two and 205 pounds, Young could dominate not only by rifling precise passes but also by darting away from charging linemen and bolting downfield with would-be tacklers in pursuit. On one characteristic play, he ignored teammates' pleas to safely run the ball out of bounds after his helmet came off and instead dashed downfield with his bare head exposed to the headhunters—in a meaningless exhibition game, no less. While Young's fearless and reckless play for the San Francisco 49ers made him the NFL's top-rated quarterback, it also put his brain in harm's way dozens of times every game.

Steinberg remembered the first time he broached the subject of concussions with Young. They were having dinner in a Bay Area restaurant one Sunday night after a game. Steinberg waited for a quiet moment, leaned forward, and asked, "So Steve, I've been wondering, how many concussions have you had?"

"Do you mean official ones?" Young responded.

"What's an *official* concussion?" Steinberg asked.

"Well, an official concussion is when you're knocked out and they cart you off the field and they use smelling salts to revive you."

"So what's an unofficial concussion?"

"That's when you're dazed or stunned and you're not quite there, but you can still play. You'll be impaired like that many times during the season."

"So how many total concussions does that make?"

Young shrugged and then said, "I couldn't even count 'em."

Steinberg found the whole exchange disconcerting. As he left the hospital the night of Aikman's third "official" concussion, Steinberg's brain kept bouncing back and forth between that exchange with Young and the disturbing visit he'd just had with Aikman. The more times Steinberg replayed those two conversations, the queasier he felt. He had just negotiated the richest contracts in NFL history for Aikman and Young, but he was now coming to the conclusion that no amount of money could compensate for the risks they were taking. At that moment, Steinberg decided that an agent owed his clients more than just making them big bucks. He would do for them what they wouldn't do for themselves: protect their brains.

Steinberg started accompanying Aikman and Young to their doctors' appointments. He would come armed with a series of questions for each neurologist: "How many concussions are too many? What are the possible consequences of all these concussions? At what point do these multiple concussions start to imperil an athlete's ability to live a normal life once he gets out of the sport?" It soon became clear that none of the doctors could answer his questions, and that only made Steinberg more nervous.

Still, if concussions were taking a toll, you certainly couldn't tell from the way the two quarterbacks were playing. Aikman and Young were at the top of their game. Through the mid-'90s, they took turns dominating the NFL: Aikman commanding the Cowboys to consecutive Super Bowl conquests in 1993 and '94, Young rifling a record six touchdown passes in the 1995 Super Bowl to lead the 49ers to the title, and Aikman cementing a Dallas dynasty in 1996 by capturing an unprecedented third Super Bowl in four years.

But that was all about to change, and the millions of fans who had been mesmerized by the two quarterbacks' parallel rise would soon be stunned to watch the pair's parallel descent as mounting concussions took a toll. In the 1997 season opener, Young suffered his third official concussion over a ten-month span. Then, midway through the season, Aikman was knocked out of a game with the seventh official concussion of his career. The following week, on the eve of a showdown between the Cowboys and 49ers, Aikman and Young joked with Steinberg that the game ought to be dubbed the "Concussion Bowl." Steinberg was not amused.

The time had come, he decided, to have the toughest talk an agent could have with a fiercely competitive athlete: he asked Young to think seriously about retiring. Even though Young still had several years and millions of dollars remaining in his golden left arm, Steinberg felt it was an agent's responsibility to step in and protect the brain of a client who had earned a law degree in his spare time between NFL seasons.

"Since no doctor can give us a precise answer, we're playing Russian roulette with your identity, your memory, your consciousness, your ability to lead a normal life once you're out of the sport," Steinberg said. "We all understand that a retired player may have to live with aches and pains from old injuries when he leans over and picks up his child, but it's another matter entirely not to be able to recognize that child."

Steinberg delivered the same message to Aikman. The warnings to the two quarterbacks grew increasingly urgent as Steinberg tracked the early retirements of other concussed stars. In the five years since Al Toon had been knocked out of the sport, post-concussion syndrome forced three other NFL stars to retire: fullback Merril Hoge in 1994 at age twenty-nine after his sixth concussion, quarterback Chris Miller in 1995 at age thirty after five concussions in just over a year, and quarterback Stan Humphries in 1997 at age thirty-two after four concussions in less than two years. As for Toon, he was still battling post-concussion symptoms.

Steinberg worried that Aikman and Young might be just one hit away from post-concussion syndrome and forced retirement. He took no comfort from their ability to bounce back from multiple concussions with no apparent signs of long-lasting damage to their brains. He wanted them to walk away while they still had a choice.

Then, in the 49ers' third game of the 1999 season, Steinberg's fears became a reality. In the waning seconds of the first half, Young dropped back to pass and was flattened by a blitzing defensive back. The blindside blow knocked Young backward, ramming his head into a teammate's leg and, then, the ground. He lay on his side, motionless, curled in a crumpled heap. Team doctors, trainers, and coaches raced across the field and huddled over their unconscious star. When Young finally came to, he was helped to his feet and then he lumbered unsteadily off the field. Little did the millions of *Monday Night Football* viewers know, this was the last time they would ever see him play.

Young spent the rest of the 1999 season on the sidelines, struggling to overcome the fallout from his latest concussion. For weeks, he was plagued by headaches and nausea; he felt dizzy, woozy, and fatigued. Even when the symptoms began to lift, a host of people advised him to quit: his doctors, his family, even his team. That spring, eight months after his ninth official concussion, Steve Young retired at age thirty-eight.

At the same time as Young was wrestling with his lingering post-concussion symptoms and contemplating retirement, Aikman was having a rough time of his own. Midway through the 1999 season, Aikman suffered concussions in two consecutive games. A week after a helmet-to-helmet hit left him woozy but able to return to play, a smaller hit had a much bigger impact. That hit knocked Aikman out of the game and sidelined him for the following two. It was the first time in his career that a concussion kept him out of the starting lineup, but it wouldn't be the last.

Before he could complete a single pass the following season, Aikman was gang-tackled hard and knocked out of the Cowboys' opener—and their next two games—by his ninth official concussion. While recovering, he reached out to Young. Though Aikman acknowledged that their talks had an air of "the blind leading the blind because no one knows what the long-term effects are," at least the two could compare notes on their shared experiences. They talked about how it took lighter and lighter hits to cause a concussion and how it took longer and longer for the symptoms to lift. They talked about how those short-term post-concussion symptoms—and the even scarier specter of permanent brain damage—might figure into a player's decision of when to retire.

When Aikman returned to play, the quarterback who once made everything look so easy was now struggling as the Cowboys plummeted in the standings. Then, in the first quarter of a late-season game, just as Aikman flicked a pass, a linebacker dove into him at full speed and slammed him to the ground. Aikman's head bounced off the unforgiving artificial turf, denting the whole left side of his helmet. He was done for the game, for the season, perhaps forever.

It would take three weeks for the headaches and dizziness to subside. It would take much longer for Aikman to finally accept the reality of his situation and the advice of his family, friends, and teammates. The following spring, four months after his tenth official concussion, Aikman tearfully announced his retirement at age thirty-four.

Just like that, Troy Aikman and Steve Young, two of the greatest quarterbacks in NFL history, had been forced from the sport within ten months of one another.

For so long, posters of Aikman and Young had papered the bedroom walls of the countless kids who idolized them. Now, whenever Steinberg looked around his office and paused to take in the life-size cutouts of his two biggest clients, he couldn't help but lament how they had ironically become "the two poster boys" for a burgeoning concussion crisis.

At least Steinberg could take consolation knowing that the pair would no longer be poster boys for playing through concussions and that their symptoms seemed to have abated with no apparent aftereffects. Their retirements would benefit not only their own long-term health, but also that of all the kids who looked up to them.

"There are millions of young kids out there taking as their model the athlete who plays with nine concussions, who goes back into the game after he's had a concussion," Steinberg said at the time in a nationally televised interview. "And I'm scared that we're going to have a group of high school athletes, collegian athletes, and professional athletes who end up having real impairment."

• • •

Leigh Steinberg wasn't the only one worried about college and high school athletes. As the string of professional retirements played out in the headlines and highlight reels, medical researchers started to wonder about the impact of multiple concussions on younger—more vulnerable—brains. Because concussions had always been dismissed as dings or bumps on the head, no one had bothered to scientifically study their aftermath. Now that it was becoming clear that concussions could produce real damage to the brain, team physicians and athletic trainers needed answers.

For Kevin Guskiewicz, the issue had taken on a particular immediacy in the '90s. As director of the University of North Carolina's education program for certified athletic trainers, he was now constantly fielding questions on concussions. While years of study had taught him how long an athlete with a twisted ankle should be sidelined, there were no data on how long a concussed player needed to rest. These days the questions were increasingly coming from the players themselves, and Guskiewicz would sometimes lie awake at night troubled by his inability to supply a concrete answer.

Early in his career, while working as an assistant trainer for the Pittsburgh Steelers, he had become friends with the team's starting fullback, Merril Hoge. Several years later, when Hoge called to chat, Guskiewicz was taken aback: the former Steeler didn't sound like himself. Guskiewicz was sure it was due to the post-concussion syndrome that had forced Hoge to retire from the NFL.

Guskiewicz didn't want the same thing to happen to any of the athletes in his care. The only way to protect them, he reasoned, was to get more information—to scientifically investigate the impact of repeated concussions in college football. So in 1999 he gathered a group of leading brain experts and sports medicine specialists, and together they set up a large-scale study that would track concussions in nearly three thousand players from twenty-five colleges over the next three seasons. At the beginning of each season, athletes would take neuropsychological exams that could then be used as a comparison to tests taken after a concussion. The groundbreaking findings mirrored what had been seen anecdotally in the pro players: the more concussions a college player sustained, the more vulnerable he was to another one. College players with three or more concussions were three times more likely to sustain a new concussion than those with no history of head injury. What's more, multiple concussions led to longer recovery times.

By the fall of 2003, when the study was published in the *Journal of the American Medical Association*, concussion research had begun to take off. Other researchers found a similar connection between repeated concussions and a heightened risk for future ones. An alarming finding came from a study that looked at both college and high school football: players with a history of concussion were six times more likely to sustain a future concussion than those with no previous head injuries. Even more disturbing were the studies showing that scores on tests of memory and mental agility dropped when athletes sustained multiple concussions.

The football studies echoed what scientists had been learning from concussed animals. Experiments in rats over the previous decade had provided insight into what happened not only after a single concussion but also after multiple ones. Researchers found that concussed rats experienced a burst of chemical changes in their brains. Those changes made the rats more vulnerable to severe, and sometimes irreversible, damage if there was another injury. For young rats, even one concussion could be enough to impair the rodents' future ability to learn. The studies also showed that rats needed seven to ten days to recover from a mild concussion.

Some of that emerging research found its way into new and existing guidelines for concussion management. The ominous findings pushed experts to make the return-to-play recommendations more conservative. Still, among the nearly twenty sets of published guidelines, there was no consensus on how to grade the severity of concussions and how to determine when it was safe to return to play. That disparity stemmed from the lack of any solid science on the impact of concussions on human beings. As a leading animal researcher was quick to point out to one of the guideline authors, you can't assume that people's brains will respond the same as rats'.

Flawed as they were, the guidelines at least offered doctors, trainers, and coaches throughout the nation advice on how to handle an exploding epidemic. The numbers were staggering. Well over a million boys were playing high school football—and studies showed that an alarming number of them were experiencing concussions. In fact, one study found that almost half of them were sustaining concussions, with over a third suffering more than one.

It wasn't surprising that a sport marked by crashing helmets and crunching tackles would produce nearly two-thirds of all concussions among high school boys. What *was* surprising was the plethora of concussions beyond the gridiron among younger kids. Once researchers started looking at the broader picture of youth sports from peewee leagues through high school, they were startled by how pervasive the problem had become. With so many younger children playing soccer and basketball in youth leagues, those two sports combined to produce nearly as many concussions as football among kids between the ages of five and eighteen.

As if that wasn't eye-opening enough, concussions were striking more females than males in soccer and basketball, the two most popular sports in which both sexes participated in equal numbers. High school girls were sustaining more than three times as many concussions as boys on the basketball court. They were sustaining almost 50 percent more concussions than boys on the soccer field, with a rate of injury second only to football among all high school sports. On the college level, women were experiencing 60 percent more concussions than their male counterparts in basketball and 30 percent more in soccer. More remarkably, women playing soccer were suffering concussions at a higher rate than men playing football.

No one had figured out why females appeared to be more vulnerable, but there were theories: their necks weren't as strong as those of male athletes; their brain chemistry and hormones were different, too. Several factors compounded the problem for women and girls. Some concussion symptoms, such as impaired memory, appear to be more severe and long-lasting in girls than boys. Concussions are more likely to be missed in girls than boys, thanks to the popular misconception that girls don't play as hard as boys. Even when concussions are noticed in girls, symptoms are more likely to be minimized because people assume the macho subculture doesn't extend to girls' sports.

Those people haven't met Jamie Carey.

The day Jamie Carey showed up for her first basketball practice at Stanford University, coach Tara VanDerveer took her aside and handed her a bright yellow jersey. Then VanDerveer gathered the rest of the women on the team, all clad in Stanford's cardinal red, and explained why Carey alone would be wearing yellow every day. "We're going to have a strict rule in our practices: nobody touches Jamie," VanDerveer announced. "And this yellow jersey is to remind you of that."

Carey's reputation for fearlessness and recklessness on the court clearly had preceded her. Short even for a guard at five foot six, she compensated for her lack of size with a fierce competitiveness: diving headlong for loose balls, hurtling into crowds of jostling elbows, planting herself solidly against charging opponents.

That scrappy style made Carey the nation's 1999 High School Player of the Year as a senior in Thornton, Colorado. But it also had a dangerous downside: a history of concussions dating back to seventh grade when an opposing player rammed into Carey and sent her crashing to the floor headfirst.

At Stanford, six years and seven concussions later, Carey reluctantly pulled on the yellow jersey that spotlighted her vulnerability. She hated the idea that she needed the yellow jersey as armor to protect her from other players. Unfortunately, it wasn't enough to protect her from herself.

Carey was wearing it during a preseason practice her sophomore year when she dove for a ball, slid across the floor, and banged her head on a teammate's shin. She tried to dismiss the incident as just another bump on the head, but this time the symptoms were debilitating and persistent. She was so dizzy and disoriented that she couldn't walk up stairs. She had so much trouble following her professors' lectures that she stopped going to class. She would start a sentence and forget how to finish it.

Now even Carey realized there was something seriously wrong. A neurological evaluation the following week confirmed it. Doctors concluded that Carey's brain had already sustained significant damage and that she'd be risking her health if she continued to play. As soon as Stanford officials received the medical report, they called Carey in and told her she was being dropped from the team.

At an emotional press conference four days later, Jamie Carey, in a quivering voice, stunned the roomful of reporters by announcing that concussions were forcing her to retire from college basketball. When asked if she could imagine herself returning to play someday should her condition improve, Carey paused and let out a sigh. "Trust me, I asked the doctors many questions like that," she replied. "I kind of got an explanation that everyone with their brain starts out on a full tank. Or like in a video game, you start out with so many lives that you can give. You can give those lives and give those lives and, with each hit, it's fine. Nothing happens. Your brain isn't affected. But, you can't get those lives back. So once you've used them and you get another hit, it's going to start affecting your brain. And that's where I'm at. I don't have any hits left."

The ones she'd already taken had derailed not only the athletic career of the Pac-10 Conference Freshman of the Year, but also the academic dreams of a former high school valedictorian. Unable to do quantitative work anymore, Carey had to change her major from computer science to sociology. That allowed her to take courses with essay-based exams, which were easier to complete now that she was coping with cognitive deficits and memory problems.

For much of the next year, Carey laid off physical activity, and her head started to clear. Emboldened, she began playing pickup games. With no yellow jersey to protect her, she found herself trading elbows with men in daily playground games that were rougher than the Stanford women's scrimmages. There were no concussions and, to her surprise, not even a headache.

Her hoop dreams thus revived, Carey resolved to fight her way back to NCAA competition. She petitioned Stanford for reinstatement to the team she once led. University officials turned her down flat, saying the risks to her brain were simply too great.

Characteristically undaunted, Carey sought a second opinion at the University of Texas. After extensive testing showed that many of her symptoms had abated, specialists there cleared her to play again and she transferred to Texas. But with brain injury experts still debating the long-term impact of multiple concussions, the university's decision sparked controversy. Things got so heated that the team physician for women's sports at Texas, Dr. Mark Chassay, felt compelled to defend the university's stance at a press conference. He cited a recent journal article that had concluded there wasn't enough scientific evidence yet to prove concussion damage could add up over the course of an athlete's career. Then he turned his attention to the media storm over the recent rash of premature retirements in pro sports due to concussions: over the past few years, post-concussion syndrome had claimed the careers of Football Hall of

Famers Troy Aikman and Steve Young as well as Hockey Hall of Famer Pat LaFontaine. "In football and hockey, there have been some articles that scare people," Chassay told the reporters, "but those probably are repetitive injuries while the players are not symptom-free."

That, he argued, was the difference between Jamie Carey and Steve Young, whose careers both succumbed to concussions the same year. Young had continually exacerbated his problem by returning to the football field week after week before his brain healed. In contrast, Chassay pointed out, Carey had allowed her brain to rest during her forced hiatus, suffered no concussions in the two years since the one that sidelined her at Stanford, and reported no symptoms for a full year. "That's a major decision point: if she had symptoms, she wouldn't play," Chassay said. "Once those things are resolved, these people are not at risk. If I evaluated her and she were playing football, I would clear her to play."

Before she could take the court for the Texas Longhorns, though, Carey had to agree to several conditions. She had to wear a customized mouthguard designed for greater shock absorption and she had to regularly undergo neuropsychological testing. On her own, she resolved to try throttling back in practices and to think twice before diving for loose balls in games.

The payoff for all those precautions was obvious to anyone watching Carey play for Texas. The newcomer nicknamed Grandma by all her younger teammates picked up right where she'd left off two years earlier, leading the longshot Longhorns all the way to the 2003 NCAA Final Four. That was only the beginning of a stunning comeback. Through three seasons at Texas, she forged a rugged reputation as one of the nation's best and boldest college players.

Graduating to the Women's National Basketball Association, Carey would need every bit of her trademark intensity against bigger and tougher pro stars notorious for pushing around even college All-Americans like her. Carey knew she'd be putting her brain at greater risk playing in a league where the women were three times more likely to have concussions than their male counterparts in the NBA. But at least she could take comfort in the knowledge that she had suffered no concussions since Stanford despite having absorbed hard hits to the head.

Through four WNBA seasons as backup point guard for the Connecticut Sun, Carey felt lucky to be living her dream. But it came at a cost.

She had to learn to cope with headaches that were more severe than ever. She had to compensate for the mild dyslexia that developed out of her concussions. And she had to deal with odd symptoms like being unable to make out the numbers on the scoreboard or opposing players' jerseys.

By the time Jamie Carey had quietly retired from basketball for a new career in sports management at age twenty-eight in 2009, Americans could not ignore the growing menace of concussions. No longer could concussions be dismissed as the natural fallout from collision sports like football and ice hockey, where head blows were as much a part of the game as tackles and bodychecks. They weren't even limited to partial-contact sports like soccer and basketball. They were everywhere: wrestling, baseball, softball, lacrosse, gymnastics, volleyball, even cheerleading. No sport was immune, no player safe, from the impact of concussions.

Ten years after second-impact syndrome derailed his life, Brandon Schultz appeared in a 2003 CDC video designed to educate the public about the dangers of head injuries in sports. After several minutes of footage showing his continuing problems with coordination and cognitive tasks, Schultz looked directly into the camera and told viewers about his life now. His speech was halting and labored, as if each sentence took intense concentration to form.

"Before I was injured, I imagined that at twenty-six—the age I am now—I would be a college graduate and living on my own," he said. "But my life is very different today. I am finally in college, but each day is a challenge for me. I use aids to help me with simple everyday activities—things most people do without thinking, like remembering what to do next and getting to class on time. And I currently don't drive a car because I have vision problems and slow reaction times. My injury didn't end my life, but it changed the choices I have today."

Schultz then explained why he was making the CDC video: he hoped it would help prevent future catastrophic injuries like his. "I wish now that my school, family, and I could have had more information on concussion injury and some guidelines about when to return to play," he told viewers. "With proper precautions, many concussions can be prevented and permanent injuries can be minimized."

Unfortunately, his message didn't travel far. Just a hundred miles south of his hometown and fully three years after his CDC warning, another Washington State schoolboy's life was derailed by second-impact syndrome.

In the case of Zack Lystedt, a thirteen-year-old junior high school student in suburban Seattle, all the damage was done in a single game. Playing linebacker late in the first half, he chased down and tackled a ballcarrier streaking toward the end zone. When the two crashed to the turf, the back of Lystedt's head was slammed into the ground. As he lay on the grass writhing in pain and gripping the sides of his helmet with both hands, the team's coaches ran onto the field to check on their fallen player. After a few minutes, though, Lystedt pulled himself up and walked back to the bench, where he sat out the final three plays of the first half.

Because there was no athletic trainer or other healthcare professional at the game, it fell to the coaches to decide whether Lystedt was OK to return to play. They figured that the injury couldn't have been serious since he had not lost consciousness, so they decided to send him back out for the very first play of the third quarter—just fifteen minutes after he had clearly sustained a concussion. From the way he was performing on the field, it initially looked as if the coaches had made the right choice. Lystedt played the entire second half, making tackles on defense and running the ball and blocking as a fullback on offense—getting jolted on almost every down. Late in the fourth quarter, with the opposing team driving for what would have been a game-winning touchdown, he forced a fumble at the goal line and clinched the victory for his team.

As everyone celebrated the win on the field, Lystedt's father looked around for his son and then spotted him standing alone, shaking his head. Victor Lystedt hurried over and asked what was wrong. Zack moaned, "Dad, my head hurts really bad. My head hurts really bad." Seconds later, the teen collapsed to the ground unconscious. As Victor sat next to his son waiting for the medevac helicopter to arrive, Zack came to briefly and said the last words he would utter for nine months: "Dad, I can't see."

Zack was airlifted to the very same Seattle trauma center where Brandon Schultz had been treated thirteen years earlier. Over the next ten hours, Lystedt had two surgeries to relieve the growing pressure on his brain. He spent a week on life support, three months in a coma, then a year at a specialized rehab facility in Dallas. It took nine months before he could utter a single word, thirteen months before he could move any part of his body, and twenty months before he could swallow food again. After he was finally well enough to return home to Washington, he still required round-the-clock care, grueling daily therapy, and a motorized wheelchair. Though he learned to stand up and sit down on his own, he could not take a single step or even move his right arm.

On February 13, 2009, twenty-eight months after his catastrophic injury, Zack Lystedt was in Washington's state capital, Olympia, with his family to testify in support of a concussion-safety bill that would bear his name. With his curly dark hair cropped short, it was easy to see the long, jagged scars reaching from the top of his head to the backs of his ears. Victor Lystedt pushed Zack's wheelchair down to the front of the hearing room and positioned it at the end of a rectangular table facing the legislators. After taking a seat between his wife and his sixteen-year-old son, Victor began his testimony.

"Twenty-one years ago today, my wife and I started our relationship as a married couple. We waited five years to have our child. We weren't able to have any other children.

"Twenty-eight months and one day ago, Zackery was perfect. He was able to perform on the football field; he was able to perform academically, socially. He was everything a child should be to a parent."

As Victor Lystedt spoke, his wife, Mercedes, periodically dabbed tears from her eyes.

"Zackery was hurt and it was a preventable injury," Victor continued, fighting to keep the emotion from his voice. "We didn't know that when it happened. We know that now. We know that if Zackery had been taken out of the game, we wouldn't be living the life we're living."

The Lystedts were lobbying for a law that would mandate the strictest concussion-safety measures in the nation: it would require that any youth athlete suspected of sustaining a concussion be immediately removed from play and then prohibited from returning without written clearance from a licensed healthcare provider trained in concussion management.

Zack Lystedt gave a human face to the hard facts presented that day by a parade of sports injury experts. One of them, Dr. Stan Herring, a rehab specialist who had treated both Zack Lystedt and Brandon Schultz, told the lawmakers that young brains are particularly vulnerable and need extra time to heal. "The same concussion I see in a middle school athlete can take four times longer to get better than it does in an adult or a professional athlete," said Herring, a team physician for the NFL's Seattle Seahawks and co-director of the University of Washington's sports concussion program. Making matters worse, he explained, the young brain is especially vulnerable while it's healing, and a second injury while it's still recovering can lead to the type of catastrophic consequences that befell Zack Lystedt.

If the experts' persuasive testimony and Lystedt's heart-wrenching story weren't convincing enough, there was a new study to hammer home the need for a law mandating proper recovery periods. The study found that a stunning 41 percent of concussed high school athletes were returned to action before their brains had time to recover. The new statistic underscored an unfortunate reality: coaches in every sport were ignoring published guidelines that defined when it was safe for a concussed athlete to return to play. What's more, the study found that 16 percent of high school football players who lost consciousness were returned to the very game in which they were injured. That figure became even more alarming when the experts pointed out that only 10 percent of all concussions result in loss of consciousness. If coaches weren't sidelining players who'd been knocked out, how could they be trusted to act on the subtler symptoms that characterize the vast majority of concussions?

A big part of the problem, the experts said, was that coaches have conflicting interests: pressure to win, pressure from kids to play, pressure from parents living vicariously through their kids—all of which compete with the pressure to protect the players in their charge. The proposed legislation was designed to take the responsibility out of the coaches' hands.

In the end, the most compelling argument was made by Zack Lystedt himself. His words came haltingly and sounded as if they were emanating from a tape recorder slowed to quarter-speed. Laboring to form each and every syllable, he began by slowly raising his left hand in a wave and introducing himself to the legislators.

"I, for one, had my life change drastically," he said, rhythmically tapping his left hand over his heart. "I flew back behind, and hit the back of my head. And it . . . it . . ."

Struggling to find the next word, he turned to his father for help. Victor Lystedt looked at his son and whispered the missing word. Zack nodded and turned back to the microphone to finish his sentence: ". . . gave me a concussion." He paused, took a breath, and told the legislators why they had to pass the bill.

"I just wanna make sure this doesn't happen to anyone else."

On May 14, 2009, the Zackery Lystedt Law was signed by the governor of Washington. It was a landmark law, designed to help prevent a preventable injury. While head injuries can't be completely removed from sports, brain damage can be minimized if players are prevented from having a concussion too quickly on the heels of a previous one.

The law was a good first step, but unfortunately it didn't do much to change people's attitudes. Americans liked their sports, especially football, the way they were. People who dared suggest safety reforms were often met with scorn and ridicule. Hard knocks were looked at as a rite of passage, a code of honor passed down from generation to generation. It was how kids learned to be tough. The macho culture permeating the country insisted that the way to deal with a bump on the head was just to dust yourself off and keep going as if nothing had happened.

Chapter 3

Head Games

Sometimes when he's driving alone late at night, Whitey Baun will start to wonder how differently things might have turned out if he'd been less of a coach and more of a dad.

He replays the weeks leading up to that awful day seven years ago when his son's life changed forever. Was the coach in him too anxious to get Willie back to play? Could he have inadvertently pushed his twelve-year-old son to ignore the lingering headaches from a concussion five weeks earlier? Did Willie mistake the daily questions about his headaches as badgering rather than fatherly concern?

Second-guessing every choice he made, Whitey thinks back to the concussion that started it all and reproaches himself for not taking the injury more seriously.

It happened during a peewee football game. Willie dove for the ball after an onside kick and collided helmet against helmet with an opposing player—directly in front of his dad. Whitey winced when he heard the loud crack. As he watched Willie stagger up off the ground and dizzily make his way to the sideline, Whitey thought, "Oh, that's not good." The EMT on the sideline checked Willie out and told Whitey, "He seems OK, but let's sit him out for a while." A few plays later, Willie seemed fine, so Whitey put him back in the game and forgot about the whole episode.

That afternoon, after the two had returned home and were playing catch in the backyard, Willie started to complain about a stabbing pain in the back of his head. Whitey was worried and took his son to the family doctor the next day. After examining Willie, the doctor diagnosed a mild concussion and then recommended that the boy take at least three weeks off and not even think of returning to play until the headaches had completely resolved. Whitey stiffened and thought, "You've got to be kidding me. He just got his bell rung."

Even though he believed the doctor was being overly cautious, Whitey agreed to sideline Willie until the headaches went away. Over the next few weeks, Whitey regularly checked his son's progress, asking simply, "How's your head doing?" Whitey was surprised at how tenaciously the headaches hung on. He couldn't believe that the lingering pain could be tied to a routine collision weeks earlier. Maybe, he thought, the headaches were caused by something else, like the stress of starting junior high school.

Four weeks after the concussion, Willie told his dad that the headaches had gone away. Just to be on the safe side, Whitey waited another week and then cleared his son to go back to practice. Willie seemed his normal self throughout his first week back—until the last drill of the last practice for Saturday's game when he tackled a teammate. The hit didn't seem particularly hard to Whitey, but then he heard his son scream, "Oh! Oh! My neck hurts! My head! My neck!" At first Whitey dismissed it, assuming that Willie had just experienced his first "stinger." Whitey could remember the first time he'd experienced that excruciating, burning sensation from a pinched nerve in his neck. He'd thought, "Oh God, did I just break my neck? What the hell just happened to me?" The sensation had passed quickly and Whitey had gone right back to play. Now, as he made his way across the field, he wondered why Willie wasn't bouncing back up. By the time Willie finally hauled himself off the ground and staggered back toward the sideline, Whitey's stomach started to churn. He thought, "Oh my God, it's another concussion." At the hospital, doctors did a CAT scan and then reassured Whitey that there was no serious damage to his son's brain. They suggested Willie rest and sent him home. Whitey breathed a sigh of relief.

The next morning when Willie came downstairs to breakfast, he was greeted by the family's two schipperkes. "Those are cute dogs," Willie said as the furry black balls of energy swirled around and between his legs. "Whose are they?"

Whitey and his wife, Becky, were stunned. "They're *our* dogs, Willie," Becky exclaimed.

Whenever Whitey thinks back to that morning, his stomach gets sick all over again. As he drives on through the darkness, he can't stop himself from reliving other heart-wrenching moments from the days, weeks, and months that followed the second concussion.

Whitey remembers seeing Willie walk up to Becky and put his hands up to her face, his fingers running over her eyes, nose, and mouth. It made Whitey think of a blind boy trying to get a sense of the person in front of him. He knew then that Willie hadn't just forgotten who the dogs were. Willie didn't recognize his parents, either.

Whitey remembers how he and his wife took photos of Willie's teachers and friends and then pasted them in a book. Without the book, Willie couldn't keep track of anyone at school. He would arrive in the morning, learn everyone's names, and then forget them by the next morning. Each day would be a replay of the previous. In a misguided attempt at humor, one of his teachers joked that it was as if Willie were living the film *Groundhog Day*.

Whitey remembers seeing his wife standing over their son as Willie tried to work problems from a second grade math book at the kitchen table. Even those simple exercises were now impossible for a boy who'd been near the top of his seventh grade class before the concussions. Whitey felt a sharp pang in his chest as his son, frustrated and frightened that things would never go back to normal, burst into tears. "What the hell did I do to this kid?" Whitey thought. "I was the father. I was the one who was responsible for keeping my son safe."

Even when Whitey remembers a happy time—like the day Willie's memory finally started flooding back a year later—it's bittersweet. The elation Whitey felt then is tempered by his realization that his son will never be the same as he was before the injuries. Now a college student, Willie still suffers from headaches almost every day. And although Willie caught up academically, Whitey worries that his son may never regain the social ease and self-confidence he once had.

One of Whitey's biggest regrets is that Willie had to give up the game they both loved so much. To Whitey, football was an indispensable part of becoming a man. It taught him self-confidence and mental toughness. It taught him to stand up for himself and not to be intimidated by anyone. As he explained to his wife, "The lessons I got from competing in sports I didn't get from any other aspect of my life."

Those were precisely the lessons he wanted to pass on to their son. Becky wasn't sure she agreed that football was the only way Willie could learn those lessons, but she had accepted the sport as a fact of her life. Even before Willie began playing tackle football in organized leagues as a seven-year-old, Becky had recognized that he was a "ball kid." Though naturally worried about his safety, she could at least console herself with the knowledge that he'd inherited his dad's powerful athletic build as surely as his sandy brown hair. For years, Becky had shown up at all of Willie's games and had even deigned to join her family for some of those long Sunday afternoons watching the NFL on TV. That all changed the moment Willie failed to recognize the family dogs. After living through his devastating concussion, Becky couldn't bear to watch another game.

Even for Whitey, football would never again be the same. He and Willie still had fun watching NFL games together, but the hits that once roused Whitey out of his living room chair now made him wince. Worse yet, Whitey no longer enjoyed coaching. He'd always loved working with the younger kids, but now he had to force himself. Any time he saw a kid make hard contact or get up slow or stagger or cry, he'd catch his breath and think, "Oh my God, I hope he's OK. I hope he's OK. Please let him be OK." After one season coaching the team his son once played on, Whitey had to quit. It was just too hard to watch kids getting hurt after what he'd gone through with his own son.

That's a loss for all the youngsters Whitey could be coaching today. His experiences have given him insight that most coaches lack. The new Coach Baun would be so much more cautious and vigilant than the old Coach Baun, whose philosophy developed while playing football in the '60s. An All-American linebacker on a small-college national championship team at Wittenberg University, Whitey was a tough guy who considered concussions to be at once a source of humor and a badge of honor. It was a point of pride that nothing could knock him out of a game, not even the hit that had sent him staggering off the field to the opposing team's sideline. His just-rub-dirt-on-it attitude was reinforced by the macho coaches who'd tell him to "just shake it off" and get back out there. Whitey had learned those lessons well and then passed them on to the kids he coached.

Now, he understands firsthand the dangers of a philosophy that promotes playing through pain, a mentality that champions winning at all costs, a culture that celebrates athletes who shrug off concussions. It's unfortunate that it takes a personal ordeal to counter what's become so deeply ingrained in the sport as well as in our national psyche.

To understand how deeply that ethos permeated American culture, you only had to switch on your TV. In living rooms all across America, millions of fans—many of them fathers and sons just like Whitey and Willie Baun—would gather each week to watch the organized mayhem that is professional football. Sometimes it was hard to tell whether they were reveling more in the thrilling touchdowns or in the crushing hits. That shouldn't come as a surprise since they'd been programmed for decades to believe that the carnage on the screen was the main attraction. They'd been sold on the violence by everyone involved in the sport, from the National Football League to the networks broadcasting the games.

The networks did their best to boost fans' taste for brutality. For years, ABC began its *Monday Night Football* telecast with a video of two helmets—each emblazoned with the logo of one of the teams playing that night in the NFL's weekly showcase event—crashing head-on into one another and smashing into smithereens. Fox, the youth-oriented network that the NFL partnered with in the early '90s to keep kids' attention focused on the sport, aired a promo that featured only brutal hits with a voiceover blaring, "The hardest hits are on Fox!" When TNT added Sunday night cablecasts to cap off a full day of NFL games on the broadcast networks, it ran an ad in magazines and on billboards exhorting fans to "Get in a few late hits." Another TNT ad was more graphic and grim. It featured a photo of a battered football player seated on the sideline in obvious distress, his mouth covered by an oxygen mask. The sobering image stood in stark contrast with the accompanying words: "Shortness of breath. Nausea. Disorientation. Memory loss. The fun begins at 8 P.M. Sunday night. NFL on TNT."

Amazingly, that ad was running in the mid-'90s not long after NFL stars like Al Toon and Merril Hoge had been forced into premature retirement by some of the "fun" post-concussion symptoms on TNT's list. Even after the roster of concussion victims swelled to include bigger and bigger superstars like Hall of Fame quarterbacks Troy Aikman and

Steve Young, the crushing hits continued to be celebrated, glorified, and promoted. The networks spliced them together into highlight reels, with ESPN cynically labeling its collection of hits "Plays of the Week." The NFL itself marketed them not only in hardcore "Greatest Hits" videos but also in farcical "Football Follies" collections, one of which famously set a series of brutal hits to the music of *The Nutcracker* Suite and was titled "The Headcracker Suite."

The bottom line: big hits translated into big ratings and big business. The NFL built itself into a multibillion-dollar enterprise and football into the nation's most popular spectator sport by exploiting a simple formula: marry an inherently violent game with the perfect medium to showcase it. Television not only put fans right on top of the multiple collisions that punctuated every play, but also allowed them to reexperience those crunching impacts over and over from every angle and at every speed through the magic of instant replay.

Before the NFL tied the knot with television, pro football was just a quaint way for local fans in a dozen cities to while away Sunday afternoons between baseball seasons. That all changed in the early '60s, when the NFL cut its first national network deal to telecast games into America's living rooms every Sunday and viewers by the millions were treated to a regular dose of football's violence. Each week, more and more new fans found themselves mesmerized by the sight of ferocious linebackers snapping receivers down like rag dolls and packs of hulking linemen flattening ballcarriers like roadkill.

One of the most enduring images from that transformative era is of a stocky, bespectacled coach in a coat and tie stomping up and down the sideline, barking orders like a general, exhorting his troops to toughen up and to crush the enemy. Vince Lombardi's approach was neatly summed up by his most famous mantra: "Winning isn't everything, it's the only thing." That philosophy made Lombardi the most legendary of all coaches and transformed a losing team into the most dominant of all dynasties with five NFL championships in seven years. By the time his Green Bay Packers triumphantly carried him off the field for the last time after the 1968 Super Bowl, his winning philosophy was accepted not just in the sport but also in the entire culture. His maxims spread from Green Bay's locker room to America's boardrooms. Lombardi emphasized the need for toughness, both physical and mental. He preached that pain was an integral part of the game, and he expected his players not only to endure it but also to inflict it. "Football is a violent, dangerous sport," he asserted. "To play it any other way but violently would be idiotic."

Coaches striving to duplicate Lombardi's success adopted his approach and built on it. They routinely sent players back onto the field with cracked ribs, punctured lungs, broken ankles. And fans seemed to accept this as just part of the game. After all, in a society that embraced the football-as-war analogy right down to the sport's militaristic lexicon, coaches were simply sending platoons of warriors into action. Fans viewed every game as a war and each down a battle to gain ground on the enemy. They expected to see troops trudging off the field caked in mud and blood. A warrior could leave in the midst of a game only if he were carried off on his shield. All of his brothers-in-arms were expected to soldier on, stoically keeping pain and broken bones to themselves.

In that ethos, it's not surprising that players also kept concussion symptoms to themselves. If coaches were sending guys back into the game with broken bones, they certainly weren't about to sideline anyone for a little dizziness or disorientation. As far as the fans were concerned, concussions barely existed. Nobody talked about them. Nobody saw them, except on the rare occasion when a player was knocked unconscious and hauled off the field on a stretcher.

Not even the increasingly dangerous nature of the game could open fans' eyes to the menace of concussions. With players getting bigger, faster, and stronger, collisions were becoming more destructive—and more spectacular to watch. Fueled by advances in conditioning and nutrition, the average weight of NFL players grew by 25 pounds over three decades to 245. More telling, the average offensive lineman ballooned a full 60 pounds to 310. Countless hours in the weight room, coupled with supplements and sometimes steroids, made players stronger. The increase in size didn't slow them down a bit. On the contrary, thanks to sophisticated training regimens, they actually got quicker.

While the physical makeup of the players was changing, the laws of physics remained constant. Most important on the gridiron was Newton's Second Law: force equals mass times acceleration. In your typical big hit, that could translate into each player banging the other with fifteen hundred pounds of force at speeds approaching twenty-five miles per hour. An NFL study, in fact, found that players were sustaining concussions from impacts that averaged ninety-eight times the force of gravity.

Making matters worse, players were changing the way they hit. With the advent of high-tech shock-absorbing helmets and better faceguards, players assumed their heads were virtually invulnerable. Emboldened, they began to use their helmets as weapons. Instead of tackling and blocking with their hands and shoulders, they targeted opponents headfirst, using their hard-shell plastic helmets as battering rams. Coaches taught the most effective head-ramming techniques and reminded their players that the point of a brutal hit was not just physical domination but also mental intimidation. By the time rigid polycarbonate-alloy helmets and steel-alloy faceguards became the norm in the '80s and '90s, the violence had ratcheted up into outright viciousness.

Much of that was aimed at the most valuable and vulnerable player on the field: the quarterback. Targeted on every down by a horde of defenders under orders to take him out, the quarterback would typically absorb dozens of bruising hits each game. Troy Aikman learned that the hard way his rookie year with the Dallas Cowboys. Two months into what was already a disastrous season, he was slammed to the ground by an onrushing linebacker an instant after releasing a pass for an eighty-yard touchdown. For a full eight minutes, fans watched in uneasy silence as Aikman lay on his back, unconscious and motionless with blood trickling from his right ear. To his agent, Leigh Steinberg, the seconds seemed like minutes and then the minutes like hours. Steinberg was nervous and scared. Here was his marquee client, the one with the Hollywood good looks and the golden right arm that had just earned him the richest rookie contract in NFL history, not even twitching a muscle. Steinberg thought, "We're not in the Roman Colosseum in the time of Nero. This shouldn't be about sacrificing our best and our brightest."

It's no coincidence that this dramatic scene was echoed seven years later in the 1996 film *Jerry Maguire* or that the movie's protagonist is a sports agent who undergoes a crisis of conscience triggered by the concussions that hospitalized one of his clients. That's because Steinberg was the model for the title character portrayed by Tom Cruise: the agent struggling to hold on to his integrity in a cutthroat business where dollars usually trump ethics. Steinberg was never exactly your typical agent, famously wearing jeans and flip-flops to negotiate multimillion-dollar deals with button-down executives, insisting that all his clients give back to their communities as role models, and worrying as much about their physical as their financial health.

Aikman's concussion spurred Steinberg into action. Steinberg started lobbying for rule changes that would make the game safer, especially for the many quarterbacks he represented. His efforts were met with ridicule. The doctor advising the NFL on concussion management dismissed Steinberg's advocacy as "fearmongering." Football purists accused him of "trying to put a dress on a quarterback." Even his own clients, worried that any mention of concussion would make them appear weak, complained about his crusading.

While some cosmetic rule changes were adopted to protect quarterbacks from hits with the helmet and hits to the head, macho attitudes remained as deeply rooted as the goalposts. With the big hits getting bigger, more and more players were sustaining concussions. And it wasn't just the quarterbacks. It was everyone involved in those spectacular head-rattling hits, from the receivers and running backs flattened by the collisions to the linebackers and defensive backs doling out the punishment. The NFL's own data showed an average of one reported concussion every other game, a stat no doubt dwarfed by the number of concussions that went unreported. If concussions themselves remained an open secret, their ramifications were becoming increasingly obvious wherever you looked: on weekly team injury reports, in boldface headlines about forced retirements, in medical journal articles written by brain injury experts.

All of that, however, couldn't make even a dent in this old-school culture where machismo can run roughshod over common sense. Players needed to be protected from their own enthusiasm, but coaches and team medical personnel were still dismissing concussions as nuisance injuries. Every week on the NFL sidelines, coaches and team physicians were making return-to-play decisions, and to anyone watching, there seemed to be no logic guiding those calls. Sometimes it was the coaches who would send disoriented players back onto the field against the recommendations of team physicians; sometimes it was the doctors themselves who would clear wobbly players to go back into the game.

Nowhere was that dynamic more obvious than on the New York Jets sideline on a fall Sunday in 2003. Early in the third quarter of a showdown against the archrival New York Giants, Jets wide receiver Wayne Chrebet was knocked out cold by a knee to the back of the head. He lay facedown on the turf, motionless, for nearly a minute. After helping him off the field, team medical personnel hid his helmet so he wouldn't be tempted to sneak back into the game before he was checked out. Chrebet had already demonstrated time and again that he was a reckless and scrappy overachiever who would try to shake off a concussion and rush back into the fray. Although Chrebet was immediately diagnosed with a concussion, he passed standard sideline evaluation tests of memory and orientation. Early in the fourth quarter, the Jets' team physician, Dr. Elliot Pellman, pulled Chrebet aside, looked him in the eyes, and said, "This is very important. You can't lie to me. There's going to be some controversy about you going back to play. This is very important for you. This is very important for your career. Are you OK?" Chrebet replied, "I'm fine," and Pellman sent him back onto the field.

Three days later, Pellman found himself in the glare of the New York media spotlight as he announced his decision to sideline Chrebet for the next game due to symptoms of fatigue, malaise, and headaches that showed up the day after the concussion. It didn't take long for reporters to put Pellman on the defensive as they pressed him to explain his decision to return a concussed player to the same game in which he'd been knocked unconscious. Pellman made no apologies: "Am I second-guessing myself for returning him to play Sunday? The answer is no. Am I concerned enough for him not to play this weekend? Yes."

A week later, Pellman had to face the press again, this time to announce that Chrebet would miss the last seven games of the season because of persistent post-concussion symptoms. Once again, Pellman found himself defending his original decision to send a concussed player back onto the field. "Wayne returned and was fine," Pellman told reporters. "He did not suffer additional injury. If he had suffered additional injury, his prognosis would be no different. At some point, you have to rest on science and intuition. The decision about Wayne returning to play was based on scientific evaluation. As we stand now, that decision made no difference as to what's happening today."

What made the Chrebet episode even more remarkable was that Pellman wasn't just the Jets' team physician—he was also the NFL's top concussion adviser. The NFL had picked Pellman to form a concussion committee in 1994 when the high-profile retirements of Al Toon and Merril Hoge at age twenty-nine made it impossible to ignore the issue any longer. Pellman's only apparent qualification for the committee chairmanship was his experience treating Toon's concussions with the Jets. His medical background certainly didn't recommend him for the position. He was a rheumatologist with no training in neurology. He publicly professed his lack of knowledge, admitting that the only concussion training he'd received was the on-the-job variety watching Toon's career fade into a fog of post-concussion syndrome.

At the same time as Chrebet was losing his own battle with the syndrome, Pellman and the NFL were still broadcasting the message that concussions were just transient events that didn't produce any long-term effects. The NFL was now justifying its position with studies produced by Pellman's Mild Traumatic Brain Injury Committee. By the beginning of 2005, seven of the committee's studies had been published in the journal *Neurosurgery*. Those studies, based on head injury data collected from the NFL's team physicians and analyzed by a group of researchers that included a neurologist and a neurosurgeon, argued that concussions were benign. The committee concluded that multiple concussions did not lead to long-term consequences and that it was safe to return certain players to the same game in which they were concussed. This flew in the face of all the accepted return-to-play concussion guidelines, of studies conducted by researchers unaffiliated with the NFL, and of the growing roster of pro players plagued by lingering symptoms.

That didn't stop the committee from suggesting that its conclusions might well extend beyond the pros to college and high school players. "Under the right circumstances," Pellman and his colleagues wrote in a 2005 study, "it might be safe for college/high school football players to be cleared to return to play on the same day as their injury. [We] suggest that, rather than blindly adhering to arbitrary, rigid guidelines, physicians keep an open mind to the possibility that the present analysis of professional football players may have relevance to college and high school players."

• • •

The implications of that controversial assertion stretched far beyond the bounds of the NFL and the medical journal that published it. For years, its impact was felt in doctors' offices around the country. Even if a physician was savvy enough to diagnose a concussion and progressive enough to prescribe rest as a treatment, some parent or child would invariably pull out the NFL's 2005 study and use it as evidence that the doctor was being far too overprotective. "They say what I tell them about it not being safe to go back in the same game is totally wrong, and they're backed by the NFL," grumbled Dr. Gerard Malanga, director of the New Jersey Sports Medicine Institute and a team physician for several colleges and high schools. "So they go to a doctor that tells them what they want to hear. And we remain the guys holding our breath that the kid doesn't get hurt again."

College and high school players didn't need the NFL's studies to tell them how to view concussions. Long before the studies were published, these student-athletes were taking their cues from what they saw on TV.

The macho culture so evident in the NFL flowed freely down to all the Americans playing tackle football at every level—from the two thousand in the pros to the seventy-five thousand in colleges to the million and a half in secondary schools to the more than three million in organized youth leagues. Kids were looking to emulate not only the skills of their NFL heroes, but also the toughness of those role models. A seven-year-old on a peewee team was just as likely to feel he needed to push through pain and ignore the dizzying effects of a concussion as the NFL player he cheered from his living room.

Kids weaned on televised football were barraged with the message that most jolts to the head were benign. They grew up not only seeing their favorite stars bounce back from head-rattling hits, but also hearing broadcasters hype that part of the game as fun and exciting. Announcers would glorify the hit that left a player woozy: "Wow, he really got his bell rung on that one!" They would extol the courage of the player who shook it off: "What a warrior—nothing can stop this guy!" At the same time, they would play down any possible ramifications from a head injury: "Oh, it's just a dinger."

Small wonder researchers found that college and high school players didn't connect dingers and bellringers with brain injury. In a study that surveyed eight college football programs from across the nation, an astounding 91 percent of players and coaches believed that concussions were different from dingers and bellringers. That ignorance helped explain another of the study's findings: less than one-sixth of concussions sustained during the 2002 NCAA season were reported immediately after the injury, and fully two-thirds were never reported by players to either trainers or coaches.

The confusion over just what constituted a concussion led to widely varying estimates of the injury's prevalence. Incidence rates reported in medical journals ranged from 15 percent to almost 50 percent of high school players surveyed. That wide spread could be explained by the way researchers asked players about head injuries: if they used the word "concussion," the rate was low; if they simply listed concussion symptoms, the rate soared. The most eye-opening study surveyed high school players from two school districts, one in Pennsylvania and the other in Ohio, about head injury symptoms with no mention of the word "concussion." It found that 47 percent of players had suffered at least one concussion during the 1996 season. Of the injured players, 74 percent said they'd sustained multiple concussions, with an average of more than three.

The studies based on confidential reports from players contrasted sharply with trainer surveys. Several studies that included information only from trainers found concussions in just 4 percent of high school players. That statistic clearly reflected the reluctance of players to own up to their concussions. When asked why they didn't report concussions to trainers or coaches, players gave researchers enough reasons to fill a playbook: didn't want to leave the game, didn't want to let teammates down, didn't want to appear weak or injury-prone to the coach, didn't want to risk losing playing time or a starting position, didn't realize it was a concussion, didn't think it was serious enough to report.

Kids were often introduced to that play-through-pain mentality in youth leagues and then had it reinforced all through high school and college. The model for all those youth leagues was Pop Warner. From its 1929 inception at a time when the fledgling NFL was barely a footnote in a society obsessed with college and high school football, the Pop Warner program became the kicking-off point for millions of boys aged five to sixteen. Pop Warner football offered little kids the trappings of the pro ranks: big games and big pressure, miniature cheerleaders, national "Super

Bowl" championships, rabid fans disguised as parents, coaches who fashioned their dictatorial style on the likes of Vince Lombardi and Pop Warner himself. The program was named for the famed coach who learned the game as a rugged lineman playing college ball for Walter Camp, the innovator universally known as "The Father of American Football."

In the late nineteenth century, Camp transformed football from a sport that resembled English rugby into something every bit as uniquely American as baseball. The regimented structure he forged looked more like a clash between warring armies than a contest between competing athletic teams. The gridiron he laid out became a new male proving ground for collegians eager to demonstrate their toughness in hand-to-hand combat and their grit in the face of the casualties that inevitably resulted. It was a game as raw and rugged as the country that spawned it. Marauding bands of collegians would slam into each other, mauling, pushing, pulling, and tackling until the play ground to a halt in a heap of writhing, howling, gouging, kicking, and punching bodies. Watching that spectacle at a Harvard-Yale game, John L. Sullivan declared football more savage than the bare-knuckled fights he'd survived during his legendary reign as boxing's first world heavyweight champion. "Football, there's murder in that game," Sullivan told an acquaintance. "Prizefighting doesn't compare in roughness or danger with football. In the ring, you know what your opponent is trying to do, he's right there in front of you, there's only one of him. But in football, there are eleven guys trying to do you in!"

Nothing epitomized the brutality of the era better than Harvard's infamous "flying wedge." Two groups of Harvard players would race full-tilt diagonally from each sideline past the quarterback and then converge in a tight V-shaped wedge flying like an arrowhead toward the line of scrimmage, its tip aimed at a single defender to literally mow him down under nearly a ton of massed momentum. Just as the wedge pierced the opposing team's line, the quarterback would hand the ball off to the halfback, who would then tuck himself behind the wedge as it left defenders bruised, battered, and broken in its wake. The play proved so dominating that many other college teams promptly adopted it and adapted their own variations on it. The play was also so dangerous that it led to a spate of crippling injuries and even deaths.

Although the flying wedge was particularly brutal, it wasn't the only source of football fatalities. Players were dying on the gridiron with alarming regularity. The deaths were mostly from head injuries like skull fractures and brain bleeds. With nothing to protect their heads in that age before helmets, players took to growing their hair unfashionably long in a futile attempt to provide some cushioning. The flimsy leather helmets that started popping up on a few heads here and there around the turn of the century afforded little more protection than the long hair.

As the death toll mounted, the public began to take notice. Clergymen denounced the sport's brutality from their pulpits. Newspapers carried sensationalized accounts of bloodbaths, players screaming in pain, spectators shrieking in horror, and, of course, the deaths. Editorialists called for the abolition of football by act of Congress. State legislators introduced bills to outlaw the sport. College administrators responded to the carnage by canceling games that featured fierce rivalries like Harvard-Yale and Army-Navy in which passions pumped up the violence. A few colleges even suspended their football programs entirely. The abolitionist movement was gaining steam and threatening to kill the sport.

Things came to a head in 1905 during a particularly brutal season that left twenty-five players dead and more than six times as many seriously injured at all levels. A graphic newspaper photo—depicting Swarthmore's star lineman staggering off the field after a merciless and deliberate beating, his face a bloody mess—caught the attention of President Theodore Roosevelt. A gridiron enthusiast who avidly rooted for his Harvard alma mater, Roosevelt was incensed. He embraced football as a metaphor for the rugged American spirit he energetically espoused, more so than his own college sport of boxing. "In life, as in a foot-ball game," he had written, "the principle to follow is: Hit the line hard; don't foul and don't shirk, but hit the line hard!" He was proud that his eldest son, Ted Jr., was a plucky lineman on Harvard's freshman team that season. "I am delighted to have you play football," the president wrote his son in a letter. "I believe in rough, manly sports."

Fired into action by the gruesome newspaper photo, Roosevelt summoned representatives from college football's three biggest powers—Harvard, Yale, and Princeton—to the White House to address how to make the game safer. Although he believed that playing through pain built character, he was concerned about the rash of fatal head and neck injuries.

Roosevelt, as vigorous a reformer as he was a sportsman, certainly didn't want to abolish a rugged game he considered an integral link to the American identity, but he wasn't shy about using his bully pulpit to save it. "I demand that football change its rules or be abolished," he blustered. "Brutality and foul play should receive the same summary punishment given to a man who cheats at cards. Change the game or forsake it!" Over lunch at the White House, Roosevelt delivered a stern warning to the powerful football figures seated around his dining room table: the sport they all loved would surely be banished from campuses without urgent reform.

As a result of that summit meeting, colleges from across America established a national governing organization to regulate athletics and reform football. Over the next several years, the newly formed National Collegiate Athletic Association would revolutionize the way the game was played through rules designed to make it safer. By outlawing lethal flying wedge formations and legalizing the forward pass, the NCAA opened up the game and cut back on the mass maulings. The advent of aerial assaults and open-field running attacks modernized football into a spectacle more thrilling for spectators and safer for players. The fatality rate dropped, but a false sense of security arose regarding head injuries. The NCAA, becoming ironically indifferent to the very injury problem that necessitated its creation, would take another three decades to make helmets mandatory. With the lack of any standardized guideline leaving return-to-play decisions up to each college, concussions would become more and more of a problem. Only now there were no Theodore Roosevelts around to command reform.

For all the rules changes designed to improve safety over the intervening century, nothing could legislate away the macho mentality. Football became the sport that defined the way athletes viewed competition, toughness, and injury. Football would drive the way everyone thought of concussions. The attitude insidiously spread to every other sport. If concussions were going to be dismissed on the football field, they would be just as easily ignored on a basketball court or a hockey rink.

If any team sport could challenge football for sheer brutality and dangerous machismo, it was ice hockey. From its inception in Canada during the latter part of the nineteenth century at the same time as football was gaining a foothold in the United States, hockey offered its own brand of violence—high-flying collisions, head-rattling bodychecks, teeth-loosening fisticuffs—along with a play-through-pain mentality every bit as ingrained as football's.

The model of hockey toughness was Eddie Shore, the dominating defenseman whose reckless and ruthless style popularized the sport in U.S. cities in the '20s and '30s. Shore was notorious for inflicting pain—a hated villain whose most vicious blindside hit drove scoring star Ace Bailey into the ice headfirst with a skull fracture that ended his career and almost his life. Taking as good as he gave, Shore was equally renowned for ignoring pain—a fierce warrior whose battle scars included the 978 stitches he took without local anesthesia and without missing a shift on the ice.

If hockey players were expected to stoically skate with freshly stitched lacerations on bloodstained ice, they were hardly likely to break stride for head injuries no one could see. Given this cultural dynamic permeating every level from the National Hockey League all the way down to the peewees, it isn't surprising that hockey's concussion history would mirror football's.

With players wielding sharp elbows, skates, and sticks on an unforgiving sheet of ice enclosed by boards and tempered glass, catastrophic head injuries were virtually inevitable. After crashing headfirst into the sideboards during a 1950 Stanley Cup playoff game, a rising star named Gordie Howe needed a ninety-minute operation to relieve pressure on his brain, save his life, and send him back on his career path to rewriting the NHL record book and carving out his legend as Mr. Hockey. In a 1968 regular-season game, an obscure rookie named Bill Masterton was skating at full speed when he was bodychecked by a defender just after sliding the puck to a teammate; he bounced off another defender and flipped backward, slamming the back of his unprotected head on the ice with such impact that blood gushed from his nose and ears. He lingered a day on life support before massive brain bleeding made him the only player ever to die from an injury suffered in an NHL game. The NHL president, Clarence Campbell, characterized Masterton's death as "a natural hazard of our business" and took pains to avert any public hand-wringing over the sport's violent nature, deflecting calls to make helmets mandatory.

Still, the tragedy did spark a gradual change in attitudes toward protective headgear. Until then, helmets brought nothing but ridicule to the odd player brave enough to wear one amid taunts of "chicken" in a league where goaltenders were still exposing their bare faces to rising slapshots that exceeded a hundred miles an hour. By the time helmets were finally mandated for any player entering the NHL from 1979 onward, they had long been standard equipment at every other level of play. By the time the last bareheaded veteran retired from the NHL in 1997, their impact was clear. Although helmets no doubt reduced the number of catastrophic head injuries, they had a paradoxical effect of making players more fearless and making concussions more commonplace.

On the rink as on the gridiron, the concussion problem grew in direct proportion to the size, strength, and speed of the players in the world's fastest team sport. As the average NHL player sprouted to six foot two and 205 pounds, the laws of physics collided head-on with the realities of neuroscience. Blazing up the ice at breakneck speeds in excess of thirty miles an hour, strapping NHL players routinely collided with impacts significantly greater than their NFL counterparts experienced. Even peewee skaters were found to deliver hits packing the same force as college football players; the thirteen-year-old hockey players in one study sustained head impacts averaging about twenty times the force of gravity and sometimes approaching a hundred g's.

By the mid-'90s, hockey's concussion epidemic could no longer be ignored, even by fans who reveled in the sport's violence. All they had to do was watch its devastating effects on Pat LaFontaine, one of the most electrifying stars in the NHL and the greatest American-born player of all time.

From the frozen ponds where he honed his sublime skills in the hockey hotbed of Michigan to the raucous NHL arenas where he showcased them, LaFontaine had always compensated for his small stature with finesse and explosive speed, fearlessly hurtling around the ice like a pinball. His deft stickhandling, playmaking, and shooting made him a perennial All-Star center, but that also made him a constant target of much brawnier opponents hell-bent on crushing him before he could outskate and outsmart them. It was only a matter of time before all the jarring hits—and the concussions that resulted from them—caught up with him.

The hit that changed LaFontaine's life, a vicious blindside elbow to the head from a massive defenseman, sent his helmet flying in one direction and his body in another. His bare forehead bounced off the ice, leaving him unconscious and knocking him out of that game and the following one. Relying on his competitive instinct and the doctors' reassurances that he was fine, LaFontaine went back to play, pushing on through seven more games despite the headaches and the beams of light particles that he alone saw on the ice. Finally, after a loss in which the action seemed to be moving faster than his mind could process, he gathered his teammates around him in the Buffalo Sabres locker room and emotionally apologized for his inexplicably poor play. The next day, when he broke down in tears during a conference with the team's coach, he was instructed to take time off and get some medical help.

LaFontaine told the first neurologist he saw about the pounding headaches and fatigue, about the tears and mood swings, about the loss of enthusiasm and motivation. The doctor attributed the symptoms to the stresses of being a family man, a professional athlete in a slump, and the captain of a floundering team. "You know," he said plainly, as if dispensing a prescription, "I'm sure if you go out and score a couple of goals, you'll feel better and everything will be fine."

A frown of despair and disbelief spread across LaFontaine's boyish face. "Doc, I don't care about scoring goals," he explained, his voice cracking. "I don't care anymore. I'm scared. Something's not right."

The neurologist replied reassuringly, "I'm sure everything's going to be fine. Maybe you just need a few days to get some rest."

What LaFontaine's brain needed was more like a few *months* or a few *years* of rest. He spent the last six months of the 1996–97 season confined to his house and what he called the dark tunnel of his life. Each day brought migraines, nausea, crying jags, cognitive problems so debilitating he couldn't read a bedtime story to his daughters, depression so crippling he couldn't drag himself out of bed in the morning. The source of those symptoms remained a mystery until doctors at the Mayo Clinic finally explained that he was suffering from the cumulative effects of his six diagnosed concussions. The only cure, they told him, was complete rest.

When his post-concussion syndrome finally began to abate in the spring, LaFontaine decided he wanted to do what hockey players always do in the face of adversity: lace up the skates and charge back onto the ice. His wife begged him not to. She reminded him that they were financially secure, especially since the rest of his multiyear contract was guaranteed whether he played again or not. She reminded him that his place in hockey history was likewise secure, his election to the Hall of Fame already assured by his fourteen glorious NHL seasons. She reminded him that his own team didn't want him to play anymore, since the same Sabres doctors who'd once dismissed his symptoms now were refusing to clear him because of his concussion history.

Still, LaFontaine was determined to play on. He rationalized that he had more things to prove to himself and the world. He got the medical clearance he needed from Dr. James Kelly, the renowned neurologist who had authored the most widely followed return-to-play guidelines, and a contract to play for the New York Rangers. LaFontaine couldn't wait to thrill the same Rangers fans who had once rocked an ambulance attempting to whisk him to the hospital after a playoff game in which he'd suffered a bad concussion while starring for the archrival New York Islanders. He instantly won them over by playing the way he always had, firing shots and flicking passes while tumbling to the ice or diving through the air.

Just six months into his comeback, however, an accidental collision with a teammate ended his season with another concussion. That summer, Kelly told LaFontaine that the risk of permanent brain damage was now too great for him to go on playing. Hard as it was to accept, LaFontaine knew that the decision had been made for him by one of the nation's leading concussion experts. He had no choice but to retire at the age of thirty-three.

Fans had barely absorbed the reality of LaFontaine's forced departure when they were jolted by the spectacle of yet another star center being repeatedly felled by concussions. This time, it wasn't another undersized finesse player in a physical sport that traditionally valued strength as much as speed. It was Eric Lindros, the imposing six-foot-four, 245-pound goliath whose rare blend of raw power and pure skill had heralded his NHL arrival as the expected successor to Wayne Gretzky, The Great One himself. For all his hype as "The Next One," Lindros would ironically succumb to the same type of punishing hits that made him such a fearsome force. He sustained four concussions over a five-month span in

2000, a career-threatening barrage that prompted him to publicly blame the Philadelphia Flyers' medical staff for minimizing and mismanaging his head injuries. By the time Lindros was forced into retirement several years later at age thirty-three, post-concussion syndrome had claimed dozens of other NHL careers.

As the concussion epidemic spread down to all levels of play, hockey was proving more perilous than football. NHL players were five times more likely to suffer a concussion than those in the NFL, according to one report. In U.S. college hockey, men were sustaining concussions at a rate 10 percent higher than their football-playing counterparts. The NCAA stats were even more astounding when it came to women's hockey: the concussion rate among females was more than twice that of male skaters and almost two and a half times that of college football players. And just imagine how much more dire those study findings might have been if not for NCAA safety reforms. Unlike the NHL, where reformers advocating safer rules were derisively accused of trying to turn ice hockey into the Ice Capades, at least the authorities at the lower levels were willing to ban dangerous acts like hits to the head.

Despite all the safety rules adopted for amateur players, nothing could banish the macho play-through-pain mentality permeating the sport. Peewees were just as likely as pros to minimize concussions and to lie about symptoms. In a study of Canadians aged eleven to seventeen, player surveys of symptoms found concussion rates up to a hundred times greater than those officially reported to youth hockey authorities.

That came as no surprise to Dr. J. Scott Delaney, a sports medicine and emergency medicine specialist at Montreal's McGill University. As a native of Montreal, the birthplace of organized hockey, Delaney understood how it was Canadians could passionately play through injuries inherent in a rough sport that defined their national identity more than football did for Americans. What Delaney had a harder time understanding was what he witnessed from the sidelines in his role as the team physician for McGill's football and soccer programs. He could see that his college football and soccer players were frequently getting concussed, but when he pressed them, they often denied or minimized their symptoms. He couldn't reconcile what he was observing on the field with the low concussion incidence reported by fellow researchers. He'd scratch his head and think, "Are they dreaming? Have they ever seen how violent this game is? Or are they just living in a lab somewhere? They can't actually believe those results."

Delaney resolved to ferret out the true incidence of concussion among his college athletes. He copied the methodology he'd used in a previous study of pros in the Canadian Football League, where he also served as team physician for the Montreal Alouettes. For that CFL study, he had initially asked players to sign their surveys but quickly discovered that few were willing to admit to concussions for fear that the information would get back to their teams. When he then made the survey anonymous and asked only about head injury symptoms, the number of concussions soared. Equally alarming, the study found that only 19 percent of the concussed CFL players recognized that their symptoms meant they'd sustained a concussion. Delaney's McGill study would yield strikingly similar results among the college athletes. Only 23 percent of concussed college football players realized that they had suffered a concussion during the 1998 season. What's more, only 20 percent of concussed soccer players realized that they had suffered a concussion.

It was clear now that the problem extended beyond the so-called collision sports like football and hockey, where hard hits—tackling and blocking on the gridiron, bodychecking on the ice—are intrinsic to the game. Indeed, the problem reached deep into the so-called contact sports like soccer and basketball, where jolts to the head are incidental yet inevitable.

In an effort to assess the risks faced by student-athletes in a wide range of men's and women's sports, University of Akron researchers screened incoming freshmen each year from 1995 to 2001 about their concussion history, their attitudes toward head injuries, and their understanding of the dangers. Remarkably, more than half of all athletes indicated that they had absolutely no knowledge of the possible consequences of a head injury. An alarming number of the athletes had continued to compete or practice while symptomatic—30 percent saying they played through headaches, 28 percent saying they played through dizziness. Though the failure to report such symptoms to coaches or trainers was more common in football than the other five sports in the study, it was a surprisingly big problem in soccer as well.

That problem trickled down to the high school level and beyond.

In a subsequent multiyear study showing that 41 percent of high school athletes returned to play before their concussions could heal, the rate of noncompliance with published guidelines was higher in boys' and girls' soccer than in football.

What made soccer's own concussion crisis so scary were the raw numbers of both boys and girls who had transformed the world's most popular sport into America's fastest-growing sport. Providing kicks for nearly twenty million kids across the United States, soccer participation surpassed all other sports on the youth level and all team sports save football and basketball on the high school level. High school soccer players were sustaining concussions at a greater rate than every sport except football, with the girls' rate 64 percent higher than the boys'. In college soccer, where men were sustaining concussions at a rate significantly higher than every sport except football and ice hockey, the risk proved far worse for women. Not only were women sustaining concussions at a rate 29 percent higher than their male counterparts on the soccer field, but they were also getting concussed at a greater rate than even football players.

Those stats should give pause to every soccer mom and dad in America.

Melissa Inzitari wasn't always a soccer mom. When she was her daughter's age, Inzitari was a "ball kid," just like Willie Baun. Although her sport was different than his, she played it as aggressively as Willie or any other boy played football. From the instant she scored her first goal in a coed league game as a six-year-old, there was no stopping Melissa on the soccer field. Soccer was what drove her and defined her, what made her feel invincible and invulnerable.

It didn't matter if she was the smallest player out there. As a college freshman shorter than the teammate already nicknamed Midget, Melissa was dubbed Toy. That nickname only fueled her competitive fire. She may have measured all of four foot eleven in her cleats, but there was nothing small about the way she played. She was a dynamo, racing headlong into the fray, sometimes literally running up the back of an opposing player to get as much height as possible.

Nothing epitomized her aggressive style of play better than the signature move she relied on to cut taller opponents down to size. Whenever the ball sailed overhead, she would zero in on its projected flight path to time her leap, soar high into the air to meet it, then drive it hard off the side of her head. She prided herself on her ability to win those headers over taller opponents. Often she would get to the ball first, but sometimes another player would invade her airspace just as she was about to head it. To Melissa, the resulting midair collisions were as much a part of the sport as kicks to the shin.

That's why she didn't give it a second thought when her head collided hard with an opposing player's in the first half of a game early in her sophomore year at the College of New Jersey. After crashing to the ground at midfield, she instinctively picked herself up and rejoined the action just as she had following countless other midair collisions. Only this time, she felt strangely out of sync and in a fog.

At halftime, as she walked shakily off the field, she confided to a teammate that something didn't feel right.

"You need to tell Coach," the teammate urged.

"No-no-no, don't tell him," Melissa begged.

She did admit to an assistant coach at halftime that something was wrong, telling him, "I feel like I don't know where I am." But she was not about to give the head coach any ammunition to pull her from the game. It wasn't only that she wanted to keep playing. As the team captain and star midfielder, she also felt that it was her duty not to let down her teammates or the coaches. So as soon as the team's halftime meeting broke, she jogged out to her position at midfield as if nothing were wrong.

Early in the second half, while her teammates battled to move the ball across midfield, Melissa was off by herself in the defensive zone, wandering in circles, staring up at the lights. The head coach promptly waved her over to pull her from the game. In a daze, she headed to the opposing team's bench. When she finally made it to her own team's bench, she bizarrely kept asking her teammates for chocolate milkshakes.

The coach called for an ambulance and told her, "We have to take you to the hospital."

"You can't take me!" she shot back, her rage rising as she reeled off reasons not to go. Finally she threw her arms up in exasperation and snapped, "Let's just go."

At the nearby hospital in Trenton, doctors examined her and ordered up a CAT scan. After reading it, they assured her everything was normal and sent her home with clearance to return to play. The next day, she was back at practice, back in her regular routine as if nothing had happened. She played through the entire 1996 season with her usual intensity, heading balls even though she was still plagued by constant headaches. As her sophomore year wore on, strange symptoms began to appear. Loud noises now made her head pound worse, and she was so sensitive to light that she took to wearing sunglasses even in dark places like movie theaters.

Over the following year, the symptoms became stranger and scarier. She would lose her car in parking lots. She would get lost driving home. She would get confused on the way to class, wandering aimlessly through a two-story building searching in vain for a third-floor classroom. Her grades plummeted, a D for one class reducing her to tears. Her moods were swinging wildly. She'd never been one to cry no matter how painful the hurt, but now she found herself weeping uncontrollably over McDonald's commercials. She'd always been buoyant and bubbly with a broad smile that attracted friends like a magnet, but now she was increasingly withdrawn and antisocial. She'd always been measured and even-keeled, but now she was impulsive and short-tempered, sometimes to the point of nastiness. The low point was the day she confronted her coach in a crowded restaurant, screaming and cursing at him over something inconsequential. Friends and family couldn't help noticing the change. After one argument with her kid brother, she overheard him say, "She's such a bitch now."

What really scared her were the physical symptoms that threatened her very identity as an athlete. She would lie in bed and the room would spin as if she were drunk. She temporarily lost the vision in her left eye and the hearing in her left ear. One day, she was at home alone taking a shower when she closed her eyes to let the water wash over her face and suddenly lost her balance and fell. She began to think she must have a brain tumor. Of course, she wasn't about to seek help for the suspected brain tumor any more than she had for the unsuspected head injury. Having endured broken ankles, fractured ribs, and countless smaller injuries, she played through these new problems dogging her every stride: the ringing in her ears, the fogginess and blurriness, the queasiness in the pit of her stomach. She would vomit at halftime, play the entire second half, then vomit again after the game.

One day after throwing up at halftime, she emerged from the bathroom to find her boyfriend, Joe, waiting with a worried look. "Enough's enough already," he said sternly. After the game, Joe did what he knew his longtime girlfriend never would: he went to the coach and told him what had been going on. In the locker room right after the game, the coach approached Melissa and insisted she get medical help. He and the team physician sent her to see Jill Brooks, the neuropsychologist who also treated the athletes from Rutgers University.

The day of the appointment, Melissa expected to be at Robert Wood Johnson University Hospital just long enough to get the medical clearance she needed to return to play. Brooks had other plans. Before Melissa could mention any of the symptoms that had brought her there, Brooks hit her with a series of questions: "Are you sensitive to light? Are you forgetting things that happened yesterday? Are you more emotional? Have you noticed changes in your personality?" With each succeeding nod of her head, Melissa felt more and more relieved that someone finally understood what she'd been experiencing.

Six hours of neuropsychological testing would confirm Brooks's opinion that Melissa had sustained a severe concussion. Melissa was perplexed by the mere mention of the word "concussion." How could she possibly have a concussion if she'd never lost consciousness, if the doctors had found nothing wrong in the ER, if she'd been cleared to go right back to play? Brooks explained how the initial injury had been continually exacerbated because Melissa kept playing without ever giving her brain a chance to heal. Melissa let out a sigh of relief. At least she wasn't losing her mind, she thought. At least she didn't have a brain tumor—it was only a concussion.

Brooks could see that the message wasn't getting through. "This is serious," she warned. "You need to stop playing. Your body needs rest—rest from soccer, rest from all activity, rest from everything."

Melissa still didn't get the message. She stopped playing soccer, but she continued to work out at the gym and to run laps with her teammates at practice until the coach would throw her off the field. She was in denial. "It can't be that bad," she'd rationalize to herself. "How bad could it be if nobody's seen anything on a CAT scan?"

Brooks had an answer for that. She sent Melissa to a neurologist for an electroencephalogram to measure her brain waves. Not long afterward, Melissa walked into Brooks's office demanding clearance to return to play. "I'm getting back on the field," Melissa announced. "These tests aren't showing anything. There's nothing out there proving there's something wrong with me, except for what's going on with my body."

"Uhhh, how about that EEG?" Brooks said.

"It's normal," Melissa replied. "When I called them, the receptionist said that if the doctor didn't reach out to me, then it's normal."

"No, it's not," Brooks said as she reached for the phone.

She dialed it and handed the receiver to Melissa. The neurologist on the other end informed Melissa that the EEG was in fact abnormal and that the squiggly lines on the printout revealed she was suffering absence seizures. He told her that the seizures explained why she would space out for a few seconds every now and then, and he recommended that she start taking antiepileptic meds immediately. When she hung up the phone, she looked shaken. Then she suddenly perked up and asked Brooks, "How many seizures am I having in a day? Because if I'm not having so many, I could probably go back to play."

Melissa couldn't understand why she wasn't getting through to this stubborn neuropsychologist. When her mother suggested that a specialist might know more about concussions than a headstrong patient, Melissa defiantly argued, "I've always gotten my way. I haven't had a doctor sideline me before. This lady's not going to do it."

As relentless off the field as she was on it, Melissa continued to lobby Brooks for medical clearance all through her senior year. She felt lost and frustrated over not being able to play. She felt like she was no longer part of the team she still captained. She felt useless to her teammates and her coaches, pushed aside by everyone as if she were invisible. Here she was, a preseason All-American selection, sitting out her entire senior season just because her neuropsychologist wouldn't give her clearance. "I'm not hurt," she'd rail at Brooks. "*You're* the one that's out of her mind. If you won't clear me, then I'll just go somewhere else and find someone who will."

Even after she graduated the following spring, Melissa couldn't give up the game she still yearned to play. When she was offered the chance to join a local semipro team that summer, she couldn't sign the contract fast enough. The only thing that could stop her was the medical release form she needed signed by a doctor. She charged into Brooks's office, waving the form and shouting, "I know you're going to sign it. I know you're going to clear me. Sign it now. I'm standing right here."

Brooks shook her head emphatically. The time had come to sit Melissa down and explain the facts of brain injury. "You're going to have to decide about your future," Brooks said. "I recommend that you don't return to play—ever." Brooks paused before driving home her point: "You can play now, or you can read to your kids someday."

Melissa knew in her heart that Brooks was right, especially since some of her concussion symptoms still lingered, but she just wasn't ready to give up the sport that defined who she was. She kept playing in pickup games and recreational leagues whenever she could. But something was missing. Gone were the adrenaline rushes of competition and the exhilaration of winning. The mere thought of heading a soccer ball now put a knot in her stomach. She didn't want to risk another major concussion and the disabling symptoms it could bring back. By now, she had married Joe and they were about to start a family. She wanted to be able to read to her kids. The child growing in her womb reminded her that she had responsibilities to others and couldn't keep playing games with her health for their sake as well as her own.

She decided it was time to quit. In her mind, that equated to losing a part of herself. For as long as she could remember, the soccer ball had been an extension of her feet; if she couldn't find a friend or sibling to kick it around with, she'd simply go off by herself and kick it against a wall. Playing soccer had given her not only confidence and self-esteem, but also an outlet that helped her through tough times like her parents' divorce. She couldn't imagine life without soccer.

Melissa found a compromise: she became a coach. She started coaching the same youth league club on which she had played as a young girl in Bridgewater, New Jersey. She began with a team of eight-year-old girls and had so much fun with them that she soon added elite squads of teens and tweens. She also coached at the same high school where she had earned All-American honors as a junior and senior. To the kids on her teams, Melissa was a role model talking from experience as both player and patient. She taught them about the dangers of concussions and the need to report all head injuries to coaches, trainers, and parents.

Before she let her girls out on the field the first day of practice each season, she would introduce herself to them and deliver the concussion lecture. Whether in team meetings or one-on-one chats, she would never miss an opportunity to share with them what she had learned the hard way. She would buttonhole the parents, educating them about the warning signs. She told everyone who would listen about the repercussions that come when young athletes play while still symptomatic.

Every once in a while, a kid would show up who presented a special challenge. None would resonate more with Melissa than the girl who reminded her so much of herself when she was twelve years old. Not only was this girl the star player on her club team, but she also exhibited the same traits that Melissa once displayed: the speed, the aggressiveness, the determination to win, the stubbornness to play through injuries without ever thinking of reporting them. So when the girl collided hard with the opposing team's goalkeeper and got up slowly and unsteadily, Melissa sensed this was just the beginning of a long-term issue. Melissa pulled the girl from the game without hesitation and without debate. That was the easy part. It would be much harder to sideline her for more than just that one game. Now Melissa could see what it was like to be on the other side, trying to spot an injury when players were doing their best to hide it and then having to stand up to athletes and parents who pressed coaches for a quick return to play. In this case, the parents turned out to need little persuading. To convince the girl, though, Melissa had to recount her own story of how playing through concussions cut her soccer career short at the age of nineteen. In the end, her own experience became her best argument.

Melissa was now preaching the gospel according to Jill Brooks. The conversion from skeptic to apostle was complete when Melissa finally embraced her neuropsychologist's mission to spread the word. Melissa had learned that the congregants who most needed to hear the sermon were already in the pews: her girls. Brooks's research had shown that high school girls knew even less about concussions than boys—and took them less seriously than boys. When Melissa sought advice on dealing with her concussed players, Brooks explained how societal attitudes complicated the subject. Females, Brooks said, often assume they can't get concussions because they were told since they were little girls that they don't play hard enough to get them. Making matters worse, she added, females tend to ignore the most common concussion symptom; because they're more prone than males to get headaches, females often dismiss them as a sign of stress or a symptom of premenstrual syndrome.

Brooks didn't have to tell Melissa what she would be up against as a coach trying to protect her players from concussions. Melissa knew from personal experience how easy it was for an athlete to rationalize away warnings, even when they came from a specialist. She was hardly the only patient who dismissed Brooks as a doctor just being overcautious, a mother hen just being overprotective. Melissa could remember many times when, in response to yet another lecture about protecting her brain, she'd tell Brooks only half jokingly, "Stop mothering me."

Brooks had been struggling for years to find a way to get through to the girls. Then she stumbled upon the most effective of all educational tools: the athletes themselves. If her patients wouldn't listen to doctor's orders, maybe they could be reached by fellow athletes who'd experienced what they were now going through. And who would make a better peer mentor than Melissa Inzitari?

Melissa had been out of school only a few years when Brooks asked her to meet with another patient, a college field hockey player who wasn't getting the message. When the two young women were introduced in Brooks's office, Melissa saw a mirror image of her younger self. The story Katrina Majewski told her that day sounded eerily familiar.

A few months earlier, in a field hockey scrimmage at the beginning of Katrina's freshman year at Rutgers, a ball had deflected off a stick and struck her in the temple. Although so dazed that she staggered to the wrong sideline after being pulled from the scrimmage, she was cleared to resume practicing the next day. Accustomed to playing through pain, Katrina ignored the migraines and the odd symptoms that began bothering her seemingly out of nowhere. She was nodding off in class, unable to focus on lectures. She sank into depression, sleeping and crying all the time. She was often irritable, sometimes snapping at her teammates. Since it was early in her freshman year, her new teammates and coaches didn't recognize how uncharacteristic her behavior was. But her mother noticed it during their daily phone conversations and she confronted team doctors, insisting that Katrina get further medical evaluation. Which is how

Katrina wound up getting referred to Brooks, the neuropsychologist for Rutgers athletic teams.

Brooks's diagnosis of post-concussion syndrome shocked Katrina, who had always assumed that a concussion required loss of consciousness. Not only had Katrina sustained a concussion in that preseason scrimmage, but she had also suffered at least seven undiagnosed ones in high school by Brooks's count. The cumulative effect explained why her symptoms now were so profound and persistent, why her cognitive deficits were so pronounced, why this honors student would need special accommodations to help with such routine tasks as taking notes and taking tests.

Brooks refused to clear Katrina to return to the Rutgers field hockey team. What's more, Brooks told Katrina to refrain from all physical activity until her symptoms completely resolved and to think seriously about giving up field hockey because of the risk of permanent brain damage. Katrina had dreamed of playing college field hockey too long to accept that concussions could stop her before she could play a single game for the Scarlet Knights. When Katrina continued to talk about how much she wanted to get back on the field, Brooks suggested she meet Melissa to get the perspective of a peer who had been through a similar experience.

As Katrina recounted her story in Brooks's office, Melissa nodded knowingly and sympathetically. Melissa told Katrina her own story and talked about the factors that influenced her decision to finally walk away from something that had once defined her. Then Melissa uttered the words that gave Katrina pause: "You can fulfill your dreams as an athlete now, or you can have a normal life and read to your kids someday."

Melissa was speaking from the heart as well as from experience, having recently given birth to her first child. Playing the "kid" card turned out to be her trump. It convinced Katrina to give up her dream and her sport, and it converted her into another of Brooks's apostles. As a mentor in this growing network of one-on-one support groups, Melissa played the kid card with all the other young women whose concussions brought them to a crossroads in their lives. "I'm past that point in my life, I have kids," she said. "If some of these athletes don't stop, they're not going to get to that point. They're not going to be able to enjoy their kids or read to them or any of that stuff."

Melissa still had some post-concussion symptoms, but at least she could read to her daughter, Alyssa. The lingering symptoms—headaches, sensitivity to light, short-term memory problems—wouldn't stop her from going back to school to become a registered nurse, raising a growing family, and continuing her concussion crusade. Nor would it stop her from being a soccer mom to dozens of girls—including her own daughter.

When Alyssa turned seven, she started playing youth soccer on a coed team. As a soccer mom, Melissa couldn't help but worry about head injuries. While other parents shouted encouragement for their kids to score goals, Melissa would be hollering, "Don't hit 'em in the head!" At Alyssa's age, the kids look more like Weebles than soccer players, the ball stays on the ground, and the goal is fun rather than winning. In a few years, when the games become ultracompetitive, the play superaggressive, and the impacts inevitable, Melissa knows she might feel differently about Alyssa's participation. At least Melissa can take comfort in knowing that her daughter will have been regularly schooled on the importance of playing safely and of telling adults about any injuries. Before Alyssa started playing soccer, Melissa sat her down and explained the facts of brain injury. Not long afterward, Melissa overheard Alyssa telling someone, "You know, Mommy lost part of her brain." That reminded Melissa about the need to tailor the message to the age of the audience.

Melissa developed a whole new perspective when she became a soccer mom. She remembers how her dad broke down in tears the day in Brooks's office when he learned about the concussion problem she had kept hidden from him and everyone else. That memory fuels her resolve to make parents allies in the war on concussions. "You can't be a friend to your kids all the time," she'll tell parents. "When my daughter cries and says, 'You're a bad mom,' it breaks my heart. But in the end, every time she goes out to ride her bicycle, I don't even have to say, 'Get your helmet.' She has it in her hand."

If Alyssa isn't growing up in the same concussion culture her mom did, it's only because Melissa Inzitari is an anomaly, an enlightened crusader at a time when brain injury is only beginning to come out of the dark ages. Most Americans still don't see concussions for the traumatic brain injuries they are.

Chapter 4

Sudden Impact

Over the past decade, it has become clear that damage from concussions can add up. And the result can sometimes be as debilitating as a severe brain injury. Scientists are beginning to believe that all traumatic brain injuries—from concussions to severe head traumas—have a similar impact on the brain; these injuries are simply at different points on a continuum. The reasons will become clear if you look at the symptoms suffered by someone with a severe TBI, be it from a wartime bomb blast or a horrific car wreck.

I

The sun was just peeking over the horizon as Sergeant Brian Radke and three other soldiers loaded their Humvee for the day's mission. A few wisps of cloud mottled the brightening Baghdad sky, and the deep reds and purples of the sunrise reminded Radke of mornings back home in Arizona. Normally, his brain would have been racing and his heart pumping as he psyched himself up to venture beyond the relative safety of the Army base. But today, the memories of home and the beauty of the sunrise brought a surprising sense of serenity.

As the team loaded the last of the equipment into their Humvee, the soldier who was supposed to man the gun turret asked Radke to swap positions. Though Radke would have preferred to keep his assignment as driver, he could see that Specialist Jeremiah Robinson was feeling queasy and clearly not up to standing in the turret on constant alert for snipers and warning signs of a roadside bomb.

The Humvee rolled slowly through the gate past the coils of razor wire that surrounded Camp Liberty, and Radke poked his head up through the turret. Once on the smooth four-lane highway, he was struck by how light the traffic was and how pleasant the cool desert air felt against his face. "This is a *nice* day," he thought.

As the Humvee powered past the broad fallow fields that bracketed the highway, Radke stood in the turret, swiveling the .50-caliber machine gun right and left, his eyes searching for any indications of danger. After several uneventful miles, he spotted the section of highway where another Humvee from his platoon had been blown completely off the road a week earlier by an improvised explosive device. The IED blast had killed a buddy from his unit, the Arizona National Guard's 860th Military Police Company.

Normally traffic was fairly heavy in this area, but today it was so quiet that Radke started to feel uneasy. As they approached a pedestrian overpass where insurgents would often toss grenades down into the turrets of passing Humvees, he looked up to check the railing for anything suspicious. The overpass was deserted, so he turned his attention back to the road. A broken-down van on the right shoulder beneath the overpass caught his eye. Because abandoned vehicles were often used as car bombs, Radke ducked down into the Humvee for safety. With his left hand holding on to the roof and his right hand clutching his M4 assault rifle, he continued to scan for danger through the windshield as they passed under the overpass.

Then he heard a click.

Everything after that seemed to pass in slow motion. He felt himself blown backward. As he lay on his back, he noticed the brilliant blue sky through the turret. He glanced to his left and saw smoke pouring in through the driver's side. He peered through the smoke looking for the driver, his close friend Jeremiah Robinson, and saw a body with no head.

Suddenly Radke realized the truck was still moving—without anyone to steer it. "We're out of control," he thought. The Humvee lumbered on through the barren fields with Radke slipping in and out of consciousness, briefly coming to each time it hit a bump. He was jolted awake when the truck crashed through a brick wall and then finally came to a stop after smashing into the front of a house. With the engine stalled out, there wasn't a sound. The unexpected quiet made him nervous. He wondered whether he was the only member of his team to survive the blast.

At first he lay on his back silently, worried that any sound might attract the attention of the insurgents who had planted the bomb. He started thinking what might happen if the wrong person found him. "If I get captured, I could end up in some video getting my head sawed off," he thought, "and then it'll be all over the Internet for my family to see."

As time passed, Radke found himself worrying less about the insurgents and more about his own condition. He could feel the blood running down his face, but he couldn't feel anything else. The blood from his head wounds had poured into his eyes, leaving him unable to see. He tried to sit up, but couldn't. He could feel panic starting to rise up. Finally, he screamed for help, and, seemingly out of nowhere, the team's medic appeared.

"Everything's OK, everything's OK," the medic said as he opened one of the rear doors. "Help is on its way. Let's get you out of here."

He grabbed Radke under the arms and tried to pull him out. But Radke was stuck. He couldn't feel his legs. He thought, "Oh my God, my legs are gone."

The medic said, "I need you to push with your legs."

"I can't feel 'em, Doc," Radke shot back.

"Just push, just push," Doc encouraged.

Radke started to think that maybe his legs were indeed still there. He willed them to push, and finally Doc was able to pull him free. For the first time, Radke screamed in pain. Then he lost consciousness.

When Radke came to, he was on the ground. Another medic was cutting off his clothes and patching up whatever wounds he could. The medic kept repeating, "Stay with me, stay with me."

A hail of molten metal from the IED had pierced whatever flesh Radke's body armor didn't cover. Five pieces of shrapnel had lodged in his brain. Hundreds of other shards had lodged in his face, neck, arms, and legs. One of them had nicked his carotid artery. His jaw was fractured. His left forearm was broken in two places and the wrist was shattered. His right index finger was hanging by a shred of skin.

As Radke lay on the ground, his squad leader periodically came to check on him and to reassure him. "You're doing good—just hang in there," the squad leader said as he knelt next to Radke's head. "The medevac is on its way. We're getting you out of here." Two soldiers loaded his stretcher onto the hood of a Humvee and climbed up beside Radke to steady him during the drive back to the highway.

His vision, which had been coming and going, had not returned for a while. He heard the rotors as the medevac helicopter approached and then felt the wind coming off its blades when it landed. He felt himself being lifted off the Humvee and carried onto the chopper. After the door slammed shut, he felt the chopper lifting off the ground. Every time he would lose consciousness during the short flight, medics would shake him awake.

When the helicopter landed, he heard the door open and then, over the roar of the rotors, he heard some female voices. He felt himself being carried off the chopper and had the sensation he was being wheeled into a hospital. In the operating room of the 86th Combat Army Support Hospital, a nurse kept prompting him for his name. He sensed a very bright light above him. For a while, he focused on the light. But then, everything started to fade to black. The bright light above him got smaller and smaller, until it was just a pinpoint. Then there was nothing.

Nova Radke had spent a restless night. Again and again, she'd been jolted awake by terrifying nightmares. Each time, she would see something horrible happening to her husband—Brian being shot, Brian being blown up, Brian being captured and tortured—and then she would wake up in a cold sweat. As morning broke and the Arizona sun rose high enough to start warming the cool desert air, Nova's terrier shot up, circled at her feet, and began to whine.

Nova woke briefly, then slipped into a kind of waking dream. She had the sensation that Brian had just entered the room and then she felt his presence, his warmth, as he came closer to her.

"I just need to come to bed," she heard him say. "I'm tired. I need to go to sleep."

She scrunched her eyes tight, and said, "No, you need to go back! Don't lie down! Go back to where you were and fight! You'll be alright."

He disappeared as quickly as he had appeared, and Nova opened her eyes. She rolled over to look at the alarm clock and saw it was exactly 9:00 A.M. She was still looking at the clock when the phone rang at 9:02. She glanced at the caller ID, saw that it was an Army number, and immediately grabbed the phone.

"Nova Radke?" a female voice asked.

"Yes," Nova answered nervously as she stood up and started walking aimlessly around the room.

"This is Colonel Spear from the Arizona National Guard. Brian's been hurt in an accident. We don't have much more information about what happened. I'm en route to your home—"

"Ma'am, is it OK if you don't come over?" Nova interrupted. "I just need to be by myself for a few moments. I *will* call you back."

She let the phone drop into the cradle and sank to the floor, weeping. She sat there for a few minutes, thinking about her life and how, in an instant, everything had changed. Still in a daze, she picked up the phone and dialed Spear back.

As soon as the colonel picked up, Nova asked the all-important question: "Is he alive?"

"Yes," Spear answered.

Nova hung up and called Brian's cell phone, hoping that someone might pick up. She called over and over again, but it just kept dumping into voicemail. Remembering that a friend's husband was stationed in Baghdad with Brian, she called him. The soldier on the other end reassured her, "Brian's at the CASH, they're working on him, and he's stable." Another friend supplied a phone number that gave her direct access to the 86th Combat Army Support Hospital. A doctor there told her about the shrapnel, the lacerations, the broken bones, and the severed index finger. He told her that Brian had lost a lot of blood, that he'd had a stroke, and that twice his heart had stopped and they'd had to shock him back to life.

A team of eight surgeons had worked on him for twelve hours to get him stabilized, the doctor continued. Because of his head wounds, Brian had been medevacked sixty miles north to the military's frontline trauma center at Balad for evaluation by brain injury specialists. There, doctors decided to leave the five pieces of shrapnel in his brain because surgery to remove them might do more harm than good.

Once Brian was stable enough to travel the two thousand miles to the U.S. military's main foreign hospital in Landstuhl, Germany, he was placed on an Air Force cargo plane specially outfitted to provide the same critical care as a land-bound intensive care unit. At Landstuhl Regional Medical Center, he coded again as doctors were getting him ready to fly back to the United States. At that point, one of the doctors called Nova and suggested she fly to Germany with Brian's parents. Nova knew what that meant: the doctors didn't think Brian was going to make it home alive. "No, I'm going to see him on American soil," she insisted.

Five days after the explosion, Brian was back on one of the Air Force's flying ICUs, headed home. He was still in a medically induced coma, but at least he was alive and on his way to Walter Reed Army Medical Center in Washington, D.C., where the most seriously injured soldiers are sent for state-of-the-art treatment.

When Nova heard that Brian had arrived at Walter Reed, she raced over to see him. As she walked across the hospital's dark and deserted parking lot, she thought, "This all feels so surreal." The silence gave the night a dreamlike quality that followed her down the empty hallways leading to the ICU. As she approached Brian's bed, the bevy of nurses bustling around him jolted her back to reality. The closer she got to his bedside, the faster her heart beat. The sight of him lying there so still suddenly brought home the overwhelming reality of his wounds. His face was so swollen that he was barely recognizable. It seemed as if there were stitches and tubes everywhere. His red and raw neck made her think of ground hamburger meat. Staples ran all the way from his right ear to his collarbone. Bandages ran from his fingertips to his armpits and from his toes to the tops of his thighs.

Nova could hear the ventilator steadily breathing for her husband. As she watched his chest rising and falling in rhythm with the machine, her own breathing started to quicken. Suddenly she had the sensation of hot water pouring over her. She felt the heat flow from the top of her head, over her shoulders, and down to her waist. Then she crumpled to the floor, unconscious. The next thing she knew, she was sitting in a chair and a nurse was asking, "Honey, are you OK?"

The following day, Nova was sitting across from the doctor in charge of Brian's care. The doctor explained that he wasn't very optimistic after looking at Brian's brain scan. He said that there was extensive damage to the right frontal lobe and that there was even a possibility that her husband might end up "a vegetable." He then asked Nova if she had any questions.

"Yes," she said. "Will he still be able to have children?"

"Oh yes," the doctor nodded reassuringly, "those muscles still work."

"No, I mean *mentally*," she exclaimed, starting to laugh for the first time since the distressing call from Colonel Spear. "What is he going to be like when he wakes up?"

"Until he comes out of the coma," the doctor said, "we just won't know."

Stunned, Nova sat silently for a few long moments, a rush of new worries tumbling through her brain. "What if he wakes up and tells me he doesn't love me anymore?" she thought. "What if he doesn't even know me?"

The doctor told her that the only thing she could do for Brian while she waited for him to wake up from the coma was to sit by his side and talk to him. So Nova essentially moved into Brian's room. She slept and showered there, going out for just a few hours each day to clear her head. Knowing how much he loved sports, Nova made sure his TV was tuned in to whatever game she could find. When there wasn't a game, she would sit next to Brian and reassure him that he was home now and that she would take care of him. Periodically she would try to bring him out of the coma by loudly calling his name.

One day, about a week after he had arrived at Walter Reed, Brian suddenly opened his eyes and looked straight at her. Even though his jaw was wired shut and he shouldn't have been able to speak with the trach in his neck, Brian somehow managed to utter the words: "I promised. I promised." Nova saw one big tear well up in his left eye, and as it trickled down the side of his face, she knew he was going to make it back to her. Then his eyes closed and he again slipped into a coma.

Brian's words brought Nova back to the day, two weeks before the explosion, when the promise was made. He'd returned from Iraq for R&R and had traveled with Nova to visit his family in his hometown of Vancouver, Washington. As they stood on the patio of his parents' house holding each other's hands in the shadow of Mount St. Helens, Brian and Nova talked about the future and their fears for his safety. Brian told her that no matter what happened, he'd come home to her, "I promise."

For the next couple of weeks while he remained unconscious, nine teams of doctors took turns putting Brian's broken body back together again—one day placing rods in his shattered forearm, another day removing the bigger hunks of shrapnel from his legs. When he finally did come out of the coma for good, he was disoriented. He thought that he was still in Baghdad and that only a day had passed since the explosion.

He was still trying to piece together memories of the blast when Nova walked into the room. She was dressed all in black, her slight five-foot-three frame swallowed up by the bulky Army-issue poplin jacket, her face, tanned dark by the Arizona sun, barely peeking out from under a scarf beanie. "Hi, honey," she exclaimed, happy to find him finally awake.

"Get out!" he screamed. "Get the hell out of my room, dammit, you little Iraqi S.O.B.!"

Nova reached over to touch his shoulder, hoping to reassure him. But Brian pulled away and yelled, "Help!" Again she tried to comfort him, and he growled, "Quit touching me! Quit touching me!"

Hearing the commotion, several nurses rushed in and took Nova aside. "He doesn't recognize you," one of them explained. "You need to go out and take your hat and jacket off." Nova left the room and shed the offending articles of clothing. When she returned, she found Brian bolt upright in the bed, his eyes wide open. He looked at her and exclaimed, "I'm so glad you're here. Some Iraqi kid was trying to take my body parts."

Relieved as Nova was to be recognized, she was frightened by the implications of what she had just seen. "Oh my God, is he going to be like this forever?" she thought. "If he's like this all the time, how am I going to live and deal with it? Am I going to lose my husband?"

It would take several months before Brian consistently recognized his wife. Even on the days he didn't know who Nova was, he was happy for her visits. "Well, I don't know who she is, but she's hot," he'd think. "She's nice. She hasn't hurt me. She wants to take care of me. I'll stick with it."

On a warm September day almost a year later, Brian Radke was in the vast physical therapy room at Walter Reed seated across the table from a therapist, working to regain strength and flexibility in his shattered left wrist. Nearby, a gaunt teenager in a wheelchair was raising and lowering an exercise ball behind his head while another soldier was flipping through the latest issue of *Amputee Golfer* magazine.

The once-muscular physique that had made Radke a star high school and college athlete—a quarterback and shortstop who went on to play two years of minor-league baseball—was now wasted by the loss of nearly sixty pounds from his six-foot-one frame. A baggy ARMY T-shirt tucked into formfitting sweatpants accentuated his unintended trimness. Shrapnel had marred his chiseled features, leaving scars slicing across both cheeks and several small dents just above his thick, dark eyebrows. He was clean-shaven and still wore his brown hair short in a military-style fade.

As he finished up his exercises, Radke started thinking about what he was going to say to the two reporters he was scheduled to meet after the morning's physical therapy session. If he was going to give them an unvarnished view of what life was like for brain-injured soldiers coming home from the war, he would have to be completely honest about how the explosion had changed his own life. That would mean being candid about the profound memory loss still plaguing him and the behavioral problems that were whittling away at his relationship with his wife. For a man with a strong sense of privacy, it was going to be a challenge.

Radke hobbled into the lounge where the reporters were waiting, introduced himself, and carefully eased his body onto a couch. As he started to tell his story, his face was expressionless and his voice so dispassionate that he could have been reciting the details of someone else's horrific ordeal. He impassively told the reporters about the click he heard an instant before the explosion, the image of his best friend's decapitated body, and the molten metal that had pierced so many parts of his own body—and his brain. Then he began to describe all the enduring repercussions from the blast, both the obvious injuries to his body and the far less visible wounds to his brain.

Since that fateful October day in 2005, Radke's body had been constantly under siege. He suffered from relentless headaches and extreme sensitivity to light. High doses of painkillers had become a routine part of his life. He had undergone some sixty surgeries. There was one to replace a damaged nerve in his arm, another to repair a mangled knee, dozens to remove the shards of metal embedded in his arms and legs. Even a year after the blast, he still had more than five hundred pieces of shrapnel in him. Every so often, his body would expel one of the small steel shards.

Last winter, on his thirty-first birthday, he was eating a grilled cheese sandwich with Nova in the hospital cafeteria when he suddenly started to choke. He brought a napkin up to his face and coughed up a small rounded hunk of steel that had worked its way through the lining of his throat and into his mouth.

As distressing as the injuries to his body were, they worried Radke far less than what had befallen his brain.

Before the blast, Radke said, he had been easygoing and quiet. Now, he was moody and quick-tempered. "Some days I'll get really emotional," he said. "This past Sunday I cried for seven hours, and I have no idea why. I don't know from one minute to the next how I'm going to feel. I'll go from being in a good mood to being upset. Some things that didn't bother me before drive me crazy now. In sixty seconds, I can go from happy to 'I wanna kick your butt.'" He said he had also lost the ability to censor ugly thoughts. Once something popped into his brain, he'd need to say it even if it hurt the feelings of those closest to him, like Nova. "It's almost like having Tourette's, I guess," he said with a smile. "That's what my wife says when we're joking about it."

Worse yet, the brain injury had left Radke with slowed mental processing and with problems focusing and organizing his thoughts. Expressing them was even more difficult. After months of speech therapy, he sometimes still had trouble stringing together coherent sentences. Occasionally he'd stumble over a word and then lose his train of thought, unable to remember what he'd just been saying. His inability to keep track of verbal exchanges was causing trouble with Nova. "A lot of times my wife and I will be talking and we'll get into an argument and she's like, 'You said da-da da-da,' and I'm like, 'What? You're crazy. I did *not* say that.' And that just fuels the fight."

Those kinds of short-term memory problems extended to every part of his life. Before the explosion, he was always able to keep his schedule in his head. Now, he needed to write down every detail in a day planner and still he'd forget the purpose of appointments or miss them entirely. In fact, he said, just this morning he'd had a typical memory lapse as he was starting the therapy for his shattered wrist. After noticing that his watch was getting in the way, he decided to bring it over to where he had stashed his belongings. By the time he got there, he'd forgotten that he wanted to drop the watch off. So he returned to the table where his therapist was waiting, only to realize that he was still wearing the watch. There would be three more futile trips across the room before he finally came up with a strategy: he took the watch off and carried it over in his hand as a concrete reminder to leave it behind.

More troubling to Radke was the loss of his long-term memory. He couldn't remember his favorite color, his favorite food, his favorite movie, his favorite football team. He remembered that Nova was his wife, but couldn't recall the past he shared with her. He remembered his parents' names, but not his childhood.

Without memories of his past, he'd lost any sense of who he was. "Sometimes," he said, "I feel like I'm just a body."

Feeling lost and empty, Radke searched desperately for clues that could help him understand who he'd been before the blast. The neurologist at Walter Reed had told Radke that his memories hadn't been completely erased, only locked away: "The filing cabinet is there. What's impaired is your ability to open it."

Radke found a key to some of those locked-away memories in his hometown. Visiting his parents while on a brief leave, he stopped by the baseball field where he'd played Little League as a boy. As he looked out across the expanse of lush green grass, images of long-past games and old teammates started flashing in his brain, like still photos. He couldn't convert those mental snapshots into a flowing narrative, but at least it was something.

He drove back to the small brick house that had been his parents' home for nearly half a century, hoping that the familiar surroundings might spark more flashes of memory. But even when his mom and dad tried to reminisce with him, he couldn't remember anything before Iraq— not his childhood, not his school years, not even the day he met Nova. Trying to help things along, his mother dug out a stack of family photo albums. As he thumbed through the stiff pages, he saw himself wearing his father's Army jacket while playing dress-up with his big sister, blowing out birthday candles, running the football in a high school game. He'd stare at a series of photos chronicling an event in his life and then try to connect the static images. But he never managed to fill in the voids between the snapshots.

Radke's luck wasn't much better on a trip back to Arizona with Nova, even though that was where they'd built their life together. They had met late one night a few years earlier and had immediately connected, sharing their most intimate thoughts and dreams. Right from the start they were finishing each other's sentences. It felt as if they had known each other all their lives. Nova would say later that it was the first time she felt she could breathe. Within a year, they were married.

Nova was now hoping that the sights, sounds, and scents flooding her heart with warm memories would spark the same for Brian. But he couldn't remember what was important about any of the places and things that meant so much to her. She rented movies they'd enjoyed together, but none resonated with him. She took him to his favorite restaurants, but he didn't order any of the foods she knew he'd loved. She would start to reminiscence about one of their shared memories, hoping he'd chime in and finish the story, but he would only stare back blankly.

It was as if a complete stranger had taken over her husband's body, one who sometimes bizarrely spoke in a southern drawl that Brian had never used before the blast. Worse yet, the man beside her was a stranger even to himself.

Nova had heard the divorce statistics—that fully three-quarters of marriages involving a brain-injured spouse fail—and now she could understand firsthand why. But she wasn't ready to give up. She was sure the old Brian was locked away somewhere in that brain, and if she kept searching, she would find him and rescue him. Only a year had passed since he'd awoken from the coma—she just needed to be persistent.

Brian wasn't as confident, and he was scared that Nova might lose patience and leave before he could figure out who he was. He kept poring over old photos, trying to use them to reconstruct his life story. It would be another two years before his mental snapshots started to connect like the film frames of a movie.

In the meantime, memories trickled back only as disconnected fragments. For Brian, it was like having a handful of pieces from a huge jigsaw puzzle—there weren't enough of them yet to get even a glimpse of the whole man. When new memories did show up, it was with no pattern or predictability. Sometimes he'd have a flash when he was concentrating hard on an exercise during cognitive therapy. Sometimes a memory would resurface when he wasn't even looking for it.

That could happen during something as mundane as eating dinner at home with his wife. One evening, while he was still chewing on a forkful of taco salad, he suddenly stopped, looked down at the tomatoes and onions on his plate, and exclaimed, "Are you trying to kill me? You know I don't eat this stuff!" Then he flung his plate across the room. Nova was taken aback. While it was true that Brian had hated tomatoes and onions before the blast, he'd been gobbling them down with gusto ever since then. Before Nova could respond, he pointed an accusing finger at her and said, "I have a brain injury and you're just trying to use that to change me into what *you* want me to be." She shook her head emphatically and replied, "No-no-no-no, I was just feeding them to you because they're healthy and good for you. I don't know, I figured maybe you like them now."

Nova didn't understand why tonight that particular memory suddenly surged back. For months, she had been watching Brian eat all sorts of things he'd previously hated and turn away from foods he'd formerly loved. She had recently taken him to a steakhouse so he could enjoy his favorite cut of beef, only to watch in disbelief as he ordered chicken.

Brian's recollection that he hated tomatoes and onions was a turning point. In the months that followed, he started to remember which foods he loved. Of far more significance to him were the bits and pieces of his past that also started to flow back. He could now recall how it was that he'd wound up in Iraq: he had decided in the wake of the 9/11 attacks to join the Arizona National Guard and hoped to parlay the Military Police training he would receive into a career in law enforcement. He remembered that before enlisting he'd coached football and baseball at his old high school. The pieces of the jigsaw puzzle were starting to fall into place.

While relieved to see improvements in his long-term memory, Brian was discouraged by the continuing problems with his short-term memory. No matter how well he remembered his past, he would never be able to function independently without the ability to create and store new memories. Sometimes the fallout from these deficits was simply tedious and vexing, with Brian repeating the same task over and over again because he'd lost track of what he'd been doing. One day, he spent the better part of an hour riding the Walter Reed elevator up and down in search of the orthopedic clinic he'd been to countless times before. On another occasion, officials contacted his case manager after Brian was found wandering aimlessly through the hospital halls and then blamed Nova for failing to care for him properly. He had simply forgotten where he was going.

Sometimes the consequences of that spotty short-term memory could be much more distressing and dire. When a new psychiatrist prescribed an antidepressant, Brian didn't remember that he had taken the drug before and it had caused confusion and hallucinations. So he had the prescription filled again. The next night Nova found him out in woods behind Walter Reed, crawling on the ground as if he were on maneuvers back in Iraq; he'd strapped a flashlight to his cane and was carrying it like an M4 rifle.

As time went on, Brian realized that the enduring problems with his short-term memory might be his most life-altering handicap. He'd pieced together enough of the jigsaw puzzle that he now had a picture, albeit a blurry one, of the man Brian Radke had been before the blast. He could remember how much he'd identified himself as an athlete and as a soldier with dreams of a future as a police officer. Now it was becoming increasingly clear how much the explosion had stolen from him. Without his trigger finger and a dependable memory, his dreams of a career in law enforcement had all but evaporated. He was becoming more and more resigned to the probability that he wasn't going to have anything like the life he'd planned. The day he finally accepted all the changes as permanent, he told himself, "You're not the same person you used to be, and you never will be."

What he couldn't know was who Brian Radke would become. With his identity and dreams wrenched away from him, it was like going back to the beginning and starting over. "Sometimes," he told Nova, "I look at it almost like being born again."

Brian wasn't telling Nova anything she didn't already know. It seemed as if the blast had sent her husband back through time. In an instant, Brian had regressed almost to the point of infancy. When he awoke from his coma, he had become childlike in so many ways. From her perspective, it was almost like raising a baby. She would see him gradually progress over the next few years from a toddler to an adolescent to an adult striving to be the man she married.

The process seemed painfully slow to Brian. Day after day, he would endure hours of cognitive therapy with barely a sign that it was having an impact. He often didn't understand the point of the various exercises he was asked to perform. Sometimes the therapist would reel off a list of words and then ask him to repeat them. Sometimes she'd show him a geometric design and then ask him to replicate it from memory with a set of children's blocks. Each session, she'd give him a newspaper article to read and then minutes later quiz him about it—but he could never recall a single detail.

Brian didn't realize at the time that the therapist was trying to help his brain rewire connections obliterated by the blast. The bits of information in his head were like the books in a library; if the card catalog were destroyed, it would be impossible to locate a specific book. The therapy was designed to reconstruct the card catalog in Brian's brain. When the therapist would give him a list of animals, for example, she'd tell him to think about which ones were pets, which ones were wild, and which ones were farm animals. Now when he'd try to remember the words on the list, he'd first think about pets that could have been on it.

Although Brian could see small improvements in his short-term memory, he still felt like a schoolboy destined to repeat first grade for the rest of his life. It didn't matter how adept he became at recalling lists of words if he couldn't remember the contents of a newspaper article he'd read minutes before. That frustration was further magnified as the improvements became smaller and smaller. Some mornings he could barely drag himself out of bed. Discouraged and depressed, he thought, "Well, maybe this is the best I'm going to get. Maybe this is *me* now. And I'll just have to deal with it."

Through it all, Nova kept encouraging him to stick with his therapy, to keep fighting like the Brian she married. "You're going to get back to a hundred percent," she'd say reassuringly. One day he just wheeled around and snapped, "Your husband died in Iraq." As Nova stood there in stunned silence, he hammered home his point by announcing that he now considered the day of the blast to be his real date of birth.

Despite his frustration, Brian slogged on, attending his therapy sessions no matter how futile they seemed. Then he had a breakthrough: he'd had to read his assigned newspaper article in the noisy, bustling lobby, and this time, despite all the distractions, he remembered every detail when his therapist quizzed him later.

In October 2008, three years to the month since the blast, doctors at Walter Reed decided to send him home to Arizona for good. "You still might see some improvements once you get home," they said, "but this is probably as good as we can get you." Brian nodded his assent. "It's time to go," he thought. "I've got to try and do this on my own."

Brian arrived home full of hope. Now that he was back among the people and surroundings that made Phoenix so comforting, he assumed everything would fall into place. He and Nova had just bought a house, and they were expecting their first baby in a few months. He still harbored aspirations of salvaging some sort of career in law enforcement; if he couldn't be a cop on the street, maybe he could find a training position or a desk job. He saw his homecoming as a chance to start over, a chance to build new dreams.

That optimism didn't last long. He had placed too much faith in the power of home and underestimated the pull of what he'd left behind at Walter Reed. There, he could lean on a ready support group of soldiers who, like him, had been wounded in the war. Back in Phoenix, despite being surrounded by family and friends, he felt more isolated and alone than ever. No one understood his frustration and anger.

With each passing day, Brian's mood darkened. His pending medical discharge from the Army left him adrift, without direction. He reached out to friends in law enforcement, but no one had any job leads. He reached out to the Phoenix Veterans Affairs Medical Center, but it seemed too much like a hospital and not enough like a community. Instead of being comforted by the warm anchor of home, he felt more disconnected than ever. Nova saw Brian losing his bearings, his confidence, his self-esteem. To her, he seemed like "a tumbleweed blowing around the desert."

Here he was, just thirty-four years old with no prospect of a job and no idea what he was good for now that his brain was broken and his body damaged. Within weeks, Brian was so depressed that sometimes he felt the only solution would be to take his own life. His despair was so deep that it couldn't be salved even by the imminent arrival of his first child. While Nova was all aglow throughout the pregnancy, Brian became increasingly distant and unresponsive. Although he knew intellectually that the baby was on the way, he never emotionally connected his wife's burgeoning belly with his own approaching fatherhood.

That all changed the instant he heard Nema cry for the first time in the delivery room, on Christmas Day of 2008. It was as if life flowed back through him again. From that moment on, Brian would tell everyone that his infant daughter saved his life.

Nema's impact on Brian is clear to everyone attending her first birthday party. Family and friends watch as Brian hovers over his daughter, trying to coach her to blow out the single candle on her cake. When Nema is turned loose on the living room carpet, Brian eases himself down on the floor despite the excruciating pain he still feels, then starts rolling around with her like a little kid. As she rips open her birthday gifts, Dad proudly snaps photo after photo. Watching all of this, Nova can't help shaking her head in wonder. "I think our little girl is what brought him out of it," she marvels. "I do believe she is what he's living for."

To Nova, it's as if Brian were a wilting plant and Nema the water that brought it back to life. Nova can see new branches shooting out from her plant as Brian reaches for things that for a long time seemed beyond his grasp. He's begun talking hopefully about doing volunteer work and going back to coaching high school baseball. As much as Nova is heartened by this recent progress, her hopes are tempered by all that's gone before.

"For so long I thought that, with all the doctors and the love and his strength, we were going to get him back to a hundred percent," she says wistfully. "I knew that we couldn't get his finger to grow back, but I really thought that somehow, some way, we could get *my* Brian back. Now I've just got to accept that's never going to happen."

Brian, too, mourns the loss of his former self. He remembers a time when he was so much more easygoing, when he and Nova rarely said an angry word to each other. Now even little things can set him off. In a flash, he'll go from talking calmly to screaming obscenities at his wife. Though he later regrets these outbursts, he hasn't figured out a way to keep them from happening. Sometimes, in the middle of a fight, he gets so befuddled and scared that he'll yell at Nova, "How am I supposed to trust you if I can't trust my own mind?"

Making matters worse, Brian still can't connect with the man Nova first fell in love with. "I guess you could say I used to be a hopeless romantic and now I'm just not very loving," he says glumly. "I care and I feel all the stuff I'm supposed to, but I just don't show her. I don't do the little things. A lot of times I forget; it just slips my mind."

Nova still loves her husband, but she misses the man she married. "They say women pick the strongest men to protect them and to procreate with, and I know that's true for me because most people couldn't survive what he survived," Nova says. "He was my knight in shining armor. It's like he got knocked off his horse and he held on to the tail and he pulled himself back up and now he's riding right along with me again. I glance over at him and he looks the same, but it's just somebody different." She pauses for a second to wipe away the tears. "I love him because in so many ways he's still the same," she says sadly, "but there's so much that's different."

II

The last thing Chari Abb remembers from the cold winter night that forever changed her life is steering onto the quiet country road that should have taken her home.

Everything else she learned from the police report: how a drunk driver swerved into her lane just after she made the turn, how there wasn't time to notice the other car before it struck hers, and how the force of the head-on collision crushed both vehicles beyond recognition.

The loud bang from the crash caught the attention of a bartender at a nearby restaurant and he raced out to investigate. He found the two cars in a tangled heap, steam rising into the frigid air, fluids streaming onto the asphalt of the deserted road. As he peered into each vehicle, he shuddered at what he saw. Between the mangled metal and the pooling blood, he couldn't imagine how either driver could have survived. Blood covered Abb's head and face; a crumpled steering wheel pinned the drunk driver against his seat. The bartender determined he could do nothing for them and raced back inside to dial 911.

Within minutes, there were flashing lights and rescue personnel everywhere. Abb jolted awake and screamed, "Help! Get me out of here!" Firefighters cut through the mangled car frame with a Jaws of Life and carefully pulled her out. Once the paramedics stabilized her, she was loaded onto a medevac helicopter and flown to the University of Maryland's Shock Trauma Center. At the hospital, Abb remained awake long enough to give nurses her mother's name and phone number. Then she lost consciousness.

A team of surgeons worked on Abb for more than twelve hours. Her chest had been crushed, both arms and both legs broken, her left wrist smashed. Most of the bones in her face had been shattered. The cosmetic surgery to repair that damage would have to wait for several days until the swelling had gone down.

The doctors opted to put her in a medically induced coma to protect her brain from swelling. They cautioned family members about the possibility of brain damage. Until Abb woke up and the painkillers had left her system, they said, there was no way to know about the condition of her brain.

When Abb finally did come out of the coma three weeks after the accident, her doctors were relieved that she was able to understand and respond to questions. Her communication skills seemed a bit off—she was having problems finding common words—but she appeared to be alert and functional. Back in 1987 virtually no one was offering rehab for the brain. Abb's doctors predicted that the word problems would soon pass and that her brain would be fine by the time she worked through the months of rehab she was going to need before she'd be able to walk again.

Abb surprised everyone by getting out of the hospital in less than five weeks and by powering through her grueling physical therapy sessions at the rehabilitation center in just four weeks. During the months following her accident, she developed a new focus and a sense of purpose. She'd been a waitress at a local restaurant since dropping out of high school. Now, in her mid-twenties, she decided to go back to school and work toward a career. She returned to the community college where she'd taken occasional liberal arts courses before the crash, this time with a plan to get a degree in education and eventually a job teaching elementary school. When the semester began, she was excited to think that she was starting down the path to a career and a new life.

That excitement was short-lived. For the first time, Abb was struggling with schoolwork. She was easily distracted and would quickly lose track of what the professor was saying. She couldn't follow complex sentences from beginning to end. She would fall hopelessly behind taking notes because she couldn't figure out which details were important and would end up trying to write down every word the professor uttered. Tests were impossible; there was never enough time and she would often get sidetracked in the middle of answering a single question.

Frightened that she was about to fail all her courses, she turned once again to the doctors at the Shock Trauma Center. Only this time it wasn't for the injuries to her body—it was for the injury to her brain.

Abb wasn't sure what to expect when she went back to the Shock Trauma Center. On the day of her appointment, she sat nervously in the lobby, hoping that someone would be able to explain the mysterious symptoms she was experiencing. Eventually she noticed a trim, dark-haired man striding toward her. He walked up to her, extended his hand, and introduced himself as Dr. Mark Sementilli, the neuropsychologist who would be evaluating her for possible brain damage stemming from her car accident.

As they walked down the long hallway leading to his office, Abb looked around and realized that she was on the very floor where she'd been treated after the crash. The acrid smell of the ward hit her nostrils, and she was suddenly overwhelmed by a rush of emotions. Her skin started to feel hot, her legs wobbly. Seconds later she crumpled to the floor, sobbing. Sementilli was taken aback. Reaching down to help her up, he said, "You haven't dealt with this, have you?"

When they got to his office, Sementilli asked Abb to detail the symptoms that had led her to seek help. She told him about the troubles she'd been having in school and described the problems she'd been having with memory, concentration, and organization. They talked about the other changes she'd noticed in her life since the accident. She told him that she'd been completely self-sufficient since moving away from home at

age sixteen, but now she couldn't even make it to her parents' house for
Thanksgiving dinner without a reminder. To get a handle on the severity
of Abb's problem, Sementilli turned to a battery of neuropsychological
tests that would take her nearly six hours to complete.

In the days after the appointment, he considered the test results and
the observations he'd made during his conversations with Abb. Although
her performance on the standardized tests of memory and verbal ability were within the normal range, he had observed signs of frontal lobe
damage while talking with her. One symptom in particular stood out: the
volatility of her moods. In a flash, she would go from happy, bubbly, and
chatty to distraught and weepy.

When she returned to his office for a follow-up, Sementilli gave her
his diagnosis. He told her that he believed the crash had caused damage
to the section of the brain located just behind the left side of her forehead. Even before meeting her, he had suspected as much based strictly
on the information in her medical files and the description of the accident. "The frontal lobe is very vulnerable because of its location in the
brain," he explained to her. "It's really packed in there against the orbital
floor of the frontal bone. You'd think that the bone would be smooth, but
it's not. There are these bony ridges. And when you have a head-on collision, where the body and the neck and the head are propelled forward
and then suddenly stop, the brain is also propelled forward and then back
in a sloshing motion. The brain rams into the skull and the orbital floor.
Those bones are not forgiving. And that's a perfect recipe for frontal lobe
damage."

He told her that the hallmark symptoms of this kind of brain injury
could explain the difficulties she was having in school. People with frontal
lobe damage often have problems with initiating, planning, and organization. They also have difficulty prioritizing and multitasking.

Abb was astounded. Finally someone had an explanation for what
was happening to her. She was at once relieved to have an answer and
anxious about what it meant. Sementilli told her that she would need
help to get through college. He recommended that she find an academic
counselor to assist with her schoolwork and a therapist to help with other
deficits resulting from her brain injury.

Then Sementilli turned to the toughest part of his prescription. He'd determined that her spatial abilities were now significantly better than her language skills, so he advised that she rethink her career goals and give up her dream of teaching. He told her she no longer had the organizational skills that teachers need. "You should find a career that involves working with your hands," he said.

Abb was devastated and angry when she left his office. She wondered what career she could possibly choose that would involve working with her hands. In the months that followed, she mulled over his advice while thumbing through the course catalog. Finally she stumbled upon the horticulture department and thought, "Maybe this is the kind of thing he meant. This could be a blessing in disguise: I love nature and working in the dirt with plants." She switched her major and went back to college with renewed motivation—and with newfound help. Her academic counselor suggested she explain her situation to her professors and tape-record lectures rather than try to take notes. Most of her teachers agreed to give her more time on tests, and the tape recordings allowed her to focus in class strictly on what the professor was saying. Two years later, she had an associate of arts degree and a career.

It seemed as if her life had finally turned around. She landed a job at a large garden center, caring for plants and advising customers on how to maintain them. On top of that, the ruggedly handsome store manager with the penetrating blue eyes was starting to flirt with her. Soon she and Chris Abb were spending most of their free time together, hiking, camping, and motorcycling through the Maryland countryside. As they became closer, Chari shared with Chris her dreams of getting married and having a baby by the time she was thirty.

The job initially seemed to be everything Chari had hoped for. She enjoyed working outdoors. The customers loved her; she was affable and always took the time to teach them about the plants. But soon she started having problems with other aspects of her job. She couldn't manage her time and seemed to have no organizational skills. She would spend an entire day deadheading a single row of plants. She'd go to rearrange a flower display, only to find herself unable to figure out where to begin. Hours would invariably pass and her boss, shocked to discover how little Chari had accomplished, would remark, "You're still doing that? What's the problem?"

Chari had no answer, and she wasn't even convinced there was a problem. She just figured she had a grumpy boss and the solution was to find a new job. But her next one didn't work out any better. Chari bounced from job to job. One thing remained constant: she brought to each new position the same old problems with organization and time management. As her résumé lengthened with a new entry every few months, she began to question whether her bosses were really to blame for all her problems. One day it dawned on her: "My God, there's something wrong with *me.*"

For the first time, she connected her work problems with her brain injury. Since she'd gotten the diagnosis of frontal lobe syndrome from Sementilli, she'd gone blithely along thinking she needed help only to get through college. Now, three years and seven jobs later, she realized that the fallout from her brain injury wasn't limited to her schoolwork—it was wreaking havoc with every aspect of her life. Not only were her cognitive deficits costing Chari jobs, but they were also exasperating friends and family. No one understood why she would show up hours late for appointments—if she remembered them at all.

Frustrated by her inability to keep track of anything in her life, Chari sought help from Maryland's Division of Rehabilitation Services. Because she could no longer depend on her brain to organize her life, therapists taught her compensatory strategies; they recommended she follow a regular schedule, keep a detailed day planner, and make to-do lists. Because she also wanted to avoid more confrontation with bosses, they suggested she try working from home.

Chari came up with a new strategy. She had recently married Chris and moved to his rolling seventy-acre farm in rural Maryland. There was plenty of room to build a greenhouse for a cut-flower business. No sooner had she bought the plants, however, than she became pregnant. What had been difficult before was now becoming impossible. Once Shelby was born, it was all Chari could do to take care of him. The house fell into disarray. The plants withered, along with her business plans and dreams. Rehab became a luxury she could no longer manage.

As time went on, Chari focused all her energy and attention on raising Shelby and his kid sister, Emma. She was too overwhelmed to do anything else. The clutter in the house grew and grew, cardboard boxes and piles of paper covering almost every inch of floor. Each night after work, Chris would clear pathways connecting room to room, like a man shoveling his way through a thick blanket of snow.

By the fall of 2008, Chris Abb decided he couldn't deal with the chaos anymore. He didn't understand why the house was always such a mess, why his wife would spend hours aimlessly wandering around supermarkets only to come home with just two or three items, why she couldn't find at least a part-time job now that the kids were in school. Chari would try to explain how the brain injury had ruined her ability to focus and to organize her life. But Chris could only understand the damage he could see: the scars on her lip, neck, and arms.

Eventually, Chris told his wife he wanted to move out of the house. He wasn't sure how things were going to turn out, but he needed some time to think. Chari was scared. She couldn't stop fretting over the prospect of being divorced and on her own. To make ends meet, she'd have to go back to work. Even if she was lucky enough to find a job, she had no confidence in her ability to hang on to it given her history of workplace failures. Making matters worse, this time she would be trying to work while also raising two kids. The idea of reentering the workplace after fifteen years' absence would have been daunting for any full-time mom, but it was terrifying for a brain-injured forty-five-year-old who couldn't multitask.

Desperate, she turned once again to Maryland's Division of Rehabilitation Services, hoping to pick up where she'd left off so many years before. Counselors there scheduled Chari for a neuropsych exam to determine whether her deficits were still debilitating enough to warrant a prescription for rehab services. She glanced at the doctor's name on the appointment card and smiled: it was the very neuropsychologist who had evaluated her back when she was in college.

The day of the appointment, Chari walked into Mark Sementilli's office and announced, "Remember me?" He looked at her, puzzled. Something about the tall, slender woman with the cascading blond hair was vaguely familiar, but he couldn't quite place her. She handed him a faded computer printout of a neuropsychological evaluation that he had written seventeen years earlier. As he leafed through the pages, a look of recognition spread across his face. "Oh, I remember you now," he said.

Chari smiled broadly and said, "You're the one who explained all the problems I was having and told me I had frontal lobe syndrome. Do you remember you also told me I should find a career working with my hands? Well, I took your advice." Chari went on to update him on everything that had happened—both good and bad—since their last meeting. "I'm back because my life is coming apart," she concluded, tears streaming down her face. "I can't seem to do anything right. The house is a wreck. I feel like I'm a bad mom. My husband's threatening to leave me. I can't be who he wants me to be: I have a brain injury. It took many years for *me* to accept me for who I am now, but *he* doesn't get it. And if he leaves, I'm going to have to go back to work, and I'm terrified I'm going to lose any job I get."

As Sementilli talked with her, he observed one of the telltale signs of brain damage: she couldn't follow complex sentences. Noticing her confusion, he would often find himself having to repeat complicated instructions or break them down into simpler components. More obvious were the mood swings he saw throughout their session. One minute she'd be laughing, the next she'd be crying. It reminded him of the first time he met with her. He could see that she was still having problems regulating her emotions. She seemed to be missing the set of "mental brakes" that stop a healthy person from blurting out every thought—evidence that her brain hadn't recovered from the frontal lobe damage.

His observations would be supported by a battery of neuropyschological tests. Chari had trouble with tasks designed to ferret out deficits in memory, organization, planning, and problem solving. In one memory test, she was asked to listen to a story and then to recall details from the narrative; minutes after hearing the story, her recall was almost perfect, but half an hour later, she could remember little of what she'd been told. Another test required her to solve a problem through trial and error; after choosing the wrong solution, she would invariably keep repeating the same mistake. As Sementilli went over the test results, he was struck by how closely they mirrored those from seventeen years earlier. Chari was still showing the hallmark symptoms of frontal lobe damage.

After explaining everything to Chari, Sementilli told her that he would be recommending to the state that she get rehab therapy and job coaching. She breathed a sigh of relief and thanked him for validating what she'd been experiencing for years. She complained that most people—her husband included—couldn't look past her healthy exterior to the deficits within. Because her appearance and speech seemed so normal, they couldn't imagine anything could be wrong with her brain. "The doctors put me back together so well that most people wouldn't know I'd been in an accident," she said, "but that creates a problem: they can't see that I have a brain injury." Sementilli told her he wasn't surprised, because people often underestimate how much lingering damage can follow a jolt to the head. "Even mild injury can result in significant impairment," he said.

Chari found that a lot had changed since she last sought therapy for her brain injury. Scientists had learned better ways to help people cope with injuries and had discovered that some damaged sections of the brain could be coaxed to rewire through the proper types of exercises. The state set Chari up with weekly therapy sessions at an independent center specializing in rehab of neurological injury. Her therapist, Tom Thompson, decided that the first priority was to help her organize her life. That meant she would have to get back to using aids such as day planners that scheduled every facet of her day in half-hour increments.

To address her deficits with planning and problem solving, Thompson turned to a computer game designed to simulate daily life. Each time she played the game, she would guide an animated version of herself through a typical day. Her cartoon self would have to go to work and solve the kinds of problems that she might encounter in everyday life. She'd get points for successfully maneuvering cartoon Chari through life, remembering for example to have her animated self do important things like cooking meals and showing up for appointments, and she'd lose points for mistakes such as forgetting things. One day she asked Thompson how the computer game could possibly help her. He explained that by repeatedly going through daily rituals with her cartoon self, she might actually be able to rewire damaged parts of her brain. Chari's face brightened. "That gives me hope," she said with a smile. "I didn't know that my brain could actually change."

Whether it was the result of the game's impact or Chari's newfound resolve, things started to turn around in real life. She got a job waiting tables at a local restaurant and enrolled in a class on how to start a small business. After losing his job as a motorcycle mechanic, Chris moved back into the house and took over the domestic chores. She was happy with the role reversal. The house was finally clean and organized. Chris was starting to grudgingly accept the possibility that the reason for all the chaos wasn't that his wife was lazy but rather that she did in fact have a debilitating brain injury. He was starting to realize that the invisible scars inside her brain were causing the host of odd symptoms he'd observed for the past two decades.

If it was hard to recognize the cognitive changes wrought by a horrific car wreck, how much harder would it be to accept that brain damage could result from a mere fender bender?

Chapter 5

Through the Cracks

Anne Forrest was starting to get scared. It had been weeks since she felt normal. She'd been plagued by excruciating headaches. She couldn't concentrate at work. She'd lose track of what friends were saying in the middle of a conversation. Though the thirty-nine-year-old economist had always been calm and measured, she found herself losing her temper and screaming at people for the most minor of infractions. Then, on the drive home one day, she lost feeling on her right side for several minutes. Somehow she managed to get the car pulled over onto the shoulder to wait and see if the numbness would pass. It did, but she was terrified that something was going horribly wrong with her brain.

The episode in the car prompted Forrest to make an appointment with a neurologist. Because hers wasn't an emergency, she would have to wait several weeks before seeing him. Worried, she pushed for an earlier date, but the neurologist's receptionist was firm. The weekend before her appointment, Forrest planned to watch the Fourth of July fireworks display with her boyfriend on the lawn near the Washington National Cathedral. Shortly after they arrived, she noticed a man making his way toward her. He came up and introduced himself, and though Forrest soon realized he was someone she worked with, she couldn't remember who he was. She was shaken.

Now, as she lay on her back in the grass looking up at the bursts of light, she couldn't get her brain to make sense of the night sky. Stars that should have been a stationary backdrop for the fireworks were whirling furiously. She tried to get the stars to stay still, but they just spun all the more crazily. Forrest started to cry, and her boyfriend suggested they walk around inside the cathedral instead of watching the fireworks. When they got there, she sat down for a few minutes and prayed that she would be OK.

When Forrest finally got to see the neurologist, he ran her through a series of neurological tests and asked her if anything out of the ordinary had happened over the past few weeks. She told him about the day she'd lost feeling on her right side, about the terrifying swirling sensation during the fireworks—and about the fender bender she'd been in a few weeks earlier. She suspected that the accident, though minor, was somehow connected to her odd symptoms.

It had happened down by the Lincoln Memorial. Forrest had been waiting to merge onto a major road, craning her neck to the left to assess when it would be safe to hit the gas. While she was waiting, an SUV banged into her Acura from behind. The hit wasn't that hard—it barely made a dent in the back of Forrest's car. She and the driver of the SUV got out of their vehicles and exchanged information. Then Forrest got back in her car and drove the rest of the way home. It had been such a minor accident that she hadn't thought anything of it, and she certainly didn't think she needed to see a doctor. Besides, since it was a Saturday, the emergency room would have been her only option.

The following Monday, Forrest woke up with chills, nausea, and a pounding headache. When she went to see her primary care physician, she told him about the car accident and he suggested that her symptoms might be due to whiplash. He told her to check in with him every few days over the next couple of weeks just to make sure she was OK. He suggested she go back to work but skip anything physically strenuous. She'd been disappointed when he told her to avoid physical activity. Volleyball season was about to start and she'd been eagerly anticipating the matches on the National Mall. Playing in the shadow of the Washington Monument and the Lincoln and Jefferson Memorials gave her the feeling that she was really a part of Washington. The prospect of missing the season altogether was disheartening. Nevertheless, she resolved to try to get her life back to normal—until the day she lost feeling on her right side. She went back to her primary care physician and asked what could possibly be wrong. He couldn't find anything even with a CAT scan, but he referred her to a neurologist, just in case.

The neurologist told Forrest that it was possible she had developed epilepsy or multiple sclerosis based on her symptoms. The most likely explanation, however, was that the car accident had left her with a mild traumatic brain injury. In most people, he said, symptoms resolve in three to six months. But a small percentage of people who suffer a mild TBI don't seem to improve, he cautioned. "If you're not better in two years," he added, "you'll never get better." Though the idea of a brain injury was scary, Forrest hung on to the word "mild." She told herself, "I'll just have to be one of the people who gets better in six months."

Forrest left the doctor's office assuming that she just needed to wait out the brain injury. In three to six months, she'd be fine. She returned to work at the Environmental Law Institute, figuring that was the best way to get her life back. When she went to fill out her timesheet two weeks later, Forrest, an internationally recognized economist with a Ph.D. from Duke University, couldn't make any sense of the blank columns and rows. The institute's CEO told her to go on disability leave. "If you can't fill out your timesheet, you certainly can't work," the CEO said.

Things didn't improve in the months that followed. Forrest couldn't balance her checkbook anymore—the math was too hard. She would wear the same clothes for days on end because changing them would mean she'd have to figure out how to match the colors. Besides, she was just too tired to make the effort. Forrest had always been energetic and sociable; now she was spending much of her time in bed, sometimes sleeping as many as eighteen hours a day. During dinners with friends, she'd just listen quietly, unable to follow the conversation well enough to participate. When an old college friend came to visit, she found reminder notes plastered all over Forrest's apartment. One on the door reminded Forrest to take her keys and wallet with her when she went out.

Friends could see something was wrong with Forrest, but they never connected her problems with the car accident. And she was in too much of a fog to explain anything to them. Forrest's own insight was limited as she spiraled downward. She was aware she was having memory problems, but didn't connect them with the concussion. She just adapted by writing herself notes and to-do lists. As skills disappeared, she found ways to compensate, never really having the wherewithal to put it all together.

Even though they didn't understand what was happening to her, Forrest's friends knew she needed help—paying bills, balancing her checkbook, making doctors' appointments, dealing with her insurance company. When she'd lock herself out of the apartment or get lost after taking the wrong bus, someone was always ready to come to her rescue. After she forgot to turn off a burner on her stove, her boyfriend bought her a toaster oven.

Forrest's short-term disability ran out after six months, and her regular health insurer denied her application for long-term disability because she lacked proof that she couldn't work. Forrest was forced to live off her savings while her lawyer tried to get the disability insurance company to reinstate her benefits. She went back to the neurologist who had diagnosed the brain injury a year earlier, hoping he could help her prove to her insurance company just how disabled she was. He referred Forrest to a neuropsychologist who told her that she was indeed struggling with TBI symptoms and suggested she get rehab. Worn out by the grind of daily living, she couldn't imagine summoning the energy to search for a rehab doctor and to negotiate with her recalcitrant insurance company. She was just too exhausted to deal with any of it.

In the meantime, Forrest's lawyer was trying to get her auto insurance company to pay for her care and expenses. Because Forrest had been hit by a driver with minimal insurance, her lawyer worried that it wouldn't be enough to cover her medical bills, let alone her living expenses, especially if it turned out that she would never be able to work again. He determined that her car insurance policy had a provision designed to help cover damage caused by underinsured drivers. But her insurance company refused to pay, arguing that she couldn't possibly have such serious damage to her brain when her car had only a tiny dent as a result of the accident. Forrest sued, but lost her case. Part of the problem, her attorney said, was that because she looked and sounded so normal most of the time, only people who knew her well could see something was wrong. Even *he* hadn't noticed her deficits initially. They only became clear to him when he asked her to help prepare for the case and she had trouble doing the simplest things, like gathering up her medical bills.

After nine months with no income, Forrest started receiving disability benefits again. But the disability insurance company insisted she go see two of its own handpicked experts, a psychologist and a psychiatrist. They concluded that she had mental problems and was a "narcissistic histrionic malingerer." She was relieved that their diagnosis qualified her for two years of disability payments, the company's maximum for mental health problems, but she was disappointed that that meant she wouldn't get a referral for TBI rehab.

On the recommendation of a friend, Forrest traveled up to New Jersey to meet with a TBI expert. After evaluating Forrest, the specialist told her she needed cognitive therapy to help her understand her deficits and to learn how to compensate for them. Back home, Forrest again made an appointment with a neuropsychologist in hopes of getting a referral to rehab. But the neuropsychologist told her she was "doing too well" for rehab to make much difference and suggested that the only reason she wasn't progressing was that she didn't really want to get better. Although Forrest knew that couldn't be true since she was still unable to work or drive a car, her brain was processing too slowly to come up with the correct response until she was on her way home from the doctor's office. The neuropsychologist did tell her that she needed more rest, so Forrest started taking naps in the middle of the day and stopped trying to push through the fatigue. That helped some. She found she had a little more energy to deal with the daily necessities of life—like making sure she got enough to eat. Still, the battles with the insurance companies and the fight to get some sort of rehab were taking a toll.

Making matters worse, Forrest was on her own most of the time because her boyfriend, Michael Crider, had moved to Texas for a job a few months after her accident. Crider did his best to help her on his visits back to Washington, but he could see that that wasn't enough. He began to press her to move down to Austin. Forrest was nervous about leaving the familiar surroundings of her Washington home. If she was getting lost on short excursions away from her apartment now, how was she going to manage in an unfamiliar neighborhood in a new city? Eventually Forrest overcame her fears and moved to Austin. She'd lost so much of her life already; she didn't want to lose Crider, too.

The move came with an unexpected benefit. Forrest finally found a rehab facility that was able to help her—three and a half years after her accident. After running Forrest through a battery of tests, therapist Liz Joiner broke the bad news: the former economist couldn't even do second grade math. Division was impossible for Forrest to grasp. She thought, "Who am I if I can't even do second grade math?"

For Forrest, rehab was like going back to elementary school. She had to relearn basic math. Her lack of organizational skills was affecting every part of her life. Writing was almost impossible because she couldn't form her thoughts into a logical progression; she had to once again learn how to start paragraphs with topic sentences.

Joiner helped Forrest work on multitasking issues and attention problems. Forrest's brain had gotten so distractible that she couldn't even make her way through a basic recipe. But the more Forrest cooked at the rehab center, the better she got. Joiner explained that sometimes you could get the brain to rewire broken connections if you did something over and over again.

While Forrest worked at getting her brain to rewire, Joiner gave her tools that would help her get through her daily life. She taught Forrest to keep a detailed day planner. The benefits of that would be twofold: helping Forrest to remember things better by writing them down and, more than that, serving as a replacement for her imperfect memory.

As part of her therapy, Forrest was encouraged to write and deliver a speech about her experience with brain injury. In doing so, she'd be using one of the few skills that had survived from her old job untouched by the TBI. There would be another benefit: by writing about her life after the brain injury, she would have to become more conscious of its impact. The exercise was painful. Though she had been working on improving her deficits, it was the first time she had thought about all of them together, the first time she'd pondered the totality of the impact of the injury on her life.

When Crider got a job offer in Washington, the couple, now married, decided to move back. Although she'd lived in the city for years, Forrest had trouble readjusting because so much was unfamiliar. At least her old neurologist could now point her in the right direction, referring her to a rehab facility that recognized her deficits. There, she started to work on balance problems that no one else had addressed. Dizziness had precluded her from using a treadmill since the accident. Her new therapist gradually got her to work up to the point where she could walk without holding on to the sides.

Even with therapy, Forrest was still too disabled to return to work. She finally recognized that some of the fallout from the fender bender was permanent, and she had learned to adjust her life to her brain's limitations. She had accepted that she would never be able to return to economics. But she found something else to fill the void. She honed the speech she had written in Texas and started giving it at TBI conferences. That caught the attention of advocates at the Brain Injury Association of America, and Forrest was added to its list of speakers. Soon she was giving regular talks about concussions and how devastating the damage could be even if the initial brain injury seemed mild.

She had learned to make adjustments to her everyday routine that compensated for her deficits. Trips to the store became strategic missions. She would decide what she wanted in advance, think about where she would find each object, and then stick with her mapped-out mission at the store. She and Crider eventually adopted a baby boy, and she decided she could be a stay-at-home mom. With to-do lists and a scrupulously filled-out day planner, she was getting by.

Though she had accepted that she would never be the same person she was before the accident, Forrest sometimes wondered wistfully how different things might have been if she'd managed to find good rehab right away. That point was brought painfully home one day in 2003—six years after her life-changing fender bender—when she attended a book reading by TBI survivor Trisha Meili, who had written a memoir titled *I Am the Central Park Jogger: A Story of Hope and Possibility*. Meili had experienced a much more severe brain injury, but she had managed to come back from it and was even able to return to her job in finance. After the reading, Forrest's hand shot up. She asked how Meili had managed such a full recovery. Meili answered that she'd gotten therapy at a top rehab center right away. What's more, she'd gotten job-skill training early on. Forrest couldn't help thinking, "What she went through was so much worse than anything I went through. Where would *I* be now if I'd had that kind of rehab?"

Unfortunately, stories like Anne Forrest's are all too common. People with brain injuries seem to just slip through the cracks, especially those with concussions. The ones who get correctly diagnosed by a doctor are often sent on their way without any referral for follow-up or rehab. Others, assuming that they simply had an innocuous bump on the head, never see a doctor and just go on with their lives without ever linking the injury to the plethora of disparate symptoms that develop afterward. Experts estimate that 20 to 40 percent of people who experience a mild traumatic brain injury never seek medical attention. Even people with more severe injuries can end up floundering when doctors focus on damage to the body and forget about the brain.

For some, the injury is the beginning of a slow downward spiral. Alterations in cognitive function, coupled with personality changes caused by the brain injury, can lead to lost jobs and crumbling marriages. The problem is often compounded by lack of insight; people with a brain injury are often oblivious to the changes that seem so obvious to others. A man who experiences a loss of inhibition because of a brain injury may frighten women he's dating because he no longer can rein in his conversation and behavior; unrestrained enthusiasm can be misinterpreted as stalking. On the job, errors due to damaged math skills can be misinterpreted as fraudulent behavior.

Those were the kind of stories that originally caught the attention of Wayne Gordon, a psychologist at the Mount Sinai School of Medicine who specializes in neuropsychology and rehabilitation. Over the years, Gordon became convinced that "hidden"TBIs were at the root of many of society's ills. Back in the late 1980s, he noticed while asking his standard intake questions that a surprisingly large number of patients had suffered jolts to the head that weren't documented anywhere in their medical records. They had come to him because they could see their lives unraveling and they were having a harder and harder time coping with relationships and job responsibilities. Some of them could trace their downhill slide to a particular event, such as a car accident or a fall, but they didn't understand what it was about the incident that had thrown their lives so out of whack.

"Over and over again, I was hearing the same stories," says Gordon, associate director of Mount Sinai's department of rehabilitation medicine. "People were being sent home from the emergency room and told that there was nothing wrong with them because they'd had a normal CAT scan. Emergency room doctors wouldn't see memory problems and executive dysfunction. No one was giving these folks a list of things to look out for. Lives were being altered by this one event."

With a clean bill of health from the ER and no education about the possible fallout from a jolt to the head, people often didn't link the strange symptoms they were experiencing to the brain injury. A mom might find that she couldn't multitask anymore; for example, she might be unable to talk on the phone while ironing or washing dishes. "She would find herself fuming at her kids for making too much noise; she couldn't tolerate the radio blaring anymore because it was too much stimulation," Gordon says. "But she never would make the connection with a brain injury."

Often, Gordon could see the huge sense of relief many patients felt when they learned that the bizarre symptoms were real and could be traced back to a specific event. But, he says, it would have been much better if they'd been told on the day of the injury what to expect so they could have found a doctor to help. Even patients who recover in a relatively short time benefit from education about brain injuries. The doctor can explain what causes the strange symptoms and can provide a framework that helps a patient understand what to expect in the weeks to come. Beyond this, Gordon says, people can get help with immediate symptoms—medications for headaches and sleep problems, for example. And if the symptoms persist and there are cognitive deficits, then rehab is a possibility.

Most of the patients Gordon saw in his New York City office were adults, but he began to wonder what might be happening to kids in the same situation. He and his colleagues developed a questionnaire designed to ferret out undiagnosed TBIs and cognitive difficulties in children. The researchers took the questionnaire into the New York City schools to get an idea of how many kids were suffering with undiagnosed brain injuries. The results gave Gordon pause. In one city school, 10 percent of the children said they had sustained a significant head injury. When tested later, these children turned out to have cognitive impairments.

It was Gordon's first hint that TBIs might be at the root of many cases of learning disability. With a grant from the U.S. Department of Education, he was able to explore the issue further. He and his colleagues surveyed children who'd been enrolled in special education classes. He was startled by the results: more than 50 percent of the learning-disabled children had experienced a sharp jolt to the head.

While the children had been identified as having some sort of learning disability, the typical curriculum in special education classes didn't help with brain-injured kids' deficits. Gordon realized that the best way to help these children was to educate the educators. He gathered up a team of Mount Sinai psychologists and, with federal dollars that had been set aside to fund TBI education, set up a project in 1995 to send them into the New York City schools.

One of those psychologists was Tamar Martin. She would meet with a school's special education teachers and explain how the fallout from a brain injury could impact a kid's class performance. Then she would show them ways to help brain-injured students do better in school. Each time she met with teachers from a new school, Martin would start by popping a video into the VCR. The video, titled *All the King's Horses and All the King's Men*, told the story of a family with a child who had sustained a TBI during a summer vacation. The child had always been a good student, but when school started up again in the fall, he was floundering. What's more, his behavior had become increasingly odd. His brain injury—sustained when he fell off a bike and hit his head—was never reported, and nobody was able to make a connection between what had happened to the child and the impairments that appeared later. "Every time I would show that film," Martin recalls, "there would be a few teachers in the audience who would say, 'I have a kid just like that in my class.'"

These were often the kids that teachers saw as having transformed almost overnight from serious students to classroom problems. They would forget to do homework, forget to bring books back to school in the morning. They couldn't seem to focus and would often drift off in class. They could be distracted by the most innocuous stimuli. Eventually, they would slink off to a seat in the back of the class, the one that was farthest from the watchful eyes of the teacher.

The children were soon labeled difficult. Their memory problems were misinterpreted by teachers as signs that the students didn't care anymore, that they lacked ambition. Their exhaustion after one or two difficult classes in a row was mistaken for lack of initiative and motivation. When kids forgot to bring their homework to school, teachers would assume they hadn't done it. When they did poorly on tests because of slowed processing, teachers would assume the kids hadn't studied enough.

Martin remembers one little girl who languished for years, her schoolwork failing, her IQ scores declining. When "Julie" started first grade, teachers had noticed that she was a little off. She was highly verbal, but also seemed unfocused, immature, and accident-prone. As time passed, Julie got worse and worse. When she was seven and a half, she was evaluated again. This time she displayed problems with short-term memory and hand-eye coordination. She was also starting to show signs of a speech impairment. School administrators decided she should be moved to a class for the learning disabled. All the while, her parents were becoming increasingly distressed, pushing the school to figure out what was wrong with Julie. Two years passed and Julie seemed to be getting only worse in special education classes. Her parents asked administrators to put her back in a regular class. But that didn't help, either. By the time Julie reached fifth grade, she had fallen even further behind and was exhibiting even more deficits: her language skills had declined; she had developed word-finding problems; she was restless, anxious, distractible, and depressed.

Having heard Martin's presentation about brain injuries in children, one of Julie's teachers began to wonder if a TBI might explain the girl's sad spiral down. By the time Martin got involved, Julie's school file contained so many tests and evaluations that it stacked a full two feet high. In an interview with Julie and her parents, Martin learned that there had been a car accident when the girl was two. Julie had been rushed to the hospital and kept there for over a week.

When Martin told Julie's parents that their daughter's problems most likely traced back to a brain injury suffered in the car accident years before, she was worried about how they would take the news. As it turned out, they were relieved. Someone had finally explained how their bright little girl could have developed so many problems. They asked if Julie's declining IQ scores meant she was getting worse. Martin explained that in young kids you don't always appreciate the extent of the brain damage immediately. It isn't until classwork becomes harder and more complicated that certain deficits become obvious because the brain can't deal with the new demands. Often that happens in fifth or sixth grade, when kids need more analytical skills and when deficits in executive function become apparent. This is when "word problems" are introduced in math class, and brain-injured kids often get stuck on these kinds of exercises.

Part of Martin's mission in her yearlong course was to teach teachers to identify the signs of a TBI and show them strategies to help brain-injured children cope better with the demands of school. Teachers learned that brain-injured kids often had trouble maintaining focus. One way to help with that was for the teacher to keep walking around the classroom, periodically tapping students on the shoulder to snap them back to attention. Teachers were also told to seat students with a TBI far from windows and doors so the kids wouldn't be distracted by outside activities or people walking past the classroom. Another strategy was to make lettering on handouts large and to limit the amount of information on a single page so students wouldn't be overwhelmed. Teachers were encouraged to provide brain-injured students with a peer note taker and a tape recorder so that the children would be able to focus all their attention on understanding what was being said.

School administrators learned that brain-injured children tended to become exhausted easily. The way to deal with that was to set up schedules that put breaks between tough classes like math and science, which would give the kids time to recharge. To accommodate damaged memories, Martin suggested that brain-injured students be encouraged to visit the resource room before and after school. That way teachers could make sure the student went home with the right assignments and had the right preparation to start each day. If books had been forgotten at home, spares could be loaned out. Teachers were encouraged to pay attention to the brain-injured children's energy levels. If it looked like a kid was flagging, then it made sense to offer a break.

Martin explained to teachers that TBIs often led to slowed mental processing. This meant that kids would need more time for tests and that timed tasks should be avoided whenever possible. "We explained to them that it was better to emphasize the quality of the student's work rather than the quantity," Martin says. "Teachers needed to provide them with extra time and to reduce homework levels."

As another concession to slowed processing, teachers were encouraged to give students more time to formulate answers to questions in class. "We taught them to avoid badgering students and to provide them with a preview of classwork for the day," Martin says. "Then the students could be prepared." Martin taught teachers about the value of day planners for brain-injured students and of color-coding materials by class; if the history text had a blue book cover, then it made sense that folders and notebooks for this class be blue as well.

Teachers were taught to break long-term projects into chunks that were more easily accomplished by brain-injured kids. Martin also had to convince teachers to be more open-minded so they would provide accommodations for students with TBIs. She encouraged the teachers to let brain-injured children use calculators in math class. Teachers, construing that as an unfair advantage, would often be pushing the kids to memorize multiplication tables. "You'd have to work with the teachers to get them to understand that this kid probably never would be able to do that," Martin says.

Over the five years that the program was in effect, Martin and her colleagues worked with more than four hundred children. Funding petered out in 2001 and no one else stepped up to keep the TBI education program going. "I'm not aware of any program in existence now that is specifically geared to the needs of children with brain injuries," Martin says. "I don't know what happens to them now."

The experience with "hidden" TBIs in the school system led Gordon to suspect that other people might be getting off track because of unrecognized brain damage. After a 2000 study showed that people with a head injury were at higher risk for depression as well as alcohol and drug abuse, Gordon and his colleagues decided to look at the prevalence of TBI in New York State substance abuse programs. The researchers interviewed more than eight hundred patients and found that 54 percent had a history of head injury. Forty percent of those with a history of head trauma had symptoms indicative of post-concussion syndrome. Further, those with head injuries turned out to have more mental illness and to be more prone to recidivism and treatment failure. "That suggests to me that these folks need a different treatment program," Gordon says. "You can't expect people with learning and memory problems to learn at the same pace as everyone else. If you see that a thirty-day program doesn't work, that may mean that these people need sixty or ninety. Maybe they need structured environments to live in, too."

The patients were all in their thirties when they were screened for TBI, and after extensive interviews, researchers learned that many had sustained multiple head injuries. Among those with multiple injuries, the average age when the first TBI occurred was fourteen. This, Gordon thought, might mean that early intervention could prevent damage down the line. "If they had been picked up and identified and treated as folks with a TBI upon that first injury," he says, "they might have gotten the services they needed to prevent them from going down the path to substance abuse."

In 2006, Gordon turned his eyes to the burgeoning homeless population. He linked up with Common Ground, a New York City nonprofit that builds houses for the homeless. Gordon and his colleagues tested one hundred homeless persons for signs of brain injury. Nearly 70 percent of the homeless people interviewed by the Mount Sinai researchers had deficits in memory, language, or attention—all indicative of a possible brain injury. Further, 82 percent reported a significant jolt to the head before they became homeless, often the result of abuse by a parent. Many of these people might be in a very different place in life had their brain injuries been recognized as serious, had they received treatment.

While the solution seems simple in theory—get patients diagnosed quickly and then give them whatever rehab is necessary—it doesn't translate into reality so easily. Most of us continue to think that if we can walk away from a collision, we're fine. Still, if there was one place where you might expect brain injuries to be spotted, it would be on the battlefield—certainly military personnel would be on the lookout for injured brains. But, as it turns out, soldiers fighting in Iraq and Afghanistan were far more likely to receive a diagnosis of post-traumatic stress disorder than traumatic brain injury even if they'd been involved in explosions.

For the longest time Major Michael Zacchea assumed his persistent headaches and nausea were brought on by the pressures of his job. He'd been sent to the Middle East to train a battalion of Iraqi soldiers for the war and then to lead them into battle. From the moment the thirty-six-year-old marine stepped off a plane in Baghdad, he was on constant high alert. Westerners were being targeted for kidnapping and torture. Attacks by Iraqi insurgents could spring up out of nowhere. And once he had arrived at the Iraqi army base where he'd been assigned to retrain soldiers, there were regular death threats to him and his men.

But when Zacchea thinks back now, he realizes that those symptoms, along with others that developed later, could be traced to the two times he hurt his head. The first incident was back in September 2004 while he was out on a reconnaissance mission near the Taji Military Complex, the Iraqi army base where he was stationed. He had gone out to assess the severity of an insurgent attack, and as he drove along the perimeter of the base, a hail of bullets from an insurgent's machine gun suddenly engulfed his vehicle. He careened off the road into a ditch and slammed his head hard on the steering wheel. Dazed and seeing stars, he pulled himself out of the truck and ran to take cover in one of the rickety wood guard towers just behind the chain-link fence that surrounded the base. He paused for a few minutes trying to shake the fuzzy feeling from his brain, then radioed back to the base to order up air support to push the insurgents back and to request help for the wounded soldiers he'd passed while driving along the perimeter. Zacchea stayed in the tower for another six hours, fighting alongside his Iraqi soldiers until the attack subsided.

In the days that followed, he began to have migraines and often felt nauseous. Because he never linked those symptoms to his bang on the head, he never went to a doctor. He just kept on doing his job and assumed that the migraines and sick stomach were symptoms of the unremitting tension he was experiencing. Since the stress wasn't about to let up anytime soon, he figured the migraines and nausea would be there for the duration.

Two months later, Zacchea and his troops were ordered to join a force of marines and soldiers storming Fallujah, which several months earlier had been ceded to the insurgents. Once they battled their way into the city, Zacchea and three other marines began a house-to-house search for insurgents. As they made their way down one street, the marines suddenly became the target of machine gun fire from the upper story of a nearby house. Taking cover against one of the stone walls lining the street, they crouched down and began to leapfrog their way closer to where the shots were originating from. When they were close enough, Zacchea and two of the others stepped out into the street to shower the house with bullets, providing cover while the fourth marine ran over and tossed a grenade up through the second-story window. As the marine turned around to face Zacchea and his comrades, he suddenly froze, his eyes wide open.

Zacchea turned to see what had so startled the marine. Then he saw them: just down the street were two insurgents positioning a rocket-propelled grenade launcher and sighting it on the marines. Without an instant's pause, Zacchea swung his rifle into position, located the insurgents in his sight, and let off a shot. As he pulled the trigger, he heard the RPG go off and then a whine and roar as the grenade streaked toward him. Everything from that moment seemed to pass in slow motion. He could see the round flying toward him. He thought, "I have time for another shot."

Then he had the sense that he was floating. The next thing he knew, he was lying on his back on the street. He couldn't move or speak. He looked up at the sky and noticed it was a brilliant blue. He thought, "OK. This is how I'm going to die. I can do this." Zacchea closed his eyes and waited for death to come. Then, through a hail of sniper fire, the two marines who had taken cover against one of the walls rushed out, grabbed him, and dragged him down the street and around the corner. As he made it to his feet and leaned up against the wall, Zacchea wondered whether he'd been hit. One of the marines noticed blood on his shirt and asked, "Whose blood is this? Who's been hit?" Zacchea, soaked from water that had spewed from his canteens and camel pack when they were shredded by shrapnel from the grenade, wasn't sure. Then he noticed the bloody body print he'd left on the wall and thought, "Oh boy, I'm in big trouble." He looked up at the other marines and said, "I think I was hit." They pulled off his clothes and examined him. There were shrapnel wounds on his shoulder, but the main damage appeared to be a fracture to the joint. They wanted to medevac him back to the Combat Army Support Hospital just outside of Fallujah, but Zacchea refused. He was afraid that if he left, his Iraqi battalion might desert en masse. So he stayed on in Fallujah fighting alongside his troops for another six weeks, never stopping to get his shoulder set.

Back at Taji again, Zacchea was having problems. His headaches had intensified. He couldn't eat. He couldn't sleep. He was constantly irritable. He still was thinking that everything was related to stress—and with good reason. His men had become targets of insurgents trying to frighten Iraqi troops into deserting. Six of them had been abducted and beheaded. Five more were kidnapped and tortured. Making matters worse, he'd been told that the 288 men in his battalion were going to have to take on sole responsibility for defending Taji in place of the brigade of more than 2,000 men that was being sent up to join the fight in Mosul. Zacchea was worried that they were now far too shorthanded to protect the base from insurgent attacks.

In January 2005, he learned of a plot to assassinate him. He decided to take a wait-and-see approach and eventually broke up the conspiracy, but all of that just compounded the tension. Zacchea was sure that the stress from the plot and the constant attacks on his men were taking a toll on his own health. Finally, he went in to the stress clinic at the neighboring Camp Cooke and met with a psychiatrist who asked him to complete a questionnaire designed to ferret out cases of post-traumatic stress disorder and traumatic brain injury. Zacchea checked "yes" to almost every question, including the ones asking if he'd been involved in a blast or vehicular accident. He indicated that he'd lost consciousness during the blast and had seen stars during the wreck. He noted that he had been experiencing headaches, sleep problems, and a constant sense of irritability since then. When the psychiatrist rendered his opinion, it confirmed Zacchea's suspicions: post-traumatic stress disorder, or PTSD. The psychiatrist thought Zacchea ought to rest. But military commanders were unwilling to let him take leave—or even take any time off. Iraqi elections were coming up soon and they wanted security to be tight. So Zacchea continued to go out on combat missions for the next two months.

When he was finally sent back to the United States, his first stop was at Quantico, Virginia, where marines are out-processed. There, physicians noted that he'd been decorated for bravery and recommended for the Purple Heart. They read the descriptions of the vehicle crash and the RPG explosion. They saw the diagnosis of PTSD. When Zacchea told them about the headaches, the sleep problems, and the anxiety, they recommended that he check everything out with his family doctor when he got home.

Zacchea had always figured that his symptoms would resolve once he got away from the battlefield. But when he arrived home in Hicksville, Long Island, his symptoms only intensified. His migraines were lasting longer. He'd spend entire days lying in a darkened room, vainly trying to ease the throbbing in his skull with regular doses of Excedrin. When his head didn't hurt, he was consumed with anxiety and anger, though he never could pinpoint what was triggering either emotion. He would sometimes become paranoid, once barricading himself in his mother's basement, and sometimes fly into a rage. His memory was starting to fail. He often couldn't remember his phone number and would get lost on short trips away from home. He would set out for the grocery store but would forget what he needed to buy by the time he got there. His fiancée was worried about him. She'd noticed that along with his other symptoms, Zacchea now seemed to have problems talking. Once a fluid conversationalist, he was talking slowly and his speech patterns had become choppy. He was having trouble finding words and he had developed a stutter. She didn't know what was wrong, but since he'd been diagnosed with PTSD, she urged him to see a psychologist.

All the while, Zacchea was making monthly visits to the Veterans Affairs Medical Center in Northport, Long Island, to get help with the pain in the shoulder that had been fractured in Iraq. He told doctors there about the headaches, the memory problems, and the irritability. They told him his symptoms were a result of his PTSD and never referred him to a neurologist.

In 2005 he returned to his job as a financial analyst with the Wall Street firm he'd worked at before being sent to Iraq. It didn't take long for his uneven moods to convince his bosses to restrict his contact with clients, so Zacchea found himself concentrating on data collection and market analysis. But even then things didn't go smoothly. He was having trouble with work that had come easily before. His brain seemed to have lost the ability to organize and analyze. He couldn't stay focused. Coworkers told him that since he'd come back from Iraq, he'd been "out in left field." By this time, he knew there was something seriously wrong with him. He was beginning to realize that even if he did have PTSD, that diagnosis couldn't explain all the bizarre symptoms he had been experiencing. He wondered if something had gone wrong with his brain, though he still hadn't connected his symptoms with the jolts he'd experienced in Iraq. He made his case to doctors at the VA, but they refused to refer him to a neurologist.

As time went on, work became even more of a struggle. He was having trouble with fairly simple math, with numbers in general. Then in 2008 he got a call from ABC News. The producer on the phone told him that Bob Woodruff wanted to interview him for a piece that would appear on the evening news exploring the stigma associated with PTSD. One of the veterans' support groups had recommended that ABC contact Zacchea for perspective on the syndrome. During the interview in Central Park, Zacchea talked about the stigma of PTSD. Within a week of the broadcast, doctors at the VA wrote Zacchea a referral to a neurologist from the Yale School of Medicine who was doing some contract work for the military.

Dr. James Hill listened to Zacchea's symptoms and examined him. His diagnosis: Zacchea did indeed have a traumatic brain injury, as well as PTSD. "You should have been in here years ago," Hill told the marine. The neurologist then explained what happened after a TBI. "Your brain is like a computer," he said. "What happens in a TBI is that the operating system gets a glitch in it. It's like you dropped your computer and then it didn't work right anymore." Hill sent Zacchea off for neuropsychological testing to confirm the diagnosis and to pinpoint the marine's deficits. The tests showed that Zacchea was actually getting worse with time.

Zacchea went to his Wall Street bosses with his new diagnosis and asked for some time to try to get rehab. He was also hoping for some accommodations that would make his job easier. But they weren't interested in that approach. In fact, they started to complain about all the medical appointments and the time he was spending on the phone with his doctors. They told him that he could get rehab while out on short-term disability and that he shouldn't expect his old job back when that was done.

The treatment he got from the military wasn't much better. He had been a career officer, having enrolled in the ROTC before starting college at Notre Dame. He had planned to stay with the Marine Corps until retirement just as his father and grandfather had done. But the Marines weren't interested in finding a place for a man with a brain injury and PTSD, even in the reserves. Once he accepted the idea that they weren't going to find a position for him, Zacchea tried to get the Navy to retire him, but that turned out to be just as complicated as everything else in his life now. Navy officials told him that despite all the doctors' reports saying that he wasn't able to continue as a marine, he ought to be able to return to work—based on his past performance. It was a classic catch-22: he was told he couldn't retire because he was healthy enough to get a job with the Navy, but there was no job there for him.

While he appealed the decision, Zacchea found rehab with a private neurological facility. Doctors prescribed medications to help with his migraines and insomnia. Therapists worked to improve his memory and make his speech more fluid. They helped him develop strategies to compensate for his problems with organization and planning.

Realizing he was never going back to the Marines, Zacchea enrolled in a graduate school program at the University of Connecticut focusing on business and policy. He planned to help design a UConn program for disabled vets. After his struggles with his job and the military, Zacchea considers his university experience "the one bright spot." Right from the start, the school was willing to accommodate his disabilities. Professors gave him extra time for tests and were understanding when he forgot assignments. They gave him time to make up work when a migraine broke through and put his life on hold.

Even with those accommodations, Zacchea is sure he wouldn't be where he is today without his wife. "She's hung in there against all odds," he says. "This is not what she signed up for. It can be really difficult at times. I forget a lot of things. Sometimes I forget to take a shower or to brush my teeth. Sometimes I forget to eat. Sometimes I eat twice because I forget that I already ate. She reminds me and sort of keeps me going. She reminds me about deadlines at school. I'd be floundering without her."

Zacchea's long-term plan is to work with disabled vets trying to make their way back into work and society. Energized to find a new path in life, he hopes that he'll be able to put his degree to use helping veterans like him who have slipped through the cracks.

As the wars in Iraq and Afghanistan ground on, reports began to crop up in newspapers and magazines describing the plight of soldiers and marines who, like Zacchea, had come back with undiagnosed brain injuries. They were struggling to adjust to life at home while having to deal with strange symptoms that no one around them could explain. Traumatic brain injury was still under the radar as far as most Americans were concerned. But some experts were beginning to warn that the issue was going to explode as the numbers of veterans from the wars in Iraq and Afghanistan grew and grew. Doctors who treated the returning vets dubbed TBI "the signature wound of the war," because they were seeing such a high percentage with lasting brain damage. At Walter Reed Army Medical Center in Washington, D.C., where many of the most severely injured soldiers were being treated upon returning to the United States, everyone got checked for TBI. Doctors there found that about 60 percent of the soldiers had suffered TBI, with more than half of those brain injuries diagnosed as moderate or severe. Wayne Gordon and other TBI experts were convinced that the brain injuries spotted by doctors at military hospitals were just the tip of the iceberg. Without routine screening, Gordon said, there was no way to prevent brain-injured soldiers and marines from slipping through the cracks.

It's not that TBIs were unheard-of in previous conflicts, but rather that the proportion of military personnel returning from Iraq and Afghanistan with significant injuries to their brains was far greater. The rise in the incidence of traumatic brain injuries resulted partly from the widespread use by insurgents of improvised explosive devices, or IEDs. Ironically, it also resulted from innovations in protective gear and emergency medicine. Soldiers who might have died in earlier conflicts were surviving this one because high-tech helmets and body armor protected the head and torso from penetrating wounds. Advances in first aid and quicker trips to sophisticated medical centers were saving soldiers who might have died on the battlefield in previous wars. But many of those who escaped death because of these advances were surviving with badly wounded brains.

By 2006, experts at the Defense and Veterans Brain Injury Center were beginning to appreciate the scope of the problem. "TBI looms large in terms of chronic consequences," said Dr. Warren Lux, a neurologist then serving as the center's acting director. "Brain injuries, like amputations, are for life."

And while the Department of Defense was counting the numbers of dead and wounded, it wasn't keeping track of mild-to-moderate brain injuries, especially those that occurred without life-threatening wounds to the body. The military still hadn't recognized that significant brain damage could result without any external signs. Nobody was systematically checking soldiers and marines for brain damage after blasts. The troops themselves weren't aware that their brains could be harmed by these invisible wounds. Many chose to stick by the sides of their comrades rather than get checked out after a blast. "A lot of guys don't want to leave their buddies after they've been injured," Lux explained. "They try to tough it out."

The issue came front and center when Bob Woodruff, the ABC News anchorman who had sustained a traumatic brain injury while covering the war in Iraq, put together a prime-time special on TBI that was broadcast by the network in February 2007. By taking Americans through his painful road to recovery, Woodruff put a face on the invisible injury. After telling his own story, Woodruff broadened his report to look at what was happening to soldiers and marines who had suffered wounds like his. He brought the military's polytrauma wards into the nation's living rooms and showed Americans the suffering of soldiers who were having an even harder time recuperating than he had. He exposed problems with the Department of Veterans Affairs' treatment of brain-injured soldiers through the heart-wrenching story of Sergeant Michael Boothby, who, after improving under the care of doctors at the Navy's premier hospital in Bethesda, had begun to lose ground when his case was transferred to the VA hospital near his hometown of Comfort, Texas. For many soldiers and marines, there was no continuity of care once they left polytrauma wards, Woodruff reported. He then took the military to task for letting brain-injured soldiers slip through the cracks, making his case with the story of a soldier who had suffered through a year and a half before he was able to convince the VA that his disparate and debilitating symptoms were the result of a TBI.

Even with all the media attention, though, there was a segment of the military pushing back. Some medical officers insisted that the majority of brain injuries were mild, transient phenomena and that screening for them might cause more problems than it would solve. In a study published in *The New England Journal of Medicine* in January 2008, Army researchers went so far as to suggest that if doctors diagnosed mild traumatic brain injuries in soldiers and marines, it would cause the service members anxiety and slow their recovery. "If you tell a soldier he's got a mild traumatic brain injury, he'll think, 'Maybe I'm brain-damaged,'" said the study's lead author, Colonel Charles Hoge, a psychiatrist and the director of the division of psychiatry and neuroscience at the Walter Reed Army Institute of Research. "They don't realize how remarkably resilient the brain is. Then they read in the papers that exposure to a blast leads to brain damage, and that elevates their alarm further."

For the journal study, Hoge surveyed 2,525 soldiers three to four months after their return from a yearlong deployment in Iraq. The soldiers were asked about a host of symptoms, including various types of pain, sleep issues, irritability, and problems with memory and concentration. The soldiers were also asked whether they'd been injured during deployment by a blast or explosion, a bullet, a fragment or shrapnel, a fall, a vehicle accident, or other means, and whether the injury involved the head. Soldiers were presumed to have had a mild traumatic brain injury, or mTBI, if they checked one of the following: lost consciousness, became dazed or confused, saw stars, had some sort of amnesia. Hoge and his colleagues also asked the soldiers to complete questionnaires designed to ferret out depression and PTSD. When the Army researchers analyzed the responses, they determined that almost 15 percent of the soldiers had suffered mTBIs and that these service members were more likely than those with other injuries to have been hurt in a blast. Further, the researchers concluded that soldiers with mTBIs were more likely than others to be suffering from concentration difficulties, memory problems, ringing in the ears, and regular bouts of irritability. Many of the soldiers who met the criteria for mTBI also appeared to have PTSD. Then the researchers took a leap in logic that many concussion and brain injury experts criticized: Hoge and his colleagues insisted that the vast majority of symptoms suffered by these soldiers could be explained by PTSD, rather than by a TBI. Because of this, Hoge concluded, it would be better to just focus on treating the PTSD.

Hoge went on to suggest that the best course would be to tell brain-injured soldiers that they had sustained a "concussion" rather than a "mild traumatic brain injury." That's because soldiers would associate concussion with an injury they knew occurred in sports, an injury that had the reputation for being mild and transient. The soldiers would expect to get better quicker than they would if they thought they had a brain injury, Hoge said, and they actually would get better quicker.

Not long after Hoge's paper appeared, a 499-page report was published that examined the toll that TBI and PTSD might be taking on service members coming back from the wars. The report, which was

compiled by the RAND Corporation, estimated that by 2008 as many
as 320,000 soldiers and marines had suffered mTBIs, while 300,000 had
ended up with major depression or PTSD. Almost 50 percent of the soldiers with depression or PTSD had not sought treatment, and almost
60 percent of those with a probable TBI had not been evaluated by a
physician. The report warned of "long-term, cascading consequences" if
service members with these health issues didn't receive treatment. Those
consequences could include drug abuse, unemployment, increased mari-
tal problems, and suicide. The RAND report figures were a far cry from
the numbers being posted by the Department of Defense: 43,779 TBIs
through the end of 2007.

When the RAND report was published, Hoge attacked it in the pages
of *The New England Journal of Medicine*. He insisted that the numbers
cited in the report vastly overestimated the number of service members
with head injuries. Further, he argued, the report's suggestion that soldiers
be screened for mTBI would have negative consequences, leading them to
think their brains were permanently injured, which would lead to slower
recoveries. Beyond this, soldiers might be diagnosed with a brain injury
when they didn't have one and then receive inappropriate medications.

This time, Hoge's writings drew an immediate reaction from some
of the nation's leading brain injury experts, including Gordon. Their response, published in the same issue of the journal, took Hoge to task
for minimizing the long-term consequences of mTBI and for suggesting
that the proper diagnosis would delay recovery. "Education after a mild
TBI has been found to reduce distress rather than exacerbate the condition," they wrote. "The opinions expressed by Hoge et al. may harm service members and civilians alike by limiting the identification of persons
who are injured and the provision of appropriate care, thereby causing
unnecessary suffering, disability, and ultimately greater taxpayer expense."

Other researchers grappled with the controversy over how TBI and
PTSD were linked in a study that took some of the wartime politics out
of the issue. That 2009 study looked at medical records of 124 randomly
selected individuals who had sustained some of the milder injuries during
the Oklahoma City bombing. Researchers pored through the survivors'
medical records to see if there was a correlation between any particular
type of injury and the occurrence of PTSD. In the end, they found that

the only type of injury that consistently predicted that a person would develop PTSD was a TBI. "The potential relationship between TBI and PTSD may therefore be one of reinforced neuronal circuits where TBI may sensitize the emotional learning or modulate memory retention," the researchers concluded.

By now, the military was beginning to accept the notion that even mild traumatic brain injuries could change lives. As the Department of Defense searched for a solution to the growing problem, it looked to the model developed in the sports world for catching and treating concussions.

Chapter 6

Playing Defense

On any given Monday, the vast waiting room at the University of Pittsburgh Center for Sports Medicine is packed with patients injured over the weekend in western Pennsylvania, where football is as tightly woven into the collective psyche as the steel mill. Some are limping, some are using crutches, some are wearing slings. But many have no obvious signs of injury. These are the concussed: a couple of dozen high school teens, a handful of collegians, even an NFL pro or two. The season after leading the Pittsburgh Steelers to the 2006 Super Bowl title, quarterback Ben Roethlisberger—fresh off his second concussion in five months—could be found sharing that waiting room with schoolboy quarterbacks who idolized him.

On this particular Monday, Mark Lenkiewicz is leaning forward in his chair, his elbows on his knees, staring down at the floor while unconsciously wringing his hands. His white baseball cap is on backward and pulled so far down that it completely covers his short-cropped brown hair and almost obscures his eyebrows. He's dressed like a typical teen, right down to the diamond studs in his earlobes, but even under an oversized T-shirt, his broad shoulders and thick neck give him away as a football player.

Lenkiewicz is abruptly brought back from his reverie when his mother taps him on the shoulder and nods in the direction of the familiar figure striding toward them. Mark Lovell, the director of the nation's leading concussion clinic, has come to collect his patient. Lenkiewicz forces a smile, stands, and follows his neuropsychologist down the long hallway to the exam room, past the framed photos and jerseys autographed by Joe Namath, Lance Armstrong, Pelé, and scores of other sports heroes.

As they're walking, Lovell is again struck by how much Lenkiewicz has grown. Five years ago, when Lenkiewicz first showed up at the clinic, he had just suffered a concussion in an ice skating accident. That concussion was so severe that Lovell had told the seventh grader to rest his brain by taking a month off from school and to protect against another head injury by completely avoiding contact sports. So Lovell was surprised when Lenkiewicz, now a high school senior, turned up in his office a week ago nursing a sports concussion. The skinny little kid Lovell remembered treating five years earlier had grown into a five-foot-eleven, 190-pound mass of muscle who'd been playing football for the past four years.

This time, Lenkiewicz had been going for a tackle at his high school's summer football camp when he tripped over a fallen teammate and landed hard on the side of his head. As he lay on the ground, he pulled his helmet off and grabbed his head, trying to dull the excruciating pain. He rolled over onto his back, blinking as the bright sunlight intensified the pain. Everything was blurry. His ears were ringing, his stomach churning. As Lenkiewicz slowly sat up, the team trainer began to ask the standard set of questions: "What's your name? Do you know where you are? Do you remember what you had for breakfast?" Then the trainer asked him to repeat three words: "Girl, dog, green." Lenkiewicz could only come up with the first two. The trainer tried again: "Girl, dog, green." This time Lenkiewicz got all three right, but in the wrong order.

The trainer helped him off the ground and then off the field. As Lenkiewicz sat on the bench, hunched over with his head in his hands, the coach appeared in front of him.

"Lenkiewicz," the coach barked, "you ready to get back out there?"

"No, Coach," Lenkiewicz replied, "I can't."

"Oh c'mon, it's just a headache," the coach urged.

"No, it's not," Lenkiewicz shot back. "I'm not going back out there. I need to see a doctor."

As soon as Lenkiewicz's parents got the trainer's phone call, they raced the seventy miles from their home in the suburban Pittsburgh town of Baldwin to pick Mark up and take him to the hospital. In the emergency room, the doctor diagnosed a concussion and told Lenkiewicz's mother that Mark could go home.

"Whoa," Diane Lenkiewicz snapped, "aren't you going to do a CAT scan?"

"He doesn't need one," the doctor countered. "It's just a concussion."

"No way," she said, planting herself in front of the doctor, arms folded across her chest. "He's not leaving here till he gets a CAT scan."

Once the CAT scan confirmed that there was no swelling or bleeding in her son's brain, Diane Lenkiewicz called the Pitt concussion clinic to make an appointment. The next day, Mark Lenkiewicz was describing his symptoms to Lovell, undergoing a complete neurological exam, and taking a neuropsychological test to measure any cognitive deficits. The computerized test showed that this concussion was almost as severe as the one five years earlier and that Lenkiewicz now had significant memory problems as well as slowed mental processing. Lovell sent him home with an admonishment to completely rest his brain and body for the next week and then to come back for a reevaluation.

This morning, as they walk down the hallway, Lenkiewicz is relieved to report that his concussion symptoms have cleared up. Now he's anxious to retake the test to prove that his brain has healed enough for him to return to play. They enter the exam room—bare except for a chair, a table, a computer, and a framed Steelers jersey autographed by former fullback Merril Hoge—and Lenkiewicz sits down to take the test that will decide his football future.

Lovell began developing the test in the early '90s while working with Dr. Joseph Maroon, the team neurosurgeon for the Steelers. Lovell and Maroon were looking for a way to diagnose and measure the severity of concussions without having to depend on athletes' self-assessments, which were notoriously inaccurate and untrustworthy.

Maroon first recognized the need for a streamlined neuropsychological test after an argument with longtime Steelers coach Chuck Noll. Before practice one day, Maroon had approached Noll in the locker room at Three Rivers Stadium to suggest that the quarterback be sidelined. Looking up at the big, burly former NFL lineman, the diminutive Maroon took a deep breath and said carefully, "He can't play in Sunday's game."

"Why not?" Noll asked brusquely.

"Well, he's had a concussion and the guidelines say he shouldn't play for two or three weeks," Maroon explained.

"Who wrote the guidelines?"

"Well, I did, as well as a few other neurosurgeons and neurologists."

"What basis did you have for writing those guidelines? Don't tell me I have to keep a player out if you can't give me some objective data."

Maroon got quiet. Noll may have been a coaching legend, having built the Steelers dynasty with a record four Super Bowl titles in six years, but he was no brain expert. Maroon thought angrily, "Who are you to know about this? You think you know more about medicine than I do?" But even before he heard Noll's verdict, Maroon knew he'd lost this battle to the aloof and hardheaded disciplinarian known as The Emperor. "He can throw the ball and knows the plays," Noll pronounced. "I see no impairment here whatsoever."

Over the next few days, as Maroon replayed the argument in his head, he realized that Noll had a point. There was no real science supporting the guidelines. A onetime major-college football player himself, Maroon could understand Noll's obsession with cold hard numbers in a sport where success is measured in yards and proven by stats. But he also knew firsthand what concussions could do to the brain, having suffered several as a smaller-than-average running back routinely crushed by bruising Big Ten linebackers.

He reached for the phone and called Lovell, who was then evaluating brain-injured patients at the same hospital where Maroon was chairman of the neurosurgery department. "Mark, he's right," Maroon said. "We do need objective information if we're going to keep people out of sports."

Both Maroon and Lovell had been impressed by a recently published landmark study that established the utility of neuropsychological testing in college football. After using neuropsych tests in players from ten colleges over four seasons, researchers from the University of Virginia determined that this was an effective way to measure cognitive deficits from concussions and to track recovery. Now Maroon and Lovell were eager to extend this protocol to the pros.

So Maroon went to Noll with a proposal. "Look, you told me to come back to you with some data," Maroon said. "Here's what I want to do." Maroon's plan to get the data had one catch: Noll would have to encourage his players to volunteer for a neuropsychological test that Lovell had devised. Noll thought it over, and realized there was no good reason to say no.

Though reluctant at first to be tested by a "shrink," many of the players eventually agreed to meet with Lovell. Since it was before the boom in personal computers, Lovell had to rely on lengthy face-to-face interviews, standardized pencil-and-paper tests of memory and cognition, and a stopwatch to measure each player's reaction time. For his breakthrough experiment in 1993, he tested twenty-three healthy Steelers in preseason training camp to provide baseline measurements, which could then be used as a comparison with tests taken during the season by concussed players.

One of those players was Merril Hoge. During the fall of 1994, soon after he'd left Pittsburgh to play for the Chicago Bears, Hoge was driven from a game, dazed and disoriented, by the sixth diagnosed concussion of his NFL career. In the locker room minutes later, he stopped breathing for fifteen seconds and briefly had no pulse or heartbeat. For three days, he couldn't recognize his wife or daughter. A few weeks after being released from intensive care, he returned to Pittsburgh for another round of neuropsychological testing with Lovell and Maroon. Not surprisingly, the player who could no longer drive his car or balance his checkbook would score abysmally on the test. Pulling Hoge aside, Lovell and Maroon dug out the baseline results from the summer of '93 and laid them down next to the latest data. "Look, Merril, here's where you were," Maroon said, pointing to the earlier results. "And," Maroon went on, gesturing toward the new ones, "here's where your brain is now." Three days later, Hoge retired from football at the age of twenty-nine.

Seated now under the framed Merril Hoge jersey in Lovell's exam room, Mark Lenkiewicz starts the computerized test that will determine whether he too will have to give up football. He's taking the high-tech version of the old pencil-and-paper test that Lovell devised for the Steelers. With the proliferation of inexpensive personal computers in the mid-'90s, Lovell saw a way to make the test widely available to athletes of all ages at all levels of play. His computerized version had the added advantage of being more like Pac-Man than a neuropsych exam.

Lenkiewicz is as intensely focused on the monitor as he would be on a rival team's linebacker, his right index finger tapping the mouse in anticipation. The test kicks off with a verbal memory drill: after each of twelve words flashes on the screen for 750 milliseconds, he's asked to identify them from a list of twenty-four. The second drill is similar, only this time twelve abstract designs flash on the screen before he's asked to recall which ones he's seen. The next part of the test seems a bit more familiar to a football player used to memorizing a playbook. A jumble of X's and O's pops up on the screen, looking like a deranged version of the blackboard X's and O's that coaches use to diagram plays. Three of them are illuminated in bright yellow. Lenkiewicz has just a split second to memorize their pattern and position before the screen fades to the next challenge. Then, in rapid succession, a series of geometric shapes flashes on the screen: a red square, a blue square, a red circle, or a blue circle. He must left-click the mouse any time a blue square appears and right-click for each red circle, fully aware he's being graded on both speed and accuracy. Suddenly the screen with X's and O's reappears, only this time the letters are all the same color. He must now recall and click on the three originally illuminated X's and O's. He's halfway home. Without taking a breather, he blitzes through the final three sections of the test.

His twenty-minute ordeal behind him, Lenkiewicz heads to a conference room to join his mother and anxiously wait for the grading of his test. No matter how much better an athlete feels physically, there can be lingering symptoms subtle enough to go unnoticed by players, coaches, trainers, and even team medical personnel. The test is designed not only to ferret out the most subtle deficits, but also to catch athletes bent on covering up symptoms so they can get back to play sooner. No wonder kids fear the test that Lovell fondly calls "the grim reaper."

Its real name is ImPACT, which stands for Immediate Post-concussion Assessment and Cognitive Testing. Since its development in the late '90s as the first computerized battery of tests to objectively measure cognitive function in concussed athletes, ImPACT has become the gold standard for tracking their healing and recovery. While there are several other computerized tests on the market, none has caught on the way ImPACT has. Lovell's test is now used by more than one hundred pro teams, more than five hundred colleges, and more than fifteen hundred high schools nationwide. And that doesn't include the several thousand patients who come directly to Lovell's clinic each year, some making the pilgrimage all the way across the country to the glistening glass structure erected on the site of a rusted steel mill hard by the Monongahela River.

In the conference room, Lenkiewicz drops into a chair next to his mother and they wait for Lovell to return with the test results. Diane

Lenkiewicz turns to her son and says, "You know, Mark, no matter what the test results are, I don't want you playing in Friday's game."

He shrugs and nods in resignation, setting his sights on the following week's game. "I just want to be out there with my friends," he explains. "If I get in for two plays, I'll be happy. I don't need another concussion. I don't even want to play college football anymore. The coach says I can get a scholarship, but I'm not going to be somebody's punching bag; if you're a freshman in college, you're just a tackling dummy. I might not wake up after another concussion, or I might be paralyzed. I just want to enjoy this season and be done."

His mother smiles proudly. "I say, good for you! You have to have that attitude. It's a healthy one."

Just then, Lovell walks through the doorway, his nose buried in Lenkiewicz's chart. Taking a chair, he nods to Mark and then fixes his gaze on Diane Lenkiewicz. "Well, Mark's definitely making progress," Lovell says. "He may feel a hundred percent back, but I don't feel he is." Lovell pulls a page from the chart and pushes it across the conference table so the Lenkiewiczes can see the test results for themselves. "All of his scores certainly have improved," Lovell says. "His performance in speed-oriented tasks is all the way back to normal, but his memory scores are not where we would like to see them. Given his concussion history, we want to make sure this completely resolves." Lovell pauses and glances at a calendar. "Let's see, the first game is—"

"He's not playing," Diane Lenkiewicz cuts in.

"Right," Lovell says, nodding. "But what I want him to start doing is ratchet up physical conditioning." Lovell turns to Mark and says, "You know the drill. Start to do some light jogging. If you get any headaches or dizziness, back off completely. The idea is not to push through it but to see if you can increase your heart rate without any symptoms. If you can tolerate the jogging for a couple of days, you can start building up gradually. And eventually I want to get you to the point where you can do full-out wind sprints and really be sweating without any symptoms whatsoever." Lovell turns back to Diane Lenkiewicz and cautions her, "I'll clear him for that—but not anything more." She leans forward, elbows on the table, and assures Lovell that she's already set the coach straight on that score.

Several days ago, when the coach told her he planned to start Mark in Friday night's season opener, the short, stocky blond dynamo got up in his face and snapped, "I'm telling you now, this is the deal: Mark won't be playing Friday."

"But," the coach sputtered, "he's our fullback."

"Well, you better find another one and train him now," she shot back, "because Mark's not playing. This is my kid, and I'm not going to have him sitting in a wheelchair eating Jell-O for the rest of his life."

As she replays the story in the conference room, Lovell smiles and then tells her that Mark will need to come back in to take the test again. Lovell explains that Mark's youth makes him particularly vulnerable to concussions because the brain doesn't finish developing until the mid-twenties. What's more, Lovell says, multiple concussions can add up and have a cumulative effect: even if Mark's scores come back to baseline, another concussion might have a more serious impact, one that could be permanent. That's why Lovell occasionally has to "retire" a kid from contact sports. But since he appreciates the value of athletic competition, Lovell assures the Lenkiewiczes that he'll do everything possible to get Mark safely back on the ballfield.

Two weeks later, Mark Lenkiewicz returns to the clinic and aces the test. Based on his ImPACT scores and lack of symptoms during cardio-vascular workouts, he is cleared to return to the football field. Still, Diane Lenkiewicz senses some reticence when Lovell says to her son, "What I can tell you is that you've had these injuries and you've taken progressively longer to get better, and that's not a good sign. But I can't tell you not to play, any more than I can tell Ben Roethlisberger not to play."

As much of a science as Lovell's test has made of concussion manage-ment, no one can say when—or even if—it's completely safe to return a player to action, for concussion remains the most mysterious and unpre-dictable of all sports injuries.

Mark Lovell came by his concussion education the hard way. It was back in the early '70s, and he was a typical eighteen-year-old with shoulder-length hair standing on the side of the road, thumb out, hitching a ride home from his high school in Grand Rapids, Michigan. When a car fi-nally slowed to a stop, he raced over, jumped in, and slammed the door behind him. As the car peeled away, he looked down and was horrified to see empty beer cans scattered everywhere. Even though the man was driving erratically, Lovell resisted the temptation to panic. But then the sirens started wailing, the police lights flashed, the driver floored it, and the chase was on. The next thing Lovell knew, he was hurtling through the windshield headfirst.

In the emergency room, the doctor stitched up all the cuts on Lovell's face and sent him for an x-ray. A couple of hours later, looking up at the x-ray of Lovell's skull, the doctor said, "There's nothing broken. You're fine. You can go."

Lovell spent the next few weeks at home, recuperating from what he now knows was a concussion. After returning to school, he still didn't feel like himself. His thinking was foggy and he couldn't concentrate. Friends kidded that he was "kind of goofy." He had memory problems for nearly a year and migraines for over a decade. Even more time would pass before he connected it all to the auto accident.

Lovell's first job after grad school was in one of the nation's busiest trauma centers, at Pittsburgh's Allegheny General Hospital. There, he was in charge of evaluating the mental status of patients with severe head injuries. What he observed as he examined those patients would jog his memory. They seemed to have the same types of symptoms he'd had after his concussion senior year in high school. He started to think that maybe people weren't taking concussions seriously enough. It was clear from his own experience that concussions were a form of brain injury—and yet, his colleagues were dismissing them as insignificant bumps on the head and disparaging concussed patients who complained of prolonged symptoms as litigious malingerers. He would often argue, "The brain doesn't know if it's been injured playing sports or in a high-velocity motor vehicle crash."

When Joe Maroon called to enlist his help studying concussions in the Steelers players, Lovell saw a chance to prove his point—and to meld his two passions, sports and brain science. Even better, the playing field would make the perfect impromptu lab. Nowhere else did people have concussions so frequently, so regularly, and so visibly. Besides, no one would accuse athletes of malingering. If anything, athletes—especially professional athletes—were more likely to minimize symptoms in an effort to get back to play sooner.

Over the next decade, Lovell began consulting on concussion management for the National Football League as well as the National Hockey League. He refined the Steelers' neuropsychological testing program and expanded that model to a few other NFL teams, and he worked with the NHL to develop and implement its mandatory league-wide testing program. In the meantime, he started researching the impact of concussions on college and high school athletes. By the late '90s, he had published several journal articles looking at concussion in sports as well as in car accidents.

All that research and experience made Lovell the obvious choice when the University of Pittsburgh went looking in 2000 for an expert to set up a groundbreaking concussion program as part of its new head-to-toe sports medicine center. Once there, one of Lovell's first orders of business was to incorporate his new computerized neuropsych test in the center's concussion management program and to introduce that software in a handful of local colleges and high schools. But his vision for ImPACT was far more ambitious: he dreamed of seeing the test in every school in the country to give coaches and trainers a more objective way to help assess when athletes could safely return to play. To get enough money and manpower to make that possible, Lovell partnered up with his colleague Michael Collins, Maroon, and the university to form a company that could promote the development and marketing of the test. Over the next several years, ImPACT would become a cornerstone of the center's comprehensive concussion program, and the software's use in high schools and colleges would spread from western Pennsylvania to other parts of the country.

Lovell now runs the program from a second-floor office that looks out past the skeletons of abandoned steel mills and the sluggish Monongahela River to the burnished skyscrapers of downtown Pittsburgh. A model brain huddles next to a black and gold Steelers helmet near his computer monitor. Several footballs, gifts from concussed players, are propped against the windowsill behind his desk. One ball sports the autographs of Troy Aikman and Steve Young, the biggest NFL stars forced to retire by concussions. Next to it is a ball signed by former Steelers wide receiver Lynn Swann, yet another Hall of Famer whose career was cut short by concussions. A third ball is covered with the signatures of Ben Roethlisberger and the rest of the 2006 Super Bowl champion Steelers.

Lovell, his hair now neatly cropped and more gray than auburn, leans back in his leather chair, gazes out the window, and reflects on how lucky he is to be working right next door to his "lab." The Steelers practice so close by that Roethlisberger could heave a Hail Mary pass and hit the Center for Sports Medicine. More to the point, Roethlisberger and his teammates have only to walk across a small parking lot to get from the team's locker room to Lovell's exam room.

The Steelers share one indoor and four outdoor football fields with the University of Pittsburgh Panthers as part of state-of-the-art training facilities on the same campus as the Center for Sports Medicine. The forty-acre complex at the base of the Hot Metal Bridge rose from the ashes of the mammoth South Side Works steel mill, which had been a fixture in Pittsburgh since before the Civil War. The green gridirons and gleaming glass buildings stand in a stark contrast to the grimy old mill that was once wedged into this narrow mile-long strip between the river and the railroad tracks built to export steel from the South Side Works.

At its peak, the mill employed thirteen thousand workers and produced more than four thousand tons of metal a day—steel that helped build a nation, from cars manufactured in Detroit to skyscrapers springing up in America's growing cities. The demise of the South Side Works marked the final collapse of the industry that had given Pittsburgh its economic lifeblood, its identity, and its nickname—The Steel City. Just when the wounded city needed it most, the Steelers, their helmets emblazoned with the iconic logo of U.S. Steel, stepped up to restore a measure of civic pride. After four frustrating decades as lovable losers, the team had caught fire under the iron leadership of new coach Chuck Noll. By the time the mill's blast furnaces had belched their last plume of sooty black smoke, the Steelers had risen up to replace steel as the city's identity.

No team in sports could better reflect its community's character. Noll built a dynasty in the city's tough, gritty image, fielding brutally physical, defense-oriented teams that embodied the blue-collar roots of their rabid fans. Powered by the smothering "Steel Curtain" defense and an effective no-frills offense, the Steelers brought the city four Super Bowl championships between 1975 and 1980. The bond the team forged with its loyal fans would endure and grow as Pittsburgh rebuilt its economy, now based on medicine, research, and technology.

That fervor for football extended far beyond Pittsburgh and the Steelers to every community and every school in western Pennsylvania. No region of the country, not even Texas, is more football-obsessed. Locals will happily boast to anyone who'll listen that western Pennsylvania has produced more legendary NFL quarterbacks than anyplace else, ticking off from their list the familiar names: Johnny Unitas, Joe Namath, Joe Montana, Dan Marino. On cool Friday nights, huge crowds flock to the high school stadiums sprinkled along the Allegheny Mountains. Like the moths glimmering in the night, the fans seem instinctively drawn to the arc lights hovering high over the vast green stage. Throughout the fall, townspeople build their entire social lives around the spectacle that's come to be known as the "Friday Night Lights."

The siren call of life lived in the spotlight is what ultimately lures Mark Lenkiewicz back to the gridiron even after Lovell, in clearing him to return to play, cautions that another concussion could lead to permanent brain damage. Even though he's already lost his position as a starter, Lenkiewicz is willing to take that risk for one last chance to hang with his teammates, to bask in the adulation of his classmates, and to feel the rush fueled by a roaring throng of twelve thousand fans. When the crowd exceeds over half the population of your entire town, the pull can be irresistible. "Knowing all those people are watching you play gives you a chill up your spine," he explains.

Western Pennsylvania's obsession with football made Pittsburgh the perfect place for a concussion clinic to take root and grow. But even there, Lovell initially encountered resistance. Parents would bring their kids in to be examined, concerned about concussion symptoms, but Lovell's advice seemed overly cautious. How could a bump on the head lead to weeks of missed practices and even classes? He'd have to explain that so-called dings could be serious and life-altering injuries if the brain wasn't given time to heal. He'd point to the NFL stars recently forced into retirement by concussions. But it was still a tough sell to parents and kids alike. What would ultimately make Lovell's job easier was his increasingly high-profile work with famous Steelers, none more so than Ben Roethlisberger.

From the moment he arrived in Pittsburgh, Roethlisberger clicked with the fans. With a working-class background, he seemed to embody the soul of the city and its surrounding factory towns. His style of play fit right into the Steelers mold: tough, bold, spare. An imposing six foot five and 242 pounds, the quarterback nicknamed Big Ben quickly became known for getting the job done efficiently if not artistically. Highlight reels were filled with footage featuring a deceptively agile and unflappable player—scrambling around as he searched for an open receiver, ducking and darting away from would-be tacklers, then throwing a pinpoint pass without breaking stride. As a rookie, he took a team that had fallen on hard times and overnight restored it to an NFL power. The next season, at the age of just twenty-three, he became the youngest ever to quarterback a team to a Super Bowl championship. By bringing the city the 2006 title—the first since before Roethlisberger was born—he seemed to be offering Pittsburgh the promise of another Steelers dynasty.

Then, just four months after a quarter of a million fans flooded downtown streets for the victory parade, that promise was almost extinguished. Roethlisberger was riding his motorcycle to practice—without a helmet, as usual—when a turning car suddenly cut him off. He hit the car broadside and was rocketed headfirst into the windshield and then over the roof onto the pavement. Along with massive blood loss, a nine-inch gash in his scalp, a broken jaw, and multiple facial fractures that required seven hours of emergency surgery to repair, there was a concussion.

Remarkably, Roethlisberger healed up fast enough to return for the next season. But in his fourth game back, just as he was releasing a pass, he took a vicious helmet-to-facemask hit that knocked him out cold. The next day, he was back at the Pitt concussion clinic to take Lovell's test. The scores that Monday were so low that he had to take the test again Wednesday, and although there was improvement, it wasn't until he took the test a third time on Friday that he was cleared to play. That Sunday, he threw four interceptions in a galling loss, turning in the worst performance of his worst season. The only person who took more criticism than Roethlisberger was the team neurosurgeon. "Where did you get your medical degree?" read a typical piece of the hate mail that flooded Joe Maroon's inbox. Another read, "Even I knew he shouldn't go back."

Faced with a similar decision on the eve of the playoffs two seasons later, Maroon knew the armchair experts would be back out in force. In the 2008 regular-season finale, Roethlisberger was gang-tackled hard and slammed the back of his helmet against the turf. He lay inert with no feeling in his arms for a frightening fifteen minutes. As he was driven from the field on a cart with Maroon steadying his immobilized head, Roethlisberger weakly lifted his left hand and gave the hushed home crowd a thumbs-up. Once again, Roethlisberger found himself in the familiar Pitt exam room. Once again, it would take several tests before Maroon and Lovell would clear him to play. But this time, there would be no second-guessing Maroon's judgment: Roethlisberger decisively led the Steelers back to the Super Bowl and then hurled a dramatic touchdown pass in the waning seconds to deliver their second championship in four seasons.

Each time Roethlisberger had one of those nationally televised head injuries, the public got a primer on this new concept of concussion management. From the constant TV and newspaper updates tracking his treatment, parents began to see why players might need to be tested and sometimes sidelined. Suddenly everyone wanted to go to the same clinic as Roethlisberger and his teammates. Parents were now coming to see Lovell with a grasp of the injury's seriousness and the complexities of its management. What's more, the newly converted wanted to commiserate over the ignorance of coaches who argued against sidelining players and of teachers who didn't understand that concussions could affect schoolwork.

With concussions getting more and more media play, the Pitt clinic got so busy that the university had to add satellite offices to accommodate all the kids coming in from suburban schools. Along with the college and high school students, Lovell started seeing increasing numbers of junior high and elementary school kids. Parents were now bringing in children as young as five.

As the public began to take concussions more seriously, Lovell could turn his attention from defending the mere diagnosis to researching better ways to treat severe and prolonged symptoms. This was a paradigm shift: Lovell wasn't just playing defense anymore—he was playing offense. Instead of simply advising patients to rest their brains until symptoms resolved, he started to take a more active approach, borrowing rehab techniques developed for patients with severe brain injuries. Now there were options for a patient who came in with a brain still slowed and foggy after weeks of rest.

. . .

Doreen Kruth was worried about her daughter. Angelica had smashed her chin on the gym floor in a fall during cheerleading practice and was now in excruciating pain, sipping food through a straw and complaining of pounding headaches. It was hard for Kruth to watch her bright and bubbly fourteen-year-old become so listless and dull.

But what concerned Kruth even more was the host of other odd symptoms that couldn't be explained by their pediatrician's diagnosis of whiplash. A straight-A student, Angelica suddenly couldn't focus in class. Her vision was so blurry that she couldn't read. She was so dizzy and disoriented that it was hard to walk down the bustling school hallways without banging into other kids; sometimes she felt so unsteady that she had to grab on to the lockers to keep from falling down. Whenever Kruth would ask her what was wrong, Angelica was uncharacteristically snappish and irritable.

Perplexed and frightened, Kruth took her daughter to another pediatrician for a second opinion. But the diagnosis and prescription were the same: a swollen jaw and whiplash to be treated with ice packs and painkillers. Once again a doctor pronounced that Angelica would be fine in a couple of days. Except that she wasn't. In fact, she was getting worse and worse with each passing day. None of it made any sense.

In desperation, Kruth turned to the renowned maxillofacial surgeon who helped repair Ben Roethlisberger's jaw after the infamous motorcycle crash fifteen months earlier. Despite x-rays and CAT scans to the contrary, she was starting to suspect that her daughter's jaw might indeed be broken—how else could you explain all those severe and disparate symptoms?

Six days after the cheerleading fall, Angelica was sitting in Dr. Mark Ochs's exam room at the University of Pittsburgh Medical Center, getting her jaw x-rayed yet again. Ochs came in, did a full examination, and then left to read the x-rays. When he came back, the look on his face made Kruth even more worried.

"That kid should have gone right to the emergency room," he said.

"Emergency room!" Kruth blurted, almost cutting him off. "Why?"

"She's got a severe concussion," he explained.

He looked at Kruth's face and saw worry turning into bewilderment.

"But how can she have a concussion when she hit her chin?" Kruth exclaimed.

Ochs told her that you could get a brain injury without hitting your head. As he dug out some pamphlets on concussion, he suggested that she take her daughter to a brain specialist. Angelica listened to the latest diagnosis with disbelief. "Oh great," she thought, "another crazy doctor with another crazy diagnosis. You're out of your mind, dude."

On the drive home, Angelica sat quietly in the passenger seat, stunned by the mere suggestion that she'd suffered a concussion. In her mind, concussions only happened to the football players she would cheerlead for under the lights on Friday nights. Whenever she'd see one of them staggering around after a big hit, she'd think, "Thank God I don't play football, 'cause I'll never be in a position where that could happen to me."

The next day, the Kruths met with a pediatric neurosurgeon. All it took was a five-minute neurological test to confirm Ochs's diagnosis of severe concussion. The neurosurgeon's instructions were firm and frightening: "Angelica shouldn't be going to school. In fact, she shouldn't be going anywhere for quite some time. You need to get to a concussion program." Kruth walked out of the doctor's office with another stack of pamphlets on brain injury. Though she finally had an answer to explain what was wrong with her daughter, she now had a million questions about what it all meant. "Oh brother, is this really going to work?" she wondered. "At least now I know she's got a concussion. But what all does that involve? And how are we going to fix this?"

Kruth would have to wait two weeks before she could get any answers. It was football season, and the Pitt concussion clinic was so backed up that it was impossible to schedule anything sooner. When the Kruths arrived for their Monday morning appointment, the waiting room was packed. Even so, Mark Lovell spotted the pair immediately. Angelica's long honey-blond hair, straight and neatly draped over her shoulders, was hard to miss. The slender, fine-featured teen was staring blankly out the window as her mother furiously scribbled down the latest of her concussion questions. Both were surprised when Lovell suddenly appeared and introduced himself. As they walked to the exam room, Lovell noted how wobbly and unsteady Angelica was. Once there, he guided her to a chair, and when she'd settled in, he asked for a description of the accident.

Angelica told him that it had happened during cheerleading practice when she was rehearsing a stunt called The Helicopter. She explained how the stunt is supposed to work. She was the "flyer," the one who gets tossed up in the air by four teammates. She would first be hoisted up in a horizontal position, with her back parallel to the floor. Her four teammates would then hold her aloft—one grasping her shoulders, another gripping her ankles, and the other two supporting her torso from opposite sides of her body. When everyone was ready, Angelica would stiffen her body and the four teammates would then fling her up several feet in the air with a twisting motion. She would rotate 180 degrees parallel to the ground and be caught by her teammates as she came back down. Only this time, the stunt went terribly wrong. The teammate who was supposed to catch her shoulders didn't. Angelica crashed to the ground, completely missing the mat and smashing her chin on the gym floor.

Wincing for an instant, Lovell asked Angelica if she remembered hitting the floor. She shook her head no. In fact, she said, the rest of the story she'd had to piece together from the scraps she remembered and from what her teammates told her later. "I really didn't know what was going on," she said. "I wasn't aware of what actually happened to me. I remember the trainer came and saw me, and the coaches were there. They took me to the bathroom and wiped all the blood off and gave me an ice pack. I just sat there, I guess, for a little bit, and I just went back ten minutes later. One girl told me that I went back out and did the same stunt without even hesitating. And I think I did it a couple of more times."

Lovell then asked her what symptoms she'd been experiencing since the accident. She told him about the unrelenting headaches so excruciating that they often kept her awake through the night. She told him about the crushing fatigue that kept her in bed all day. She told him about the dizziness, the nausea, the balance problems. She explained that she couldn't read anymore because she couldn't get both eyes to focus on the same spot on a page.

Considering how debilitating her symptoms were, Lovell wasn't surprised when Angelica bombed on her first run-through with ImPACT. Once the test results were printed out, Lovell spread them across a small conference table for Angelica and her mother to see. He explained that Angelica would have to take it easy for the next month or so. Her scores revealed that her mental processing was now slower than that of 95 percent of the kids who take the test and her memory was almost as dramatically impaired. Lovell looked at Doreen Kruth and said, "By Pennsylvania law, she's legally handicapped."

Noticing the frightened look on Kruth's face, Lovell immediately tried to reassure her. The good news, he said, is that most kids got better after a month or so of rest. For the minority who didn't improve on their own, he could offer newly developed rehabilitation techniques, including medication and physical therapy. Kruth asked why they couldn't start the rehab right away. "She's not ready for that yet," Lovell replied. "Her brain needs time to calm down. Right now, rest is the best medicine. She needs to stay home from school. She should have a quiet room with no bright lights. She shouldn't do anything even remotely taxing to the brain. The most I'd allow her to do is watch TV."

After a month of rest, Angelica's symptoms were still so severe that she could watch TV only when the sound was off. It seemed as if the most innocuous stimuli could spark a headache. Some days even the twenty-minute drive to the clinic was enough to make Angelica's head throb so intensely that Kruth would have to turn the car around and return to their suburban Munhall home. In an effort to get the headaches under control, Lovell began experimenting with medications designed to prevent migraines.

The drugs helped ease the headaches enough for Angelica to start working on her vision problems. At first, her vision was so impaired that if a page contained a single word, like "cat," she could tell that there were letters but she couldn't make out what they spelled no matter how large they were; the harder she tried to read the word, the harder her head would pound. To help her relearn to focus her eyes, therapists held a pencil inches from her nose and asked her to follow it only with her eyes as they moved it several feet away. In another exercise, she was told to stare at a word on the wall and turn her head from side to side without taking her eyes off of it.

As her vision began to improve, Angelica was able to start working on her balance problems. For months she struggled to make it through a rudimentary obstacle course. Therapists would place a shoebox in the middle of a hallway. Sometimes she would be asked to walk around the box, sometimes she'd be asked to step over it. Often that was too much of a challenge and she'd trip. In another exercise, she would have to grab an object off a shelf. Invariably, as she reached up, she would get dizzy, lose her balance, and start to fall.

For Angelica, the process was all the more frustrating because she had been an accomplished competitive diver before the accident. She took great pride in the exquisite sense of balance and body control she'd developed through years of practice. Now, whenever therapists asked her simply to stand with her eyes closed and arms extended, she'd start to topple over. Sometimes she'd bemoan the loss of those diving skills to her therapists: "It's like getting a really good gift for Christmas and then having to take it back."

Doreen Kruth watched her daughter struggling day after day through hours of grueling therapy and saw only the subtlest signs of improvement. During the day, Kruth would sometimes be overcome by a feeling of helplessness. At night, she'd lie awake in bed for hours, staring at the ceiling, wondering whether Angelica would ever get better. She still didn't understand exactly what had gone wrong with her daughter's brain and how they were going to fix it. Some nights the anxiety got so intense that she would climb out of bed, find a hiding place where no one could hear her, and just let it all out. She would sob quietly and pray that everything would eventually turn out all right. When morning came, Kruth would push the doubts and fears from her mind because she knew she needed to be the cheerleader's cheerleader.

When Kruth took her fears to Lovell, he reassured her that Angelica would eventually get better. "We've just got to hang in there," he told Kruth. "Time heals most of these injuries, but there are some people we see, particularly kids, whose systems need to be nudged along. Sometimes people really do need that nudge."

Research had shown that a medication called amantadine could speed recovery in people with severe brain injuries, and Lovell wanted to try it with Angelica. A mild stimulant, the drug had been shown to speed mental processing and to sharpen concentration. For the first time in months, Angelica started to feel like her old self. Her symptoms began to abate gradually. She was still getting headaches, but she'd get more work done before one would terminate a rehab session. Words were now coming into focus, and she felt less dizzy. Six months after the accident, her ImPACT scores had improved enough for Lovell to clear her to go back to school on a limited basis.

Kruth knew she would need to do a lot of educating before her daughter could return to Steel Valley High School. In the Pitt waiting room, she'd met many frustrated parents who told her horror stories about schools that didn't grasp the seriousness and severity of concussions. Sometimes it was administrators who refused to make any accommodations; sometimes it was teachers who put impossible demands on kids whose brains were still foggy and slow.

In an attempt to avoid problems like these, Kruth set up a conference with school administrators and teachers. She walked into the meeting clutching a folder stuffed with Angelica's medical records. Laying the folder on the conference table, Kruth pulled out the first of Angelica's ImPACT tests and said, "This is where my daughter started. With scores like these, under Pennsylvania law, she was legally handicapped." Kruth then pulled out the most recent test and said, "Here's where she is now. As you can see, she's still not at one hundred percent and that's where we need to get her. Now I know that's a pretty tall order, but we are very determined people."

Kruth left the meeting with a sheet of paper detailing a plan for her daughter's transition back to school. To ease back in, Angelica would be allowed to attend school for half days. To minimize the risk of another concussion, she would be allowed to go late to classes—after hallways had emptied of other students.

Some of her teachers got it, and would come up with their own ways to make Angelica's job easier; if there was a book assigned to be read, for instance, they would allow her to watch the movie instead. Other teachers grumbled about the new plan and privately suggested that Angelica might be faking her symptoms to have an excuse to skip class and still get good grades.

One time, after Angelica became dizzy from constantly looking back and forth between the blackboard and the notes she was taking, she raised her hand and asked to be excused. Clearly irritated, the teacher responded, "If you don't want to do anything in this class, then get out. I'm not going to have somebody who sits here and complains. Kids come through my class every day with a concussion. If you don't want to work, just get out."

Dealing with the doubting and disbelieving teachers was hard enough, but what distressed Angelica the most was the response of her friends and classmates. Sometimes as she was walking down the empty halls to her next class, she'd overhear students talking about her through half-closed classroom doors: "She's just wasting our time, 'cause nothing's even wrong with her."

When Angelica stopped by cheerleading practice to visit, some of her teammates just glared. They'd taken to shunning her in the lunchroom, insisting she was being melodramatic and trying to grab attention. They'd all fallen at one time or another and none had sustained a concussion. Besides, they'd seen football players bounce right back from concussions and they couldn't understand why a cheerleader would be out of school for six months after the same type of injury.

Angelica got even less sympathy from the football players themselves. One of them told her, "I don't understand. I had a concussion. I was even knocked out and had to have a facemask with oxygen—and I was back the next day. What's *your* problem?"

While Angelica was struggling to make it through her half days at school, she continued with her rehab program in the afternoons. Three days a week, she'd go over to Pitt and work on her balance and coordination. She could walk on the treadmill now, but she'd have to hold on to the sides to keep from losing her balance and toppling over.

There were days when she'd come straight home from school and just sit, staring at the walls, too exhausted to do anything after only four classes. "I'm never going to get back to where I was," she'd tell her mother with a sigh. "I'm never even going to be able to go a full day." Even though Kruth secretly worried the same thing, she never let on to her daughter. "You can never give up," she'd say. "You have to go to therapy. You have to fix this. You can still get back."

Angelica kept at it, telling herself that even if she couldn't make it all the way back, it would be an accomplishment to make it through a full day at school, to be able to walk up and down stairs without worrying about falling. "If I could just sit here for eight hours and just have it on the attendance record that I was here, maybe that's what I have to settle for," she'd think.

Angelica *was* getting better, but the signs were too subtle for her to see—until the day she managed a short walk on the treadmill without holding on to the sides. The speed was set at just 1.5 mph, but she was beaming. It had been nine months since her fall and for the first time she started to think she might make it back. The pace picked up after that, with each week bringing a tiny victory. Angelica's sense of balance returned and she was able to actually run on the treadmill.

Thirteen months to the day after the fall, Angelica and her mother were back at the concussion clinic, meeting with Lovell. "When we first met," he said to Angelica, "I told you that we'd know you were done when you had no symptoms at rest, no symptoms with exertion, and a good ImPACT test. Now that your symptoms are gone, I could clear you for diving if your test scores are where they should be."

Angelica was so confident she'd ace the test that she ventured, "What about cheerleading?"

"If you want, you could go back to cheerleading," he replied. "You could even be a flyer again if you want, but I don't think *that* would be smart. Before we even get to that, let's see what your test scores are like."

After Angelica finished the test, she rejoined her mother to wait for the results. When Lovell returned with the printouts, he was smiling and shaking his head.

"This is amazing: you got a hundred percent on two of the sections," he said. "That's not even supposed to be possible. I designed the test so that nobody gets a hundred on it."

Angelica punched her fist in the air and hissed a barely audible *"Yes!"* She could barely resist the temptation to jump up and do a little victory dance.

After letting it all sink in, Doreen Kruth turned to Lovell and asked, "Does that mean we're done?"

Lovell leaned back in his chair, stroked his goatee, and paused for a few seconds. "Yes," he said, breaking into a grin, "I think you are."

Chapter 7

Anatomy of a Brain Injury

For most people who sustain a concussion, there is no way to document the damage, no way to explain the bizarre and wide-ranging symptoms they experience each day, no way to prove beyond any doubt that there's actually an injury. Conventional brain imaging methods—MRI machines and CAT scanners—will show no indication of damage. The same is also

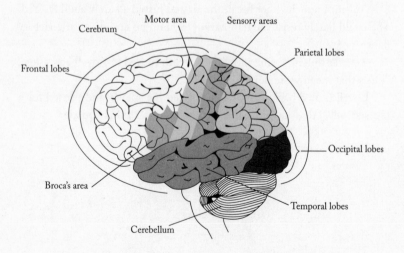

Figure 7.1: Architecture of the brain

true for many patients with severe closed-head injuries. The only way doctors can determine that something serious has happened to the concussed brain is by cataloging the patient's deficits. Even without visible proof, specific symptoms can be linked with damage to localized regions of the brain. When a patient's short-term memory becomes muddled, for example, doctors can assume that something has gone wrong with a deep brain region called the hippocampus.

The profound discovery that brain functions were localized came about over the last couple of centuries as scientists studied patients with damage that was both visible and limited to a discrete area of the brain. Prior to the discovery of localization through those famous patient studies, many scientists thought that the whole brain participated in every function. Three classic case histories provide a window into some of the most common concussion symptoms.

I

By all rights, Phineas Gage was a dead man the instant he dropped his custom-made tamping iron down into the blast hole and accidentally ignited the gunpowder he'd just poured. The iron rod—weighing 13¼ pounds and stretching 3½ feet from its pointed tip to its flat base 1¼ inches in diameter—blasted back upward like a missile, pierced his head just under his left cheekbone, ripped through the left frontal lobe of his brain, and burst out the top of his skull above the hairline. Gage was instantly thrown flat onto his back, and as the iron clanged to the bedrock a hundred feet behind him, the workers in his construction gang rushed through the smoke to his aid, stunned to find him convulsing and conscious. They watched in amazement as he slowly sat up and then, after a few minutes, started to speak while blood poured down his face.

Since it was 1848 in the middle of the Vermont countryside, the workmen had to transform an oxcart into a makeshift ambulance to take their fallen foreman to the small town where they were all staying while building the railroad. Gage propped himself upright in the flatbed for the ride back to his hotel. Once there, he stood under his own steam, walked up onto the porch, and sat himself down on a chair to await medical attention.

If his men were shocked by everything they'd witnessed in the half hour since the blast, the first doctor on the scene would be positively astonished.

Before he could alight from his horse-drawn carriage, Dr. Edward Williams was struck by the gaping wound in the head of the man chatting away on the porch, the brain's pulsations visible even from that distance. Observing the wound up close, Williams couldn't believe the man was still breathing, much less talking and joking. The raised shards of bone atop Gage's head reminded Williams of "an inverted funnel," brain matter oozing up through its apex and hanging in shreds on his matted hair. Throughout the examination, Gage related details of the accident clearly and entertained questions from curious onlookers. No matter how rational and lucid Gage sounded, Williams couldn't believe this tale. When Gage insisted that a rounded tamping iron had indeed shot through his skull, Williams shook his head in disbelief. Finally, one of Gage's workmen offered the doctor eyewitness testimony. "Sure it was so, sir," the man asserted in an Irish brogue, "for the bar is lying in the road below, all blood and brains."

About an hour later, when Dr. John Harlow arrived at the hotel to take over the case, Gage recognized him instantly as the town's regular physician and told him, "I hope I am not much hurt." Anxious to begin treatment at once, Harlow offered to help Gage to his bed. Gage stood up on his own, walked inside the hotel, and climbed the flight of stairs to his room without assistance. As Gage lay on the bloodsoaked bed, Harlow removed about an inch of brain matter protruding through the fracture and several shards of bone that had been pushed up by the iron, exposing a rectangular hole in the skull more than three inches wide. Looking for loose bone fragments, Harlow passed the length of his left forefinger down through the opening in the skull and passed the length of his right forefinger up through the cheek wound until the tips of both fingers met in the brain somewhere behind Gage's left eye. Then Harlow gently pressed the two largest bones back into place as if piecing together a jigsaw puzzle and sutured the scalp to secure them. When he checked on Gage later that night, Harlow found him surprisingly clearheaded and optimistic. When Harlow asked if Gage wanted visitors, the patient declined, saying he'd see them when he returned to work "in a day or two." Harlow hardly shared that optimism. His prognosis wasn't just grim—it was so hopeless that Gage would later be measured for a coffin.

Phineas Gage's long-term recovery from his injury would be as miraculous as his immediate survival from the iron's explosive impact had been. Barely two months after the accident, he was well enough to endure a carriage ride home to New Hampshire. When Gage returned to Vermont for a follow-up examination five months later, Harlow found the patient's appearance healthy, his gait steady, his movements rapid. Gage appeared almost like Harlow remembered him before the accident: strong and active with an iron will as well as an iron frame. The doctor pronounced Gage cured, his physical recovery complete.

Gage's psychic recovery was another matter. Remarkably, the brain injury that destroyed much of his left frontal lobe had virtually no deleterious effects on his memory, his speech, his intelligence, his learning ability. But just as remarkably, his personality had been so radically changed that his friends and acquaintances no longer recognized him. Gage, they said, was "no longer Gage."

It was as if his body had healed up only to be inhabited, at age twenty-five, by some alien presence. Before the accident, Gage had been quiet, respectful, temperate, rational. After it, he became fitful, impatient, irreverent, impulsive, capricious, obstinate. His language, once polite, was now so grossly profane that women were advised to stay away from him. His grasp of social conventions had vanished, leaving him suddenly unable to get along with anyone.

Gage had returned to Vermont, his cherished tamping iron in hand, determined to go back to work building the railroad. His bosses had always regarded him as their most efficient and capable foreman, while his men had always deemed him a great favorite. But when he reapplied for work, his bosses considered him so changed that they refused to give him his job back.

Once dependable and trustworthy, he now had no sense of responsibility. Where the old Gage had been viewed as shrewd, smart, and capable, the new Gage couldn't follow through on anything. He had lost what scientists now call executive function: the ability to plan, to organize, to troubleshoot, to reason. Harlow had discovered this with a practical little test he had given Gage. The doctor offered to trade $1,000 for a few pebbles that Gage had picked up from the riverbed near the worksite. Though Gage's math skills had survived the accident intact, he adamantly rejected the deal. Harlow realized then that a patient whose reasoning and decision making were thus impaired would have trouble holding down the kind of management position Gage had once held.

No longer able to work as a construction foreman, Gage set off on a bizarre odyssey, wandering the Americas with the tamping iron as his constant—and lone—companion. He traveled around New England from town to town exhibiting himself and his iron. He became an attraction at Barnum's American Museum in New York City, joining General Tom Thumb and the Bearded Lady of Geneva among P. T. Barnum's collection of human oddities. Billed as "The Only Living Man with a Hole in the Top of His Head," Gage would part his hair so skeptics could see his brain pulsating under a thin sheath of skin. A series of odd jobs followed: working in a livery stable in New Hampshire, driving a stagecoach in Chile, plowing farmland in California.

As time went on, Gage bounced more and more often from job to job, sometimes fired because of his quarrelsome nature, other times just quitting in a huff. His behavior was becoming increasingly bizarre. His health was failing rapidly, and he began having epileptic seizures. While visiting his mother in San Francisco during the spring of 1860, he suffered a severe convulsion followed by several more seizures in quick succession. The next day, eleven and a half years after the blast that should have killed him, Phineas Gage was dead.

His accident had made headlines in medical journals and New England newspapers, but his passing didn't occasion so much as a death notice anywhere. Harlow would not learn of his former patient's death for another six years. By then, of course, it was too late to autopsy the brain—but not too late to examine the skull. Harlow persuaded Gage's mother to exhume the body. The coffin was dug up and opened to reveal a skeleton and, alongside it, the tamping iron that Gage had carried everywhere, even to his grave. The skull, marked by its unmistakable fractures, was removed from the body and delivered to Harlow along with the iron.

On a spring day in 1868, Harlow stood in front of his colleagues at a meeting of the Massachusetts Medical Society in Boston, held aloft the skull of Phineas Gage, and revealed the inside story of its owner's miraculous recovery and mysterious transformation. Harlow couldn't resist chiding all the city doctors who two decades earlier had so doubted his initial report that they insisted he provide affidavits from lawyers and clergymen before they would accept what most had regarded as a physiological impossibility. It wasn't until a year after the society's prestigious journal published his original case history that Harlow had found an unlikely ally against the skeptics: Dr. Henry J. Bigelow of Harvard University. Bigelow himself had initially been among the chief skeptics, but he changed his mind after he extensively examined Gage and made a plaster lifemask of his head. Bigelow presented his findings to the Boston Society for Medical Improvement in 1850—his evidence including the tamping iron, the mask, and Gage himself—but the distinguished Harvard professor of surgery had little more success than the inexperienced country doctor in persuading skeptical colleagues that the case was neither a fraud nor an exaggeration.

Only in death would Gage's skull begin to play a role in unraveling the mysteries of the broken brain. Harlow had perceptively correlated Gage's cognitive and behavioral changes with damage to the frontal region, making this the first case to suggest the link between the brain and complex personality characteristics. It was an idea that was ahead of its time. Doctors back then found it as controversial as it was unbelievable. Unsupported by the anatomical evidence of autopsy results, Harlow's discovery was easy to dismiss. Many decades would elapse before further scientific consideration would be given to figuring out what brain damage the tamping iron had wrought.

In the meantime, Phineas Gage's skull found the kind of permanent home that he never could in life. Harlow donated the skull to Harvard's Warren Anatomical Museum, where it would eventually become more of an attraction than Gage himself ever had been at Barnum's American Museum. Its fame would grow with each passing discovery of brain function, until it achieved landmark status in the annals of medicine. Today the skull rests in a glass-enclosed exhibit case at Harvard, sharing shelf space with the tamping iron under the watchful gaze of the bearded Bigelow's life-size portrait. It is the centerpiece of Harvard's collection, the holy grail of skulls, drawing pilgrimages from some of the world's most renowned brain researchers.

One of them was Dr. Hanna Damasio, a neurologist who wanted to know how Gage compared to her own patients with frontal lobe damage. In the early 1990s, almost a century and a half after Gage's accident, Damasio resolved to take advantage of space age technology to retroactively study the most famous of all brain injuries. After generating a three-dimensional computer model of Gage's skull from x-rays, photographs, and measurements, she and her colleagues projected the trajectory of the tamping iron and simulated its passage through the brain. With the top of the skull open to reveal the simulated cortex, the 3-D image plotting the iron's path revealed something scientists had only theorized: the iron misses the brain regions controlling motor function and language, but plows right through areas responsible for planning, rational decision making, and sociability. The reconstructed brain even correlated with the scans of Damasio's patients whose frontal lobe damage had left them with symptoms resembling those of Phineas Gage.

II

On April 18, 1861, Dr. Paul Broca walked into a meeting of the Anthropological Society of Paris with a glass case containing a pinkish-colored brain tucked under his arm. Broca told his fellow scientists that this was the brain of a patient named Leborgne, who had died just the day before. What was interesting about the man, Broca said, was that he had completely lost the ability to talk some twenty-one years before. Broca was convinced that this man's brain would prove to the world that language ability was located in a tightly circumscribed area.

In the mid-1800s, Parisian scientists were passionately arguing over the question of whether the power of speech lay in a specific region or whether a person's ability to access words and construct conversation came from cells scattered throughout the brain. The scientific debate had gotten so heated at one point that another leading researcher, Jean Baptiste Bouillaud, offered 500 francs (a tremendous sum at the time) to the scientist who could come up with an example of language loss without damage to the frontal lobes. Broca, a physician with wide-ranging interests that included anthropology and brain science, was in the camp arguing that language ability was localized to the frontal lobes. He was sure that with the right patients, he could prove it.

He had come across Leborgne fortuitously. Though the onetime shoe-last maker had been living for the past twenty-one years at the hospital where Broca worked, the physician didn't meet him until Leborgne was in his declining days. Broca was excited when he heard about Leborgne. This was exactly the kind of patient he'd been looking for: someone who had started out in life perfectly normal, but who had lost the ability to talk without having lost the ability to comprehend and communicate.

As he examined Leborgne, Broca quickly determined that the patient had normal hearing and the physical ability to speak. Equally important, the patient appeared to understand most of what was said to him. Leborgne was also very much aware of his speech disability and would often get frustrated when he could utter only the meaningless syllable "tan" in response to questions. Leborgne was, nevertheless, able to communicate with the world through gestures. "Numerical answers were his best," Broca wrote later in a scientific paper. "He gave them by opening or closing his fingers. I asked him several times how long he had been ill, and his reply was either five or six days." When asked how long he had been at the hospital, Leborgne held up his left hand, opened it and closed it four times, and then held up a single finger to designate twenty-one years. Even when questions were more complicated, Leborgne found ways to communicate. He had become adept at finding gestures to make his thoughts known—signaling with a small movement of his left index finger to indicate when he understood something, for example.

Over the years, Leborgne had experienced a series of "attacks" that left his right side weak and eventually paralyzed. By the time Broca met him, Leborgne was, at age fifty-one, bedridden and dying from gangrene. Immediately after Leborgne died, Broca went to work on an autopsy of the patient's brain. He found plenty of damaged tissue, but one area in particular—a spot toward the back of the left frontal lobe—showed a deep lesion and signs of having been injured about the time Leborgne lost his ability to speak. To Broca, this was clear proof that language abilities were localized to an isolated region of the brain. Not everyone else was convinced, however, especially since there was so much widespread damage. Broca realized he would need to find other, hopefully clearer, examples to make his case beyond a doubt.

Broca didn't have to wait long. Before the year was out, he found an old man named Lelong, who like Leborgne had developed problems with language in adulthood. Lelong had been healthy up to age eighty-three when he suddenly collapsed with a stroke. He recovered within a few days, except that he was having problems talking. His daughter at first thought there was something wrong with his tongue, but soon realized that it was his language ability that had suffered. He just couldn't come up with words. Eighteen months later, Lelong fell and fractured his femur. He was brought to Broca's hospital. When Broca met him, Lelong could utter only five words: "oui," "non," "toi," "toujours," and "Lelo." Translated, they meant "yes," "no," "three" ("toi" was a mispronunciation of "trois"), "always," and his own name mispronounced. Lelong often used those words indiscriminately, especially "toi." When asked what he did before coming to the hospital, he answered, "Toujours," but then gestured with his arms and hands as if he were grasping a spade, pushing it into the ground, and then digging with it. Broca asked if he had been a digger, and Lelong answered, "Oui."

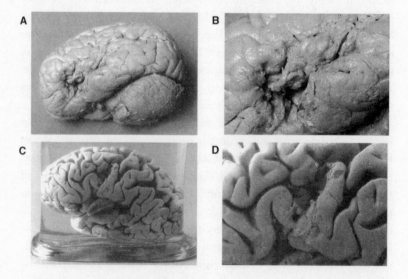

Figure 7.2: Photographs showing the brains of Broca's two famous patients. *A* is a side view of Leborgne's brain, and *B* is a close-up of the lesion in that brain. *C* is a side view of Lelong's brain, and *D* is a close-up of the lesion in that brain. (Reprinted with permission from N. F. Dronkers et al., "Paul Broca's Historic Cases: High Resolution MR Imaging of the Brains of Leborgne and Lelong," *Brain* 130:1432–41, 2007.)

Twelve days after he arrived at the hospital, Lelong died. Broca was eager to examine Lelong's brain, but nervous. The fact that Lelong could say a few words might mean that the damage to his brain was in a different region from Leborgne's. When the autopsy was completed, Broca had more ammunition to make his case. Lelong not only had a lesion in the same place as Leborgne, but it was much more clearly defined. Further, there was no other brain pathology confusing the situation. Broca concluded that the differences he saw between the two patients were not explained by the site of the brain damage, but by its nature. Broca presented his findings at a meeting of the Anatomical Society and then submitted them for publication. He wrote, "I will not deny my surprise bordering on stupefaction when I found that in my second patient the lesion was *rigorously* occupying the same site as the first."

Broca preserved the two brains in alcohol and donated them to the Musée Dupuytren, where they were exhibited until the walls of the museum collapsed in 1940. For years after that, no one knew where the brains had gone. Many thought they were lost forever. But in 1962 the brains turned up in the basement of the École de Médecine in Paris, where they had been sitting on a shelf since 1940. The damage to what had become known as "Broca's area" was clearly visible: an actual crevice in one brain and a pitted surface on the other.

In 2007, an international team of researchers led by Nina Dronkers at the University of California–Davis got together and decided to pop the brains into an MRI machine to see if they could get more detail on exactly what had been damaged in the two patients. Broca's research on Leborgne's and Lelong's brains had provided the foundations for modern neuropsychology and cognitive neuroscience since it gave credibility to the theory of localization of brain function. But studies in the late twentieth century had shown that a more extensive lesion than what Broca described would be needed to completely extinguish speech. Dronkers and her colleagues wondered just how accurate Broca had been. With the MRI scans, they constructed a computer map of the two brains and determined that only a small part of Broca's area had been injured. Further, they found that the damaged area extended beyond what Broca could have seen without dissecting the brains.

"Though the current findings provide additional anatomical information, they by no means detract from Broca's phenomenal discovery," the researchers concluded. "Because he elected not to slice the brains, Broca could not have known the extent of the underlying damage in his patients and the role it might play in their speech disorders."

III

Henry Gustav Molaison went into the hospital for an epilepsy cure and came out with a broken memory.

Molaison had been suffering from increasingly severe seizures since an accident when he was nine. By the time he was twenty-seven, in 1953, his seizures had become so frequent and so intense that he had to give up his job as an electric-motor repairman. Desperate to get his life back, Molaison made an appointment with a neurosurgeon at Hartford Hospital who was curing epilepsy through surgery. That appointment would completely upend his world.

Back in the 1940s and '50s, neurosurgeons were convinced that they could fix any brain-related illness—from depression to schizophrenia to epilepsy—with an operation. Just scoop out some faulty brain tissue and, presto, the patient would be cured with no ill effects. Lobotomies had become the rage as the cure for a host of mental disorders and even for criminal behavior. While there had been a few disastrous cases involving personality changes, neurosurgeons for the most part believed they were helping their patients by removing brain tissue.

Molaison's surgeon, Dr. William Scoville, had done his share of lo-botomies and was mostly happy with the results. They seemed to quiet unruly mental patients. But he'd heard about the personality distortions associated with destruction of the frontal lobes and had recently opted to focus on a different part of the brain: the hippocampus. It was a small structure located deep within the brain consisting of two seahorse-shaped lobes. At the time, no one knew what role the hippocampus played, but scientists suspected that it was somehow involved with the sense of smell because it seemed to connect directly with structures that originated in the nose. Scoville figured it would be better to lose your sense of smell than to have your personality distorted.

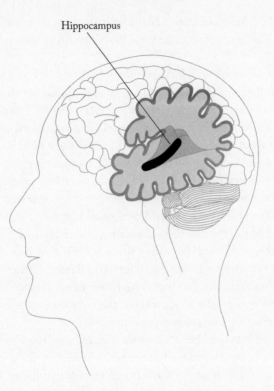

Hippocampus

Figure 7.3: Location of hippocampus

Molaison lay awake during the entire operation. Scoville anesthetized the area above his patient's eyes, cut a flap of skin to expose the skull, and then, with a hand drill, bored two holes through Molaison's forehead. Scoville slid a thin metal spatula through each hole so that he could lift the front part of Molaison's brain out of the way. Then the surgeon inserted a long metal straw attached to a suction device into Molaison's head and sucked out nearly all of the man's hippocampus.

The unintended impact of the surgery was immediately obvious. After the operation, Molaison could no longer recognize any of the hospital staff or find his way to the bathroom. He couldn't seem to keep anything that occurred after the operation in his head. And yet, the patient seemed to remember the most trivial details from the days leading up to his surgery. Further, memories from his life before the operation had been undisturbed.

Scoville was horrified. He'd never seen anything like this. He quickly realized that the problem might be that he had suctioned out all of Molaison's hippocampus. He'd done operations before where he'd suctioned out the left or right lobe of the hippocampus and there hadn't been any serious repercussions—of course, it was difficult to tell in some cases because the patients who had the surgeries were psychotic and weren't particularly revealing when interviewed by specialists. But now, he had a patient whose ability to form new memories seemed to have been destroyed. Scoville put in a call to Dr. Wilder Penfield, a renowned professor at Montreal's McGill University who had years of experience with brain surgery.

Penfield was shocked and angry when Scoville told him about the surgery. He thought it was reckless to have completely removed a part of the brain whose function was unknown. Nevertheless, he saw Molaison's disaster as an opportunity to learn about the hippocampus and immediately dispatched a young researcher to study the case.

Brenda Milner had been looking for patients who'd received surgeries to remove or destroy limited regions of the brain. She was hoping that these cases might help extend the existing research that linked localized areas of the brain to specific functions. Milner grabbed a few memory tests and hopped the next train from Montreal to Hartford. First thing the next morning, she was talking with Molaison.

Milner's tests confirmed Scoville's worst fears. Molaison appeared to have completely lost the ability to form new memories. At first meeting, he would seem perfectly normal. He could keep up his side of a conversation and would even make jokes. But if his new acquaintance got up and walked away, he wouldn't remember a word they'd exchanged—he wouldn't even remember meeting the person in the first place. Milner saw this for herself after lunching with Molaison. Half an hour after they left the cafeteria, Molaison not only had forgotten what he'd eaten for lunch, but also that he'd eaten lunch at all. It was as if a computer suddenly lost the ability to transfer what appeared onscreen to its hard drive. So long as information was on the screen, it existed; once it disappeared from view, it was gone forever.

Strangely, Molaison's memory of the past was perfect. He could remember his childhood. He could remember the day before his surgery, but nothing that came afterward. The operation didn't appear to have affected his ability to think, however. He actually had gained a few IQ points after the surgery. Milner would later tell a magazine reporter, "This was an intelligent, kind, amusing man. But he couldn't acquire the slightest new piece of knowledge. He lives today chained to his past, in a sort of childlike world. You could say his personal history stopped with the operation."

Milner realized that Molaison could provide science with enormous insights into how memory worked. Prior to his operation, scientists thought that multiple parts of the brain participated in the process through which new information is permanently filed away. From her research on Molaison, Milner deduced that the hippocampus played an essential role in transcribing experiences or episodes from a person's life into permanent memory. This is the kind of memory that accounts for our being able to summon up specific scenes from the mental video collection that makes up our past. Scientists in the 1970s would dub this kind of remembrance "episodic memory."

Milner wondered if her subject's memory loss extended to all kinds of learning. Would the loss of the hippocampus mean that Molaison wouldn't be able to pick up new skills? A simple experiment answered that question. Each day, Milner would ask Molaison to perform an exercise: he was given a sheet of paper with the outlines of two five-point stars, one inscribed within the other, and asked to draw a line that ran in between the outlines of the two stars. The tough part was that he couldn't look directly at his hand or the stars while drawing. He had to do everything while watching his progress in a mirror. It's the kind of task that practice can improve and, sure enough, Molaison got better with each passing day. But each day he needed to have the task explained to him because he had no recollection of having ever done it before. So, theoretically, Molaison could have learned to play the piano by having a lesson a day. He wouldn't be able to remember having taken any of the lessons—so he'd be surprised that he could actually do it. This kind of *skill* memory was later labeled "procedural memory."

In another series of experiments, Milner tried to determine how long

Molaison could keep information in his head before it evaporated. If she gave him a list of words and immediately asked him to spit it back, he could. On one occasion she asked him to remember a number, waited fifteen minutes, and then asked him what it was. Milner was surprised to see that he was able to remember for that long. Molaison told her that he kept repeating the number in his head. Milner had discovered "working memory."

In the fifty-five years he lived after the operation, Molaison gained an odd sort of fame. Research paper after research paper described the insights his brain had provided, with the credit given to the man known to neuroscientists only as "H.M." The knowledge he gave to scientists was something he himself would never be able to learn.

When brain damage is visible, as it was with Henry Molaison and Phineas Gage, it's a straightforward task to correlate a specific set of symptoms with injury to a certain part of the brain. When damage to the brain can't be seen—as is the case with most concussions and even severe closed-head injuries—it's a lot harder to tie the wide-ranging, and sometimes very subtle, symptoms to the jolt to the head. Not until the 1980s would scientists begin to understand how the brain could be damaged by an injury that was, for all intents and purposes, invisible.

Chapter 8

Deciphering the Damage

John Povlishock peered through his microscope at Virginia Common-wealth University and was stunned by what he saw. The tiny black bulbs of protein ballooning near the ends of the nerve cells under his lens were proof that much of the damage to the brain in a TBI occurred not at impact, but hours after the initial injury.

Just a short time earlier, Povlishock had been on the verge of giving up. He'd been trying to duplicate the findings of a recent autopsy study by Scottish researchers that had found scattered damage to nerve cells throughout the brains of patients with severe TBIs who'd died within months of their injuries. But when Povlishock looked at tissue from the brains of recently concussed rats, he hadn't seen anything like the damage described by J. Hume Adams and his colleagues at the University of Glasgow. Their study had shown photos of axons—the long threadlike structures that emanate from the center of a neuron and function like phone cables to carry information to other cells—stopped up by black balls of protein. Adams's landmark study, which was published in 1977 in the journal *Brain*, had gone a long way to explain the disparate and profound symptoms experienced by people who didn't have any obvious signs of injury to their heads. It was clear now that there could be significant damage to individual cells, and because that damage was scattered throughout the brain with no one focal point, it wouldn't show up on brain scans or on autopsies that didn't include inspection with a high-powered microscope.

One of the most astounding findings from Adams's study was the presence of healthy neurons and blood vessels running right alongside the dead and damaged cells. That meant the damage wasn't being caused by a direct hit to the cells. Something else must be going on. Adams and his colleagues suspected that the bulbs of protein suggested that the axons had been torn when the brain slammed around in the skull.

The study cleared up another perplexing question: How could so many different areas of the brain be affected by a TBI? The answer was in the ubiquity of the injuries. Adams and his colleagues found damaged and dying axons all over the brain. Each one of them signaled a broken connection. It was as if the plugs in a house had been pulled willy-nilly from their wall sockets. You wouldn't know which plug had been disconnected until you went to use the device that was on the other end of the wire.

Povlishock's first attempts to duplicate Adams's results were a dismal failure: not a single protein bulb could be seen on the slide. At first he thought the problem might be that the rats' concussions were too mild an injury for them to develop the kind of damage that Adams had observed in his patients with severe TBIs. But as the months passed, he started to wonder if he was just examining the rat brains too soon after the concussions. Perhaps, he thought, a jolt to the head kicked off a sequence of events that culminated in those black bulbs ballooning out hours after the initial injury. Povlishock decided to do his experiment again. Only this time he would wait a day before examining tissue from the concussed rat brains.

Sure enough, when he peered through his microscope, he saw the same balls of protein that Adams had seen in the human study (Figure 8.1). And just like Adams's brain-injured patients, the rats had damaged axons scattered all over their brains. What made Povlishock's study even more compelling was that he had seen damaged axons even in a mild brain injury. By extension, that might mean that concussions created some lasting damage to the brain. Perhaps the difference between a mild brain injury and a more severe one was simply the number of axons that got injured.

The most profound implication of the research may have been Povlishock's realization that the axonal damage seemed to occur in slow motion after the original jolt to the head. That meant there was a possibility

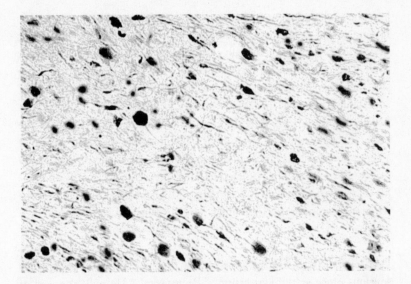

Figure 8.1: Axons with protein bulbs following a brain injury. (*Courtesy of Douglas H. Smith, M.D.*)

that scientists could find a treatment and bring the process to a halt before all the damage was done. There wouldn't be a lot of time to get patients treated, but if researchers could find the right drug, they might be able to save some people from permanent brain damage.

Povlishock wrote up his findings and they were published in 1983 in the *Journal of Neuropathology & Experimental Neurology*. Because the study involved mild TBI, its impact was huge. Newspaper reporters and lawyers deluged his office with requests for interviews and expert testimony. Suddenly there was proof that a bump on the head could cause damage you could see with a microscope.

Povlishock's study also fit nicely with some research from the University of Pennsylvania published just a year earlier. Dr. Thomas Gennarelli and his colleagues had shown in animal models that you didn't need a blow to the head to cause brain damage. All that needed to happen was for the head to rapidly accelerate or decelerate, as it might in a car accident or in an IED explosion. Because the brain isn't really anchored to anything and floats in fluid, sudden movement could send it slamming into the skull and wrench the axons so severely that their internal scaffolding would be damaged. Gennarelli and his colleagues showed that that kind of damage could result even from a simple rotation of the head, similar to what often happens to boxers when they get punched in the jaw. The researchers coined a name for the damage: "diffuse axonal injury."

Though scientists had their theories, they still didn't know exactly how axons were being hurt. In animal studies, they had examined the brain at various time intervals after a TBI, but that was like looking at a series of snapshots. You couldn't really understand the process unless you could watch it happening in real time. Then University of Pennsylvania researchers found a way to simulate TBI damage in individual axons while the axons sat on a slide under a microscope.

Dr. Douglas Smith keeps a lump of Silly Putty in the desk drawer of his spacious office at the University of Pennsylvania. He pulls the wad of squishy stuff out whenever he's asked to explain how brain cells could be injured when there isn't even a hit to the head. "If you stretch the Silly Putty out slowly, it gives," he says while pulling the wad into a long, thin thread. "It's the same in your brain. When you sat down, your brain was wiggling like a Jell-O mold. And because the movement is slow, it's OK." Then he gives the wad a yank and it breaks into two pieces. "I can take the same material and stretch it the same amount but faster, and it disconnects because it becomes stiffer with rapid stretching," he says. "Your axons behave the same way. When they're rapidly stretched, their internal skeletons can be destroyed." That, in a nutshell, he says, is all there is to the concept of "fast stretch" and "slow stretch."

Years ago, when other scientists were convinced that axons were being torn during a head injury, Smith began to suspect that the real damage was being caused by stretching. He had come to TBI research completely by chance back when he was a postdoctoral fellow in biochemistry. A family friend who had fallen while skiing and hit his head on some ice wasn't getting better after a concussion—weeks passed and his thinking was still foggy, his memory muddled. Knowing Smith's medical background, family members had reached out to him for an explanation, and for help. When Smith started looking at the TBI literature, he was shocked to see how little was known, and embarrassed that he could provide no direction. "I couldn't give them any kind of answer because there was nothing there," Smith says. "The more I looked into it, the more I realized there really was nothing. Here you had these huge numbers of people who were affected and there was so little knowledge. It didn't make any sense."

Smith was amazed that late in the twentieth century, on the eve of "The Decade of the Brain," there was an area of brain research that was still in its infancy. While there were plenty of scientists working on stroke, which disabled far fewer people and at an older age, he quickly realized that there was only a small cadre of dedicated researchers teasing out the mechanics of TBI. To a scientist just starting out in his career, this seemed to be the perfect fit. "I saw what a huge challenge it was," he says. "It was a new field. There was a need that had to be filled."

In the early '90s, Smith came to work with Gennarelli's group at Penn. "It was the mecca of brain injury research," Smith says. "They had a multidisciplinary approach to studying TBI; they had bioengineers working with neurosurgeons, neuroscientists, and neurologists, all studying traumatic brain injury with a focus on diffuse axonal injury." After arriving at Penn, Smith designed the experiments and apparatus to study what happened to individual axons when you pulled on them. Gennarelli left Penn, and Smith eventually took over as director of the Penn Center for Brain Injury and Repair.

Smith's lab has been studying axon stretch, both fast and slow, for almost two decades now. He and his colleagues have learned that when axons are stretched gradually, they just grow in length, like the slowly stretched Silly Putty. This explains how a single axon that connects a baby whale's brain to its tail can lengthen to hundreds of thousands of times its original size as the seafaring mammal matures. That seemingly simple concept may eventually hold promise for people with spinal cord injuries. In a lab setting, Penn researchers have shown that they can coax individual axons to grow longer and longer by gently—and slowly—tugging on them. The theory is that if you can get axons to grow several inches in the lab, you might be able to use these axons as a living bridge to span regions of damaged axons in a person with injury to the brain or spinal cord.

At the other end of the spectrum is fast stretch. To discover the details of what happens to axons in a closed-head injury, Penn researchers devised a way to subject individual axons to a quick stretch while they observed the process through the lens of a microscope. They start by placing two groups of neurons on a sheet of film, which is fairly stiff but will flex if it's given a hard, fast push. One group of neurons is lined up in a row on the far left side of the sheet and the other in a row on the far right side. The two rows of neurons are then encouraged to shoot their communication cables—the axons—toward one another across the empty space separating them. Once the left- and right-side neurons have connected, the experiment can begin.

As the researchers peer through a microscope, a puff of air is blown up from beneath the film, causing it to bend upward in the middle. The force of the air puff on the film is enough to make axons rapidly stretch just as they would in a car wreck. Immediately upon injury, many of the axons go from straight to wavy, which indicates that something broke inside the axons. Although the axons gradually straighten out and appear normal within hours, they begin to show signs of damage that's more permanent. In particular, they develop black bulbs of protein just like those seen in autopsies of humans and animals with a TBI (Figure 8.2).

Over the years, Smith and his colleagues have been able to tease out the details of what leads to the wavy axons with the bulbous lumps. They learned that if the initial stretch had enough force behind it, axons wouldn't rip but would sustain damage to specific internal structures. Axons get their shape and structure through an assembly of cellular "girders" called microtubules. When the axon was tugged hard and fast enough, the girders were pulled out of alignment, which is what gave the axon a wavy appearance. But the damage wasn't confined to the axon's internal scaffolding. Microtubules serve as a sort of conveyor belt to carry supplies and nutrients from one end of the axon to the other. When the axon was tugged hard, the conveyor belt would break, dumping all of its cargo at the site of the break. From the outside of the axon, the expanding pile of protein cargo looked just like the black bulbs seen by Adams and Povlishock. The end of the axon, starting at the bulb, would then wither away and completely detach just like those observed by Povlishock in animals (Figure 8.3). Eventually the axons with the blobs of protein would shrivel and die because they no longer could move supplies up and down their length.

One thing the Penn researchers didn't know was the eventual fate

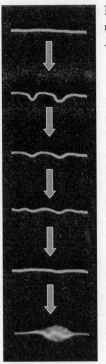

Figure 8.2: Sequence of photos following an axon from right after it's stretched until two hours later. (*Courtesy of Douglas H. Smith, M.D.*)

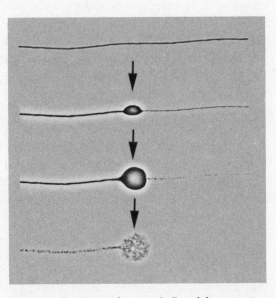

Figure 8.3: Evolution of an axon bulb and disconnection of the axon following a brain injury. (*Courtesy of Douglas H. Smith, M.D.*)

of the wavy axons. If you watched the axons long enough, some would eventually straighten out and not develop swellings. But was this because there had been internal repairs to the wrenched girders? Or were they just limping along transmitting garbled signals like a frayed, staticky phone line? The answer is important, Smith says. If an axon can self-repair, then researchers might be able to find treatments to speed up the process. But it's also possible that some of the axons are beyond repair and are just garbling communications, so it might make sense to find a treatment that would finish them off. Smith compares the damaged axons to phone lines. "I lived in an old house and the previous owner, who worked at the phone company, had jacks installed everywhere," he says by way of explanation. "Every once in a while, I discovered every phone in the house had a staticky noise problem. That's because one faulty phone wire was contaminating all the rest. By simply disconnecting the bad wire, I could clear up the signal on all the others. So by analogy, if you get a couple of axons that are not only dysfunctional but also corrupting the whole system, making communication staticky, then you might consider therapies that both rescue axons that can be repaired and at the same time get rid of the guys that are just limping along and mucking everything up."

All of Smith's findings so far were in axons stretched by forces similar to those in a severe TBI. He began to wonder whether the same kinds of damage would be seen in milder brain injuries, like the concussions so prevalent in sports. There was evidence from an autopsy study that this might be the case. Australian researchers had looked at the brains of five people who had suffered a concussion and then died from other causes, such as pneumonia, days to months after their head injures. The study, which was published in 1994 in *The Lancet*, found the same kinds of axon damage—including bulbs of protein—that Adams had found in the brains of people with severe TBIs.

Over the years, Smith had seen plenty of cases in which people with concussions—so-called mild traumatic brain injuries—had taken a long time to recover or had never completely recovered. "I like to say that the expression 'mild traumatic brain injury' is an oxymoron," he says. "It's only mild compared to the train wreck of severe TBI that can leave you in the hospital for years. But for people with concussions that just want to get back to being themselves, it's not at all mild."

Smith figured he had all the tools to answer an intriguing question: Do mild traumatic brain injuries cause permanent changes to the axons? He was very familiar with post-concussion syndrome, so he knew that something serious could occur even in mild head injuries. He started to wonder whether a first concussion might lead to axonal damage so small that it was difficult to detect. Subtle changes in the axons might predispose them to significant damage if they were stretched again soon after the first stretch. Maybe, Smith thought, post-concussion syndrome was due to an accumulation of axonal injuries. The damage from the first jolt might simply make an axon more vulnerable to a second hit.

He came up with a new experiment. He designed a stretch study that scaled back the intensity of the tug to approximate what an axon would experience in a concussion. When he and his colleagues examined the lightly stretched axons, they found no damage to the microtubules, and the axons outwardly appeared completely normal. The axons were then stretched a second time, twenty-four hours later, in exactly the same way as the first. Smith's suspicions turned out to be right. When axons were stretched lightly two times in a row, they began to deteriorate. Some took on a wavy appearance. Some developed bulbs of protein. Some eventually died. Smith had proven that the damage from two light stretches could be equivalent to a single strong stretch.

Now he wanted to know what it was about the first stretch that seemed to make the axons more vulnerable. So he and his colleagues took a closer look at what happened to the axons after an initial light stretch. They found that although the axons appeared to be structurally undamaged, there were subtle changes that might predict increased vulnerability to a second stretch. The researchers noticed there was an increase in the number of the tiny pores that line the outside skin of the axon and allow charged particles, like sodium and calcium, to come inside. When the axon was stretched a second time shortly after the first tug, huge amounts of sodium and calcium rushed in. Other scientists had shown that high levels of calcium in an axon could spark a process that would result in the cell eating away at its own structure. The effect, Smith says, "is like throwing salt water on live circuits."

Smith's results, published in 2009 in *The Journal of Neuroscience*, added to the rapidly accumulating evidence that even concussions could cause permanent changes in neurons. They also went a long way toward explaining earlier research by University of California–Los Angeles scientists that showed there was a period of time after a concussion in which the brain was extremely vulnerable to a second hit.

UCLA scientists have been looking at the impact of TBIs in both humans and rats for over two decades. Though they have studied a wide range of brain injuries, much of their research has focused on the aftermath of mild TBIs, or concussions. That approach made sense because at the outset all TBIs look like a concussion, explains David Hovda, director of UCLA's Brain Injury Research Center. The difference between a mild and a severe brain injury, he says, is in the magnitude of the brain's response and the length of time that response goes on.

A tall, stout man with a round face that easily breaks into an impish smile, Hovda roams the hallways of the Brain Injury Center perennially clad in a white lab coat that immediately marks him as one of the researchers. Within a short walk from his office are both the ICU, where severe brain injuries are treated, and the brain scanners—normal-sized ones for patients and miniature ones for the rats. In the basement several floors below Hovda's office is the rat behavioral lab. On the fourth floor is a lab with shelves of bottles containing preserved human brains, and on the fifth floor is the lab housing rat brains. Both labs have a tissue-dissection area where brains can be thin-sliced with a device that is uncomfortably reminiscent of the meat slicer in the deli department of a grocery store.

Back in the 1990s, when coaches and team doctors were still puzzling over return-to-play issues, Hovda ran an experiment to see if he could determine from brain chemistry how long the effects of a concussion lasted. Earlier studies had shown that glucose metabolism soared right after a jolt to the head. Since glucose is the fuel that powers the brain, this indicated that there was a burst of activity in the brain right after a concussion. Hovda suspected that changes in glucose metabolism might provide a window into how long it would take for a brain to recover from a jolt to the head. He decided to run an experiment in which glucose metabolism would be carefully monitored in rats for ten days following a concussion. He figured this might give a concrete answer to how long it takes for brain chemistry to return to normal in rats.

Hovda observed glucose metabolism rise immediately after a concussion, just as earlier studies had shown. But six hours later, glucose metabolism plummeted. This, Hovda realized, could easily explain the slowed mental processing that rats—and humans—experience after a concussion. What surprised Hovda was how long glucose metabolism remained depressed in the rats: an average of five days, but for as long as ten.

Hovda's study was quickly picked up by concussion experts seeking scientific evidence upon which to hang return-to-play guidelines. They used his finding that the average recovery time was five days as a justification for sidelining concussed athletes for at least a week. At a scientific meeting, Hovda corralled one of the guideline authors and asked how the one-week rest period had been determined. Dr. Robert Cantu pulled out a reprint of Hovda's journal article and said, "From *your* paper." A mischievous grin spread across Hovda's face as he responded, "You're making recommendations from rat data? People aren't rats. Well, maybe some of them are, but . . ." Turning serious, Hovda asked the neurosurgeon, "Don't you think we ought to do a study in human beings?" Cantu pointed out that such a study would take time to complete and in the meantime coaches and trainers needed some sort of guidelines so that concussed athletes weren't sent back to play too soon.

The episode did get Hovda thinking about the impact of concussions on developing brains. He wondered if there might be any permanent impact from mild-to-moderate TBIs in children. To study this, he tapped into some research from the '60s showing that stimulating experiences could spark brain growth in the young.

Researchers from the University of California–Berkeley suspected that a stimulating environment, if it was offered early enough in life, could make kids smarter. To see if this was possible, the researchers had compared rats raised in a standard setting—three to four animals per cage with a dull-colored background and no toys—to those raised in an "enriched environment"—fourteen to twenty rats in a big, colorful, two-level cage with ladders, wheels, tunnels, and a wide assortment of toys. The researchers found that rats raised in the enriched environment not only got smarter, but also grew measurably thicker cerebral cortexes compared to rats reared in a standard setting. That finding prompted the push to get kids into school at an earlier age.

Hovda wondered whether TBIs might get in the way of this kind of intelligence enhancement. He'd seen studies showing that children often developed behavior problems and learning difficulties after a TBI. Other studies had shown that brain-injured kids were more likely than other children to be put in a special education program. One particularly striking study compared concussed athletes to kids who never hit their heads. All the students were tested at the beginning of the school year to provide a baseline measurement. When they were retested at the end of the school year, the concussed athletes had all returned to baseline. What was disturbing, however, was the realization that the nonconcussed athletes had improved beyond *their* baseline measurements. That meant that even though the concussed athletes had gotten back to where they started, they'd lost ground compared to their peers. It might also mean that the concussed athletes lost some capacity to expand their brains through life experience, that their brains weren't as "plastic" anymore. "If you got back to where you were before the brain injury, you might think that is recovery," Hovda says. "It's not. I don't know one person who says, 'I'm going to stay right here, at this level.' If you have an injury and as a result you lose plasticity, you haven't fully recovered even if you're back to where you were before the injury."

Knowing that young brains are especially plastic, Hovda wondered whether you could see something similar in young rats that had experienced a TBI. One way to test this theory would be to see if a TBI blocked the effects of an enriched environment. If the TBI created learning difficulties, then rats raised in an enriched environment would be no smarter than those raised in a standard cage.

Hovda and his colleagues designed an experiment with three groups of young rats: one group would be put into an enriched environment after a moderate TBI, another group would be put into an enriched environment with no TBI, and the third group would be put in a standard cage, again with no TBI. Before they put any rats into enriched environments, the researchers compared the concussed rats to the uninjured ones. "We tested them all," Hovda says. "And there were no deficits in the concussed rats. None. Zippo. Nada." Then the researchers put some of the concussed rats and some of the uninjured rats into an enriched environment. "They all played with each other and did what they were supposed to do," Hovda says.

After two and a half weeks, the researchers looked for differences between the rats, using a standard test of rodent intelligence called the Morris Water Maze. At UCLA, researchers have built their maze in a large circular aluminum tub that sits on a table in the corner of a room in the rat behavior research lab. They place a little platform somewhere on the floor of the tub and then add water until the top of the platform is an inch below the surface. The water contains dye so the rats won't be able to see where the platform is located, and it's deep enough that the rats will have to swim around until they locate the platform by feel. On the wall to the left of the tub is an abstract ink drawing. On the wall to the right of the tub is a poster of Albert Einstein. The idea is that the rats will be able to use these posters to orient themselves.

For several days the researchers bring the rats in and put them, one at a time, into the tub and wait about forty-five seconds to see if the rat finds the platform. If the rat doesn't locate the platform on its own, it is picked up and put on the platform, allowed to stand on it for a full minute, and then put back in the water to locate the platform on its own. When the rats can find the platform within five seconds, it is assumed that they have learned where it is with respect to the posters. The smarter the rat, the fewer tries before it learns where the platform sits.

The earlier research had shown that rats raised in enriched environments took fewer attempts to learn the location of the platform compared to those reared in standard cages. The UCLA researchers found that this was true with the uninjured rats. But when it came to those rats with a brain injury, the enriched environment didn't appear to help. Concussed rats that had been raised in an enriched environment took as long to learn the location of the platform as the rats reared in a regular cage. This meant that while the concussion hadn't affected skills the rats had previously acquired, it did impact their ability to profit from a stimulating environment. "The ones with a concussion couldn't expand the cortex," Hovda says. "They couldn't grow to be smarter. They had lost brain plasticity."

The story turned out to be even more complicated than that. Other experiments showed that a concussion didn't have the same impact everywhere in the brain. While certain areas of the brain became worse at learning, others became better at it. In another experiment, UCLA researchers looked at whether a concussion affected a rat's ability to link experiences with emotions, like fear. They used a test that is similar in some ways to the Morris Water Maze. Uninjured rats and concussed rats are put in a box that can deliver a mild shock through the floor. During a training period, whenever the shock is sparked, a light is flipped on. The normal rat reaction to shocks is to freeze in place. Eventually, when rats learn to associate light with a shock, they will freeze as soon as a light is turned on, even if there is no accompanying shock.

When the UCLA researchers ran their experiment, they discovered that concussed rats learned to link light with fear much more quickly than uninjured ones. This meant that the amygdala, the area of the brain that links stimuli with emotional responses, had become more efficient. What's more, the concussed rats weren't able to forget the link as quickly as the healthy rats. This meant that rats with mild TBIs were more prone to PTSD. The finding was a surprise, since the researchers had assumed that all learning would be adversely impacted. It meant that certain areas of the brain were slowed down by a TBI and others were tuned up.

At the same time as he was looking at the impact of concussions on brain plasticity, Hovda was trying to tease out the details of the neurochemical changes that occurred after a jolt to the head. The work by UCLA researchers, when coupled with that from several other centers, began to bring the changes in brain chemistry that followed a jolt into focus. The scientists saw a consistent sequence of events that they dubbed the "metabolic cascade."

Studies showed that after a jolt to the head, cells and pathways all over the brain are pulled and twisted. That physical movement inevitably leads to a chain of events that always starts with cells sparking and spewing out their neurotransmitters in a kind of mini-seizure.

Normally the brain uses these chemical messengers frugally. Neurons shoot neurotransmitters back and forth as a way of passing signals to one another. If neuron A has a message to communicate to neuron B, it tosses out a specific chemical. Neuron B grabs the neurotransmitter with a structure called a receptor. What happens next is comparable to what occurs after a key turns in the ignition of a car: once the neurotransmitter locks into its receptor, some very specific machinery in the cell switches on.

The sudden release of neurotransmitters that follows a jolt to the head prompts neurons to open the door to two types of charged molecules— calcium and sodium. The sodium electrifies the cells, while the calcium chews away at their internal structures if it stays too long. Making matters worse, the initial mechanical pulling and twisting stretches the tiny pores lining the cell's outer skin. That results in bigger openings, which allow potassium to rush out of the neurons while even more calcium and sodium flood in. If enough sodium pours in, the results can be catastrophic because sodium brings water with it and that can cause a cell to bloat, just as a person's hands and feet swell when a large quantity of salt is consumed. Too much bloating can result in a dead neuron.

In an attempt to get their internal chemistry back to normal, the neurons turn on machinery designed to pump potassium back into the cell and sodium out of it. Potassium serves as a set of brakes to the effects of sodium, by turning off the electricity. But the ion exchange takes a lot of energy, which the cell gets from its internal power plants, the mitochondria. Just as power plants need uranium or coal to produce energy, the mitochondria need glucose to create energy for the cells. It doesn't take very long for the glucose supply to run low and for the cellular power plant to experience a brownout, which then leaves the brain running at very slow speed. This, Hovda says, explains the slowed processing and fatigue that people experience shortly after a concussion. The situation can worsen if high levels of calcium have entered the cell. Then the brownout can turn into an actual blackout, because calcium will clog the machinery in the mitochondria, disabling them even further. Eventually, if the power plant completely fails, the neuron can die.

At the same time as the brain needs more and more energy, its blood supply becomes compromised. Blood is what brings glucose to the brain. When the brain needs more energy, the cells fire and send out a message to the body to increase blood flow so that more glucose will be delivered to the mitochondria. But somehow, after a jolt to the head, that message gets garbled, and no matter how many signals the neurons send, there is no increase in blood flow. In severe cases, cells can die because they aren't getting the fuel they need to run. In response to all of this, the brain releases high quantities of potassium in an attempt to calm things down. The result of that is an even slower and foggier brain.

One question scientists still haven't answered is whether there are permanent, though subtle, changes to the brain from mild hits. Some researchers suspect that each hit causes a small amount of permanent damage that is not enough to produce symptoms but might eventually add up to something more severe if the hits keep coming. The theory is that tiny gates positioned at various spots up and down the length of the axon are corroded a little more with each hit. Since the gates play a role in the propagation of an electrical signal up the length of an axon, damage to them can make the axon nonfunctional.

You can think of the axon as a canal with a series of locks. An electrical impulse, like a ship moving up the canal, starts at one end of the axon when sodium is allowed in. The gate to the next section opens and allows the sodium, and the electrical current, to move into the next segment of the axon. The gate then closes behind it. The process continues until the current has sparked the entire length of the axon.

One of the consequences from a jolt to the head is the rush of calcium into the axon. This can activate enzymes called proteases, which act like a set of scissors. They will chop away at the gate, leaving it frayed and leaky. Some scientists believe that each mild hit results in a small amount of damage to the gates. They still work, after a fashion, but not as well. As the hits add up, the gates become increasingly more damaged until they're completely broken. That theory could help explain why people who sustain a concussion are more susceptible to another and why each succeeding concussion seems to result in worsening symptoms. Douglas Smith compares the situation to an airplane losing its engines. "One falls off and the plane might fly fine and the passengers probably wouldn't even notice," the Penn scientist says. "But if you lose another one, that's an entirely different thing."

For years, scientists had no way to "see" the effects of a concussion in a living TBI survivor. But once researchers recognized that glucose metabolism reflected the brain's response to a jolt, they realized they already had a tool that might allow them to watch the concussed brain at work. PET (positron emission tomography) scanners, which had been used for years to look at brain function, are designed to detect and interpret emissions from radioactive substances to produce an image. Much of the early work with PET had been done using radioactive glucose, which is injected into the arm of a person shortly before scanning. The glucose eventually wends its way into the brain and then researchers can watch as various regions power up, their activity highlighted by red, orange, and yellow hues on scans. In a typical experiment, researchers might want to see which parts of the brain activate when a person remembers a distressing event. Researchers can ask the person in the PET scanner to concentrate on a traumatic episode and then watch to see which brain regions light up.

Colors on the scan range from dark blue to deep red, with blue signaling no activity and red signaling the most.

Scientists in Hovda's lab at UCLA had begun using PET to look at a broad spectrum of TBI, from mild to severe. One day Hovda had a fortuitous and stunning insight. He'd ordered up two PET scans: one from a TBI survivor who was in a coma, the other from a concussed football player. When he pulled the scans out and started to examine them, he was sure there had been a mix-up. The two sheets of film he had in front of him looked almost identical. He thought they must both be from the coma patient. Both scans were mostly blue in color with faint smudges of light green scattered here and there. An image from a normal brain would have been marbled with reds, oranges, and yellows. The minor amount of glucose metabolism in both these brains was signaled by the weakly glowing smudges of green. Hovda's assistant assured him that the scans were the right ones. They were indeed from two separate patients—one in a coma, the other wide awake and recovering from a concussion. Hovda realized that the implications were profound. An athlete recovering from a concussion had the same diminished glucose metabolism as a comatose patient.

To see if this was a fluke, Hovda and his colleagues scanned forty-two other patients whose TBIs ranged from mild to severe. The researchers found that 86 percent of the patients with severe brain injuries and 67 percent of the patients with mild-to-moderate injuries had the same low levels of glucose metabolism. What was remarkable, the researchers wrote, was that concussed patients who walked up to the scanner on their own power often had the same impaired glucose metabolism as the comatose patient who had been wheeled into the PET-scanning room breathing through a ventilator.

Other researchers started to examine brain-injured patients with an imaging technology called functional MRI, or fMRI. Like PET, fMRI looks at brain function rather than structure. In the case of fMRI, scans show blood flow, which in turn tells researchers about oxygenation. When a particular region of the brain is working hard, it will need more oxygen and, therefore, higher blood flow. So, if the activity in a particular area of the brain is turned up, it will shine bright on a scan. Researchers at the University of Pittsburgh found that in the days after a concussion, brain activity in an area called the posterior parietal cortex was depressed in some patients. The patients with slowed brain activity turned out to be the ones who had been experiencing the most symptoms. After a concussion, they had reported a host of both cognitive and physical symptoms, such as drowsiness, fatigue, difficulty concentrating, memory problems, blurred vision, headache, and light sensitivity.

While PET and fMRI can give a clear picture of the brain's biochemistry, they don't provide any information about small-scale structural changes, such as diffuse axonal injury. For that, scientists turned to a developing scanning technology known as DTI (diffusion tensor imaging). The technique uses an MRI machine but a different method of analysis that exploits the fact that water tends to flow in the same direction as the structures in the brain. So, if you can follow the water with a brain scanner, you should be able to see structures like the bundles of axons that run through the brain. And if these structures are disrupted in some way, that should show up, too.

The method didn't always turn up axon damage in symptomatic patients, but some of the scans were stunning in what they revealed. You could see whole groups of axons that appeared to be sheared off. Most of the initial work with DTI was done with severely injured patients, but in 2010 researchers at the Albert Einstein College of Medicine ran an experiment to see if symptoms from mild TBIs could be correlated with actual damage to axons. The researchers focused on executive function, which is known to be seated in the frontal lobes. Before scanning anyone, the researchers tested the executive functions of a group of uninjured volunteers and a group of concussed patients. The test, which was run on a computer, looked at how well people learned from trial and error. "It's admittedly not a real-world situation," says Dr. Michael Lipton, associate director of the Gruss Magnetic Resonance Research Center at Albert Einstein. "But it does pick up people who have problems with multitasking and following multistep directions. A secretary, for example, has to manage several things at the same time. She has to plan new activities while keeping in her mind a list of things to do that day; she has to keep track of what she's finished and what she hasn't finished. These are the kinds of things we rely on our brains to do, without thinking about it."

Lipton's scans from patients who had problems with the computer test showed damage to axons in an area known to be involved in executive function, the dorsolateral prefrontal cortex. Before there was DTI, he explains, you couldn't see any of these changes; on traditional scanners, their brains would have looked completely normal. "This shows that there is clearly something wrong with the brains of these people," he says.

So far, no one has used DTI to follow concussed patients over a long period of time to see if the missing connections are repaired. No one knows how much rewiring actually takes place. One thing that is becoming increasingly clear, though, is the possibility that a TBI in some patients kicks off a degenerative process that continues for the rest of that person's life.

Douglas Smith's axon-stretching experiments, coupled with autopsy results from his lab and others examining patients with severe brain injuries, would eventually yield insights into TBI consequences that could show up decades after a head injury. His research showed how a head injury might spark a lifelong process of neuron degeneration. It also provided a possible explanation for the well-established link between TBI and a heightened risk of Alzheimer's disease: the researchers found that a single stretch could lead to the accumulation of amyloid beta, the sticky protein that clogs the spaces between neurons in the brains of Alzheimer's patients. The new discoveries came after Smith and his colleagues decided to watch axons for a longer period of time following the initial stretch.

Chief among the proteins shuttled up and down the length of an axon is one called amyloid precursor protein (APP), the stuff from which amyloid beta is made. In a healthy axon, proteins moving along the microtubules are kept separate from one another, like boxed products moving on a conveyor belt. When axons are damaged by stretching and the microtubule conveyor belt is broken, all the boxes dump over the end, smash together, and rip apart, allowing their contents to intermingle. In the jumble with APP are enzymes that can slice it up and convert it into the sticky amyloid beta. As the axon bulb swells, increasing amounts of amyloid beta are created.

Eventually the bulbs burst and disgorge their contents, including heaps of amyloid beta, into the area surrounding the axon. This observation helped explain something that the Scottish researchers had discovered years earlier: the brains of 30 percent of TBI patients who died shortly after a head injury were riddled with the same kinds of plaques found in the brains of people with Alzheimer's disease. Alarmingly, many of the TBI patients had been fairly young. "It was clear that the plaques were forming within hours of the injury," Smith says. "In many of the cases, there weren't as many plaques as you'd see in a case of full-blown Alzheimer's, but the pathology was startling, especially in relatively young patients."

When the Penn researchers first discovered the amyloid beta plaques in the brains of TBI patients, they suspected they'd found a direct connection to Alzheimer's disease. But the story got more complicated as they took a closer look. When they had the opportunity to examine the brains of patients who survived six months to a few years after a TBI, the researchers found continuing axon deterioration—complete with newly formed protein bulbs—but no plaques. Smith and his colleagues were perplexed. Study after study had established a link between TBI and Alzheimer's disease. Plaques seemed to sprout prodigiously in the hours after a brain injury, but then mysteriously disappear in the months and years following the TBI.

A few years earlier, Japanese researchers had discovered that an enzyme called neprilysin was able to slice up amyloid beta and dispose of it. In fact, certain forms of the gene that produced the enzyme seemed to be protective against Alzheimer's disease. Smith had a new hypothesis. Perhaps TBIs kicked off a degenerative process in the brain that was kept in check by neprilysin. As dying neurons spewed out heaps of amyloid beta, neprilysin would come in and sweep up the gunky protein and recycle it into nontoxic substances. You wouldn't see plaques as long as the neprilysin was able to keep pace with amyloid beta production. When they checked for differences in the neprilysin gene in the patients who died shortly after a brain injury, the researchers found that all of the patients who developed plaques also had one specific form of the neprilysin gene.

Smith suspected that this was a less efficient form of the gene, one that allowed the rapid formation of amyloid plaques shortly after a brain injury. Although the plaques seemed to disappear over months, it was possible that the balancing act between amyloid beta production and destruction could eventually be thrown out of whack. The trash heap would grow faster than the street-sweeper enzyme could clean it up, and the result would be a brain clogged with amyloid beta plaques.

There was a way to test the hypothesis: examine the brains of TBI patients who had survived for many years after their injuries. Smith and his colleagues located the brains of seventy-four patients who died from three hours to forty-seven years after a TBI. The researchers autopsied these brains and then compared them to brains from forty-seven people with no history of brain injury. This time the researchers looked not only for amyloid beta, but also for tau, the protein that makes up the stringy tangles found inside the neurons of people with Alzheimer's disease. The earlier studies had shown no tangles in the brains of patients who died within weeks of a brain injury.

Once again, the researchers found clumps of amyloid beta in the brains of about 30 percent of the people who died shortly after a TBI, while very few plaques were seen in the brains of patients who survived a few months to a few years after an injury. But plaques seemed to reemerge with time. The researchers found far more of them in people who died at least four years after a brain injury. And this was true even in people who were in their thirties, forties, and fifties when they died. Even more startling, the researchers also found extensive tau tangles in the brains of many patients who survived multiple years after a TBI. When they examined the brains of people with no history of a TBI, the results were very different: Alzheimer's pathology was evident only in the brains of people who died when elderly.

"This is clear evidence that with a single brain injury, you can get both pathologies," says Smith. "It's provocative and frightening. These patients have the hallmark pathologies of Alzheimer's disease even though they are young."

Smith's findings were profound. One moderate-to-severe head injury could kick off a neurodegenerative disease that could come back to haunt people many years after they'd "recovered" from a major jolt to the brain. What Smith's work couldn't answer was whether lesser hits could have a similar effect. But there were suggestions from studies of boxers that had been done over the previous several decades. In boxers, at least, it looked like repetitive jolts to the head might set in motion a process that would eventually culminate in dementia and changes in the brain that looked very much like Alzheimer's disease.

Chapter 9

A Pocketful of Mumbles

Jerry Quarry always had too much heart for his brain's own good. That's how it had been ever since he laced on boxing gloves at the age of three and began living by his father's family motto: "There's no quit in a Quarry." Raised to be a fighter by his hardened father in the migrant labor camps of California, Quarry used boxing to escape a hardscrabble heritage he described as right out of *The Grapes of Wrath*. By the time he'd grown to a powerful six feet and 195 pounds, he had the tools to be a top heavyweight contender: a mean left hook, a crafty counterpunching ability, a granite chin that could take any punch, and, above all, a gritty tenacity.

What Irish Jerry Quarry lacked was the luck connoted by the green shamrock on the robe he wore into the ring. It was his bad luck to be merely good in a golden age of heavyweight greats defined by Muhammad Ali and Joe Frazier. Twice Quarry fought for the heavyweight championship of the world only to end up broken and heartbroken. He fought Ali and Frazier two times apiece, bravely battling through bloody beatings even after defeat had become as inevitable as it was predictable. Quarry took everything they had without flinching, but his most dangerous and destructive foe wasn't Ali or Frazier—it was Jerry Quarry.

The very traits that made Quarry a prime contender—his one-two punch of toughness and stubbornness—would also undermine him both in and out of the ring. His opponents knew they had little chance of knocking him down and no chance of battering him into submission; his granite chin could shake off pulverizing punches that had knocked out lesser specimens, his big heart could will him through all fifteen rounds of a title fight despite a broken back. With no quit in this Quarry, the best way to conquer him was to bloody his face so that the referee or ringside doctor would have to stop the carnage for the fighter's own good. Quarry knew just as well as his foes that his tendency to cut so easily was his Achilles' heel—the one head injury too obvious for even him to ignore— but that didn't keep him from fighting with a reckless disregard for his own safety and best interests.

Never was that clearer than in his 1969 championship bout with Frazier. Right from the opening bell, Quarry charged like a bull, inexplicably abandoning the cautious counterpunching style that had earned him the title shot and might have given him a fighting chance against the swarming champion aptly nicknamed Smokin' Joe. For the entire three minutes of the most savage first round ever fought by heavyweights, the two men stood toe to toe in the center of the ring, like bulls locking horns, and rained blows down upon one another, punch after punch caroming off their skulls. As if it wasn't astonishing enough that Quarry was taking the fight to the ultimate aggressor, he was also somehow managing to outslug the consummate slugger. By the third round, however, it was clear just how doomed that strategy—of trying to beat Frazier at Frazier's own game by turning a boxing match into a barroom brawl—had been all along. Frazier proceeded to relentlessly roll over the challenger like a tank, smothering him into the ropes and firing a barrage of blows that pounded his face to a swollen, bloody pulp. When the doctor mercifully stopped it after the seventh round, Quarry was left alone in his protest, stalking inconsolably and blindly around the ring.

The following year, Quarry stepped under the klieg lights in the longer shadow cast by the most famous of all athletes. It was Muhammad Ali's much-anticipated return to the ring after three and a half years in exile, having been stripped of his title belt and boxing license for refusing induction into the Army as a conscientious objector to the Vietnam War. In his comeback fight against Quarry, Ali was determined to prove to the world that he was still what he'd always proclaimed himself to be during his undefeated reign as undisputed heavyweight champion: "The Greatest." Though obviously rusty, Ali picked up right where he'd left off, using the canvas like an artist, dancing circles around Quarry, flicking sharp left jabs, rifling left-right combinations. In the middle of the third round, Ali snapped a cracking right that split a deep gash over Quarry's left eye. Like a shark scenting blood, Ali peppered the cut with twisting jabs that intensified the rivers of red pouring into Quarry's eye and down his face. At the end of the round, as the referee examined the cut slicing right down to the bone, Quarry begged him, "No, no, don't stop the fight!" While his own trainer pleaded with him to quit, the ref stepped in and did what Quarry never would, waving the fight over.

Minutes after the cut had been closed with eighteen sutures, Jack Quarry—the hard-nosed patriarch who'd forged and hammered home the family motto, "There's no quit in a Quarry"—beseeched his tearful son to quit for good. "Jerry, you can't go on like this or pretty soon you'll be walking on your heels," Jack Quarry lectured in the darkness outside the Atlanta arena. "It's going to be another cut or another punch in the head. You've got the money now. Go do something. Buy yourself a service station or an apartment house or a McDonald's or something. Anything. Just get out of it."

But Jerry Quarry had learned his father's hard lessons too well to quit now at the age of twenty-five. He angrily parted ways with his father, who had also served as his co-manager, and kept right on fighting. In rematches, Ali surgically carved him up through seven rounds and Frazier brutally bludgeoned him through five. After that 1974 Frazier fight, Arwanda Quarry caressed her son's bloody face and pleaded with him to "get out of it." Jerry sobbed and promised his mother he would. But nine months later, he was back in the ring absorbing yet another five-round bludgeoning. That one would finally convince Quarry it was time to hang up the gloves at twenty-nine.

He retired with a bittersweet legacy as "the best heavyweight never to win the world championship" and found a safer way to stay in the spotlight. His Hollywood good looks—the mop of dirty blond hair, the twinkling blue eyes, the mischievous smile—helped land him a regular gig as a network boxing commentator as well as guest-starring roles on such hit TV series as *The Six Million Dollar Man*. But none of that could challenge the fame and fortune that prizefighting had brought him as the most popular of fan favorites. After two years he was back in the ring basking in the adulation of the crowd. Moments after rescuing himself from a defenseless drubbing with a lucky knockout punch in the ninth round of his comeback fight, he grabbed the ring microphone and shouted, "Let's hear it for the old Quarry!" In his heart, though, he recognized the fallacy of those words and reluctantly faded back into retirement.

This time he stayed out of the ring for nearly five years. It wasn't just the Quarry family motto that made it impossible for him to quit for good. It was the fatal flaw known as the prizefighter's curse: the inability to resist the siren call of the boxing bell despite the mounting toll on body and brain.

While training for that latest comeback in 1983, Quarry got a call from *Sports Illustrated* asking him to undergo neurological testing for a special report the magazine was preparing on brain damage in boxers. Decades before Quarry turned pro, the occupational hazard of his chosen profession already had been formally described and named by doctors: "dementia pugilistica" or "punch-drunk syndrome," depending on which medical dictionary you thumbed through. Call it what you will, the definition was the same: degenerative brain damage that resulted from repeated head blows, leading to cognitive decline, memory loss, bouts of confusion, slurred speech, wobbly gait, poor coordination, tremors. Studies showed that up to 90 percent of boxers eventually developed some degree of brain damage, many of them warranting a diagnosis of dementia pugilistica years after retirement. For its special report, *Sports Illustrated* wanted to take advantage of a new scanning technology that would allow doctors to look inside the brains of longtime boxers like Quarry and Ali.

Given Ali's transcendent fame and feats through a glorious pro career that spanned twenty-one years, sixty-one fights, and an unmatched three reigns as world heavyweight champion, he was naturally the magazine's first choice. It had been barely a year since he'd announced his retirement with a simple explanation: "I don't want to be one of them old fighters with a flat nose saying 'duh-duh-duh' before a fight." By the time *Sports Illustrated* invited him to join Quarry and two other boxers for neurological testing, rumors were swirling that Ali was indeed becoming punch-drunk. The finely tuned athlete whose ring motto had been "float like a butterfly and sting like a bee" was now so fatigued that he would sometimes nod off in the middle of a sentence; his movements, once so catlike and graceful that his fists and feet were all a dazzling blur, had become slow and tremulous; his speech, once as crisp and cutting as his signature left jab, had become thick and slurred. Still, Ali wasn't about to let some magazine go rummaging around for more signs of brain damage. "Why do you want to check my brain?" he railed at a *Sports Illustrated* reporter with vintage Ali loquaciousness. "They want to say I have a brain injury, that I'm crazy. I won't be no guinea pig."

In contrast, Quarry was as willing to step into the lab as he was into the ring. He was experiencing no noticeable symptoms, and he expressed confidence that nothing would be found amiss. At his rural training camp north of Los Angeles, he passed a neurological examination but performed poorly on neuropsychological tests, which exposed problems with short-term memory and hand-eye coordination. What was worse, his CAT scan showed abnormalities commonly found in longtime boxers. Dr. Ira Casson, the neurologist retained by *Sports Illustrated* to conduct the testing, showed Quarry the scan, pointing to the atrophy of the cortex and to the tunnel-like hole in the septum between the cerebral hemispheres. After explaining that CAT scans could reveal brain damage as it developed and before it manifested in symptoms, Casson urged Quarry to abandon his comeback plans and hang up the gloves for good.

Quarry, who never did know when to give up, was not about to do so now. Facing financial ruin from failed business ventures and failed marriages, he needed the money prizefighting afforded. But more than that, he craved the accolades. He'd go around proudly announcing to friends and family, "I'm going to be a hero again." Trouble was, he no longer possessed the tools that had made him the latest contender to be dubbed "The Great White Hope" in a weight class dominated by black champions. He had always hated that label—"I'm not a white hope, I'm just a fighter"—but now he was barely even a fighter. His reflexes dulled, he managed to win both of his comeback bouts against no-name pugs and then retired once again.

Over the next few years, Quarry began to show the obvious effects of brain damage from his sixty-five professional fights and his more than two hundred amateur bouts, not to mention all the rounds he'd sparred in sweaty gyms and the brawls he'd fought in beery bars as a youth to win his father's grudging approval. He was now walking on his heels, just as his father had predicted after the first Ali fight, using ring parlance for the unbalanced stagger characteristic of dementia pugilistica. And his short-term memory problems were becoming pronounced enough to worry his mother.

None of that could deter him, of course. If George Foreman could come out of a ten-year retirement on his quest to recapture the heavy-weight crown that he'd won from Frazier and lost to Ali, then why couldn't the only challenger he ever admitted to ducking—Jerry Quarry? In 1992, nine years removed from his last fight, Quarry decided to stage a come-back of his own at the age of forty-seven. Some friends had talked him into believing they could get him a movie deal, a book contract, maybe even another title shot—if he could just beat a couple of palookas.

Twenty-three years after he'd challenged Joe Frazier for the heavy-weight title at Madison Square Garden, Quarry agreed to fight a trivial six-rounder at a glorified gym in Colorado, the only state with no regula-tory commission to deny him a boxing license on medical grounds. So it had come to this: Jerry Quarry, the popular crowd favorite who'd once fought Muhammad Ali for $338,000, taking on a ham-and-egger named Ron Cranmer for a paltry $1,050. For the few hundred hardcore fans in attendance, it was a sad sight. His reflexes shot, Quarry was battered and bloodied by a clumsy club fighter through all six rounds, losing two teeth and a one-sided decision, then requiring a hundred stitches to piece his face back together.

The next morning, Quarry woke up and couldn't remember anything from the night before. Overnight, he had plummeted into the shadowy throes of full-blown dementia pugilistica. The last fight had triggered the latent time bomb that had been ticking in his brain for decades, launch-ing him on a three-month plunge into oblivion and incapacitation. He was weepy, dazed, confused, unable to recognize familiar faces. He was halluci-nating, hearing voices no one else heard, talking to people who weren't there.

No longer able to care for himself, he moved in with his big brother, Jimmy, who became his full-time caregiver. Jerry needed help shower-ing, shaving, combing his hair, putting on his shoes and socks. Mealtime became a particular problem. He had to be coaxed to eat anything other than the Apple Cinnamon Cheerios he loved for breakfast. At dinner his meat had to be cut into little pieces so he wouldn't choke on it. He was lost and disoriented, often unable to find the bathroom in the small house. He would wander off four or five times a day, sometimes necessi-tating the police to search for him through the rural roads in the shadow of the San Jacinto Mountains and bring him back home.

The magnitude of the change over such a short time was stunning. By his fiftieth birthday, Quarry was smiling like a little boy but shuffling like an old man. His speech was slow and slurred. The steely blue eyes that once stared down Ali and Frazier during prefight instructions now appeared alternately vacant, scared, and bewildered. His thoughts were random, his memories muddled. He remembered he was a boxer, but thought he'd won all his fights. He would sit on the couch watching videos of his flickering past, the memory of those unforgettable fights lost in a haze caused by too many punches from the likes of Ali and Frazier.

A neurological examination showed just how much devastation those punches had wrought. Quarry couldn't tell the doctor where he was, what month it was, what year it was. His CAT scan showed why: a severely atrophied cortex and a gaping tunnel-like hole in the septum. With each succeeding exam, the worsening results mirrored the relentless march of the disease through his shriveling brain.

Every once in a while, the fog would roll out just long enough to yield a flash of lucidity, of the old Quarry. When people recognized him, his face would light up like a little kid's, his eyes smiling beneath thick slabs of scar tissue, and he'd extend the beefy right hand with the battered knuckles of his lethal trade. He had always loved shaking hands and signing autographs, but he could no longer pen his name. At the black-tie dinner celebrating his 1995 induction into the World Boxing Hall of Fame, he tried signing his autograph on a boxing glove but had to give up after one letter. Surrounded that night by other ex-fighters shuffling slowly and slurring their words, the undersized heavyweight with the big heart reflected on what boxing had given him and what it had taken away. "I'd do it all again, same way," he'd later tell a reporter, his speech so slow that the words would become intelligible only when speeded up on a tape recorder.

His $2.1 million in ring earnings long gone, Quarry was broke and living on a $614 monthly Social Security disability check. As he regressed through a second infancy, his mother took him in so she and his sisters could care for him in shifts, supervising him round the clock to keep him from wandering off. It wasn't long before he could no longer recognize his parents, his four sisters, his three brothers, his three children, his five grandchildren, or even himself.

When he died in 1999 at the age of fifty-three from complications of dementia-related pneumonia, Jerry Quarry left a legacy that extended far beyond the confines of the ring and the sport that destroyed his brain. His losing fight against a foe that looked a lot like Alzheimer's disease was a grim echo to Muhammad Ali's parallel struggle against a condition that looked a lot like Parkinson's disease.

On May 10, 1928, Harrison Martland stood before a rapt audience in New York City and delivered a blow as devastating as the punches Jack Dempsey himself threw during his long reign as the most menacing heavyweight champion the world had ever seen. Martland wasn't a boxer; he was a beefy, bespectacled, middle-aged scientist from New Jersey. He had come to the New York Academy of Medicine, fifty city blocks north of the boxing mecca named Madison Square Garden, to introduce his fellow pathologists to something that fight enthusiasts had long known but dismissed. The mere title of the landmark paper he presented that day should have jolted the medical community: "Punch Drunk."

"For some time, fight fans and promoters have recognized a peculiar condition occurring among prizefighters which, in ring parlance, they speak of as 'punch drunk,'" he began. "Fighters in whom the early symptoms are well recognized are said by the fans to be 'cuckoo,' 'goofy,' 'cutting paper dolls,' or 'slug nutty.' The early symptoms of punch drunk are well known to fight fans, and the gallery gods often shout 'Cuckoo' at a fighter. I know of one fight that was stopped by the referee because he thought one of the fighters intoxicated."

Thus did Dr. Martland usher his colleagues into a netherworld populated by pugilists and other colorful characters right out of a Damon Runyon yarn. Though not much of a fight fan himself, Martland had managed to blend right in at the smoke-filled arenas and sweat-filled gyms where he'd recently taken to hanging out. Chain-smoking cigarettes and appearing somewhat disheveled with necktie askew, the renowned forensic pathologist cut a figure every bit as gruff as the Runyonesque eccentrics he encountered in the fight game. Even in the relative refinement of his Newark City Hospital office, he would think nothing of urinating into a hand basin during staff meetings and then explaining to scandalized interns that "any guy who pisses into a toilet is a sissy." Unlike most pathologists, he performed his autopsies—all thirty thousand of them—without gloves, fishing organs out with his bare hands as a lit cigarette dangled from the corner of his mouth. Dubbed "The Sherlock Holmes of Medicine" by newspapermen because of his uncanny ability to solve sensational murders with forensic clues, he once delivered a scientific lecture at the New York Academy of Medicine dressed like the famous fictional detective right down to a deerstalker hat and a calabash pipe.

For his "Punch Drunk" lecture at the academy, though, Martland was all business. Just the year before, he had been vexed by the lack of attention accorded another important paper he'd presented on concussive brain trauma. As chief medical examiner for Essex County, he had begun that investigation by autopsying all 309 persons who died of closed-head injuries and wound up at his Newark morgue over a two-year period. The resulting paper advanced the medical literature on the mechanism of nonpenetrating head injuries but garnered no headlines. Pondering what it might take to get publicity for such significant research, Martland needed only to open his morning newspaper and read all about heavyweight kings who were held in higher esteem than royal monarchs and presidents. Through the Roaring Twenties, "The Golden Age of Sports," nothing was bigger than baseball and boxing and nobody bigger than Babe Ruth and the only superstar capable of dwarfing even him in worldwide fame and fortune—Jack Dempsey. It occurred to Martland that prizefighters, especially sluggers like Dempsey who punched and were punched with mayhem in mind, often developed symptoms similar to those suffered by brain injury survivors. Martland saw the ring as not only the perfect vehicle to get publicity for his brain injury research, but also the perfect lab to study the impact of repeated concussions and to extend to the living what he'd observed in the dead.

Promptly turning his attention to the ring, he started by seeking out fight promoters because he knew they had a knack for judging the physical and mental fitness of boxers. One promoter provided a list of twenty-three former fighters he considered punch-drunk. Of those, Martland was able to locate ten and personally examine five.

What he found in those examinations, coupled with descriptions of other fighters' symptoms gleaned from boxing aficionados, informed his definition of the condition. The early symptoms, he observed, often manifested themselves in an unsteady or unbalanced gait and sometimes in slowed movement and periods of slight mental confusion. As the condition progressed, movements slowed further, hands developed tremors, legs dragged, heads nodded involuntarily, and speech became halting. In severe cases, symptoms included vertigo, a staggering gait, a marked dragging of one or both legs, and the blank facial expression often seen in Parkinson's patients. Sometimes, dementia and mental deterioration became disabling enough to require commitment to an asylum, as was the case with four of the ten punch-drunk fighters Martland had tracked down.

"The occurrence of the symptoms in almost fifty percent of fighters who develop this condition in mild or severe form, if they keep at the game long enough, seems to be good evidence that some special brain injury due to their occupation exists," Martland declared in his presentation, hammering home his considered opinion that "in punch drunk there is a very definite brain injury due to single or repeated blows on the head or jaw."

That was hardly a fashionable opinion during the Jazz Age, when boxing's popularity soared to unprecedented heights with each furious flurry of Dempsey's fists. In challenging the status quo, Martland found himself faced with skepticism from all corners. That included one noted sportswriter who, Martland scoffed, "recently stated that punch drunk was greatly exaggerated and that he had consulted eminent neurologists who had assured him that such a condition did not exist."

To show its existence to the eminent pathologists seated before him, Martland presented "one case of advanced parkinsonian syndrome due to punch drunk," that of an ex-fighter he identified only by the initials N.E. A sturdy lightweight who began fighting professionally at age sixteen, Nathan Ehrlich was forced to retire at twenty-three because of a tremor in his left hand and an unsteadiness in his legs. Though he seldom drank, he was often wrongly accused of being intoxicated, thanks to the tremor and unsteadiness that plagued him the last year of his career after a knockout punch had rendered him unconscious for an hour. As the symptoms gradually worsened following his retirement, Ehrlich sought treatment in numerous clinics where doctors told him that the condition had nothing to do with the fifty-three pro bouts he'd fought. He was just thirty-eight years old when Martland examined him and observed that his gait was staggering and propulsive, his speech stammering and hesitant, his facial expression masklike.

Such case histories enabled Martland to deduce what factors might put certain boxers at greater risk. "Punch drunk most often affects fighters of the slugging type, who are usually poor boxers and who take considerable head punishment, seeking only to land a knockout blow," he reported. "It is also common in second-rate fighters used for training purposes, who may be knocked down several times a day. Frequently it takes a fighter from one to two hours to recover from a severe blow to the head or jaw."

Martland, who had built his national reputation as a crusading forensic pathologist by alerting the public to the lethal effects of radioactive poisons on factory workers, submitted his groundbreaking "Punch Drunk" paper to the *Journal of the American Medical Association* in an effort to reach the widest possible audience. It was a clarion call as clear as the ring bell. "The condition can no longer be ignored by the medical profession or the public," he wrote. "It is the duty of our profession to establish the existence or nonexistence of punch drunk by preparing accurate statistical data as to its incidence, careful neurologic examinations of fighters thought to be punch drunk, and careful histologic examinations of brains of those who have died with symptoms simulating the parkinsonian syndrome."

Martland concluded his paper by quoting Gene Tunney, the cerebral champion who had shocked the world by wrenching the heavyweight crown from Dempsey two years earlier. Shattering all the stereotypes, Tunney famously read Shakespeare between sparring sessions in which he mastered a scientific style designed to turn boxing matches into chess matches. His clear-cut 1926 decision over Dempsey, who'd ruthlessly ruled the heavyweight division for seven years as The Manassa Mauler, was hailed as a triumph of brains over brawn and brawling. In a sparring session for their ballyhooed 1927 rematch, Tunney was dazed by an accidental head butt and then rocked by a hard right to the jaw, dispatching him into a bout of amnesia so profound that he didn't even know who he was for forty-eight hours. The episode wasn't enough to keep him from retaining his title with another decision over Dempsey, but it did scare Tunney into resolving to retire. "From that incident was born my desire to quit the ring forever, the first opportunity that presented itself," Tunney would explain, providing the quote with which Martland chose to close his paper. "But most of all I wanted to leave the game that had threatened my sanity before I met with an accident in a real fight with six-ounce gloves that would permanently hurt my brain."

By the time Martland's landmark paper had been published in October 1928, Tunney was already two months into retirement, having abdicated his throne in the prime of his career. Tunney may have been smart enough to get out by the age of thirty, but few others appreciated the danger to their brains. It was easy for most fighters, trainers, managers, promoters, and even ringside doctors to discount Martland's message. They were willing to admit that the occasional fighter did indeed become punchy, but they continued to insist that boxing was not the cause. Furthermore, no one—not even the pathologist Martland—had shown them that there was actual brain damage involved. But what Martland had indisputably accomplished, by coining the medical term "punch drunk" as a condition that would soon find its way into diagnostic manuals as well as popular dictionaries, was to open the floodgates for a wave of future research into the phenomenon.

Gradually, what he had observed in a handful of ex-boxers would be extended through increasingly larger population studies. Researchers expanded the narrow list of symptoms Martland had found in his physical exams to a much broader one that emphasized cognitive deficits. And they replaced the "punch drunk" label he'd co-opted from boxing aficionados with terms they deemed more clinical and less insulting. The term "dementia pugilistica" was coined in 1937 by a U.S. Navy surgeon, Dr. J. A. Millspaugh. Two decades later, an eminent British neurologist, Dr. Macdonald Critchley, introduced the phrase "chronic progressive traumatic encephalopathy of boxers."

For a 1957 study published in the *British Medical Journal*, Critchley examined sixty-nine boxers with chronic neurological disease and determined that most were suffering from the condition. He observed a spate of mental symptoms: dementia, memory loss, slowed thinking and speech, mood swings, irritability, violent behavior. He found that mental and physical symptoms insidiously developed an average of sixteen years after the beginning of a boxer's career and that they progressed inexorably and irreversibly. He found the condition more common among professionals than amateurs, among sluggers than "scientific boxers," among those who were "slow on their feet rather than nimble," among those who were "notorious as being able to 'take it,'" and among those who were knocked out more often or, just as importantly, "knocked out on their feet." Though his research had proved beyond a doubt that the condition existed, it still gave no inkling as to how prevalent the problem was.

That question festered another five years before reaching a boiling point in the British House of Lords during a heated debate over a 1962 bill that sought to ban boxing throughout the commonwealth. Thirty-four years to the day after Martland's "Punch Drunk" presentation, Lord Walter Russell Brain—Britain's most eminent and fortuitously named neurologist—stood in the ornate Palace of Westminster and urged his peers to commission a scientific inquiry to determine the scope of the problem. Led by Lord Brain, who had authored the standard textbook on neurology, the Royal College of Physicians resolved to tackle the issue by appointing an enthusiastic research scholar named Anthony Herber Roberts to conduct a large-scale survey of prizefighters and the long-term effects of their perilous profession.

For the most comprehensive study ever undertaken on the subject, Roberts randomly selected 224 men from among the 16,781 who had been licensed to fight professionally by the British Boxing Board of Control for at least three years between 1929 and 1955. His neurological examinations of the former boxers were detailed and thorough, including EEGs and neuropsychological tests. Thirty-seven of them—17 percent—had clear evidence of dementia pugilistica as manifested in varying combinations of slurring, drooling, tremor, vertigo, unsteady gait, memory loss, disorientation, slowed thinking. In thirteen of those cases, the cognitive and physical symptoms were already permanently disabling. In addition to the thirty-seven cases attributable directly to boxing, another eleven ex-fighters evidenced brain damage that could have been explained by causes outside the ring. Whether the condition was directly caused by head blows or merely exacerbated by them, that brought the overall prevalence of clear brain damage in the population studied to 22 percent, with an unspecified number of others showing "disturbed neurological function."

All told, Roberts's prevalence data established the condition as a true epidemic. Perhaps even more telling, all but 2 percent of the study volunteers interviewed by Roberts reported seeing fellow fighters they described as "punchy" or "puddled." And they estimated that up to half of ex-boxers were clearly symptomatic, generally from "too much punishment about the head for too long."

From his data, Roberts was able to tease out a host of risk factors that explained such cause and effect: length of career, number of bouts, number of losses, fight frequency, sparring exposure, number of knockouts suffered, poor performance, poor skills, age at retirement. He found the correlation between brain damage and boxing exposure to be striking. Half of the ex-fighters over fifty who had boxed at least ten years showed signs of brain damage, as did half of those who had fought at least 150 bouts. The longer a boxer's career, the likelier he was to have symptoms that were more conspicuous.

When the report was presented in 1969, the Royal College of Physicians was impressed enough to publish it in book form. The 132-page book—titled *Brain Damage in Boxing: A Study of the Prevalence of Traumatic Encephalopathy among Ex-Professional Boxers*—concluded that "the accumulated sum total of these lesions, each perhaps of negligible importance in terms of function, may eventually produce a clinical syndrome bearing some resemblance to those in which there has been one severe traumatic episode causing diffuse destruction of cerebral axons." But even while linking the pathology of those two conditions, Roberts was careful to acknowledge that "there has been no specific pathological evidence to confirm the assumption that boxing is causally related to the clinical syndrome described."

Dr. Nick Corsellis read Roberts's book with intense interest. A respected neuropathologist, Corsellis had been collecting the brains of former boxers in his London lab for over a decade. To study the pathological effects of head blows on the brain, he focused on fifteen men who had boxed in their youth, twelve of them professionally, eight of them national or world champions in their weight classes. All fifteen had died of natural causes. Piecing together case histories from their friends and families, Corsellis determined that all fifteen had developed the classic symptoms of dementia pugilistica. The autopsies revealed striking abnormalities and cerebral atrophy in fourteen of the fifteen brains—changes that would become widely accepted as the hallmark pathology of dementia pugilistica.

Corsellis and his colleagues documented damage in a variety of brain regions. The septum, a vertical membrane separating the left and right sides of the brain, was ripped, and in some cases only shreds remained. The cerebellum, a structure located toward the back of the brain that controls movement, was scarred and atrophied, explaining such punch-drunk symptoms as staggering, spasticity, and tremor. The substantia nigra, a deep brain structure associated with Parkinson's when damaged, had been so decimated that the injury could be seen with the naked eye. Even more intriguing were the tangles of protein scattered in the hippocampus and other brain regions—the same kinds of tangles found in Alzheimer's patients.

The 1973 publication of those findings in the journal *Psychological Medicine* would have a profound impact, proving once and for all the existence of documentable brain damage, fueling debate on the medical ethics of boxing, and leading to safety reforms in the most controversial of sports. While noting that medical controls had probably improved since the era when his study subjects would fight upwards of a thousand career bouts as well as take on all comers in fairground boxing booths and tents, Corsellis warned, "There is still the danger that, at an unpredictable moment and for an unknown reason, one or more blows will leave their mark. The destruction of cerebral tissue will have then begun, and although this will usually be slight enough in the early stage to be undetectable, it may build up, if the boxing continues, until it becomes clinically evident. At this point, however, it could already be too late."

Millions of people, many more than had ever seen Slapsie Maxie Rosenbloom box professionally, found themselves rolling in the aisles of movie theaters across America as they watched him spoof the stereotype of the punch-drunk fighter on the silver screen. Rosenbloom was still lightheavyweight champion of the world in 1933 when he launched his second career—as a character actor playing the punchy pugilist in B-movie comedies. It may have been his penchant for cuffing opponents with open-fisted slaps that had inspired Damon Runyon to dub him Slapsie Maxie, but the nickname took on a whole new meaning once Rosenbloom discovered he could make people laugh in the gym by parodying the slaphappy figure fight fans knew so well.

Once Rosenbloom took his punch-drunk act to Hollywood, his Runyonesque pugs became as familiar to movie audiences as he had been to real-life fight crowds through his 289 professional bouts. With his splayed nose and cauliflower ear, he was easy to typecast as the punch-drunk pugilist. He certainly had all the symptoms down pat, from the slurred "dese," "dems," and "does" of his heavy New York accent to the tipsy, lurching gait of a fighter walking on his heels. He honed his portrayal of them at his Hollywood nightclub, Slapsie Maxie's, stumbling onto the stage, rocking back and forth on his heels, and slurring his punchlines.

After a while, as the symptoms he portrayed grew more pronounced, people began to suspect that it wasn't just an act. In a case of life imitating art, Rosenbloom ironically became the punchy character he'd played onscreen throughout the '40s. His speech thickened, he would repeat tales from his colorful past without realizing he'd just told them, and he stopped recognizing his friends. He lived out his final years destitute and demented, committed to a sanitarium in his sixties, his doctor attributing his decline to too many head blows from too many fights.

By the time Rosenbloom died, three years after Corsellis's study was published, the punch-drunk punchline was no longer a joking matter. A new tool that enabled doctors to peer inside the skulls of living patients—the CAT scanner—revealed clear cerebral atrophy even in asymptomatic boxers. In fact, by the early '80s, studies were finding brain damage in the majority of professional boxers scanned and correlating the degree of damage to the number of bouts fought.

The damage evident on those scans was as clear as the symptoms exhibited by two of history's most celebrated champions, Joe Louis and Sugar Ray Robinson. The two friends had captivated America like no other sports heroes in the middle of the twentieth century: Joe Louis reigning as the world heavyweight champ for an unheard-of twelve straight years, Sugar Ray Robinson earning the title of "the greatest pound-for-pound boxer of all time" with his dominance of the middleweight and welterweight divisions. Both retired as champions at the top of their game only to fall victim to the prizefighter's curse, returning to fight on long past their primes and fading away with ignominious career-ending defeats. Ultimately, both would suffer mightily from the cruel blows of the sport they had ennobled. Given Louis's role as a Las Vegas casino greeter, it was easy for fans to trace his descent from the Brown Bomber they had long cheered into the forlorn, punchy, paranoid, demented shell he would become by his death at sixty-six in 1981. In contrast, Robinson's parallel descent into the shadowy darkness of dementia would be much more private, if no less heartrending.

Once the world's most flamboyant celebrity both in and out of the ring, Robinson gradually withdrew from public view after retiring for good at age forty-five in 1965 after 202 professional fights. In 1984, he was finally diagnosed with Alzheimer's, joining Rita Hayworth as the most famous victims of a disease the American public was just becoming aware of. He would watch live fights featuring current superstars like his namesake Sugar Ray Leonard on TV and exclaim, "I beat that guy!" When Gene Fullmer visited him, Robinson failed to recognize the middleweight he'd battled through four memorable title fights. Alzheimer's had erased his memories of not only his greatest triumphs but also his closest friends.

When Sugar Ray Robinson died at sixty-seven in 1989, his brain and body ravaged by Alzheimer's and diabetes, there were many who implicated boxing as a cause of death. Head trauma had long been associated with Alzheimer's. Studies showed that people who had sustained head injuries were more likely than others to develop the disease. When head injuries resulted in a loss of consciousness, the risk for Alzheimer's rose by 50 percent. Of all nongenetic risk factors, brain injury was found to be the strongest.

For decades, researchers going back to Martland had suggested that dementia pugilistica was most likely to strike second-rate fighters, sluggers who lacked the technical skills of scientific boxers, and heavyweights whose heads were pounded with the most force. Sugar Ray Robinson, all 155 sculpted pounds of him stretched over a five-foot-eleven frame, broke the mold. Of all the practitioners of the sport long known as "The Sweet Science," Sugar Ray was the sweetest. In that mano a mano subculture prizing the knockout punch as the pinnacle of accomplishment, Robinson had brought the manly art of self-defense to a new level. He boasted an unrivaled blend of speed, power, and the creativity of a Picasso, his skills so sublime that a precocious teen named Cassius Clay resolved to model his style on the mentor he called "the king, the master, my idol."

If Robinson wasn't immune to the ravages of brain damage, could any boxer be safe?

It seemed as if no amount of artful, scientific skill could protect a boxer from paying the price of glory. Willie Pep, nicknamed Will o' the Wisp for his elusiveness and fleet-footed agility, and hard-punching Sandy Saddler traded the world featherweight title through four classic confrontations at mid-century, then lived out their final years in nursing homes suffering from dementia pugilistica. Wilfred Benítez, a stylish prodigy whose skills and speed made him the youngest world champion in ring history when he won the welterweight title at seventeen in 1976, kept finding places to fight long after the government of his native Puerto Rico banned him from boxing on medical grounds. Stumbling, slurring incoherently, flying into rages, Benítez would be living in a nursing home by the age of thirty-eight.

The list of demented champions goes on and on. Paradoxically, the best boxers were often the ones at highest risk because they had longer careers, faced more quality opponents, and showed the most ability to take a punch. Not surprisingly, the heavyweight ranks, where researchers measured punches equivalent to a thirteen-pound weight swinging into the face at twenty miles an hour with a force exceeding a thousand pounds, were even more decimated by dementia than the lower weight classes. For too many, the reward for achieving the most coveted title in sports—heavyweight champion of the world—turned out to be a requiem for the brain. For the public at large, brain damage became as much a part of boxing lore as the championship belt itself.

In the opening scene of the 1962 film *Requiem for a Heavyweight*, the washed-up fighter Mountain Rivera, played by an aging Anthony Quinn, has been brutally knocked out in the seventh round. After examining him in the dingy locker room, the doctor tells Rivera's manager that the battered boxer's career is over because he's just a couple of punches away from needing a tin cup and some pencils. As Rivera staggers off to the shower, the manager, played with sleazy desperation by Jackie Gleason, reflects for a moment and tells the cutman with a shrug, "Maybe he's lucky at that. At least he walks away with his brains. That's better than most." The fighter who ends Mountain Rivera's career was portrayed by a brash young up-and-comer who played himself in the film: Cassius Clay.

· · ·

Two decades after winning that fictional movie fight in a dreary New York City armory and then capturing the real-life heavyweight title to turn Cassius Clay into a household name he'd soon change, Muhammad Ali returned to the same upper Manhattan neighborhood where *Requiem for a Heavyweight* was filmed. In September 1984, Ali checked himself into Columbia-Presbyterian Medical Center, right across 168th Street from the armory, hoping doctors there would tell him that he was one of the lucky ones who, in the words of Mountain Rivera's manager, "walks away with his brains." The bravado that defined his celebrated persona had given way to a subdued anxiousness. "I've been in the boxing ring for thirty years and I've taken about a hundred and seventy-five thousand hard punches," he mused, "so there is a great possibility something could be wrong."

For years, that prospect had hung over his head like a sword of Damocles. Despite his unmarked face and his elusively agile boxing style, Ali had endured a lot more punishment than it appeared on the surface, especially later in his career. Upon his 1970 return from his forced ring exile, three and a half years slower than the dazzling young champion whose tap dancer's footwork had made him hard to catch and harder to hit, he needed to compensate by adding another tool to his repertoire: the ability to take a punch. He would demonstrate this toughness in training sessions, laying on the ropes and letting sparring partners pound his body and head as a show of machismo, and in bouts against champions who punched with malice and left damaged brains in their wake. When his aura of invincibility was shattered in "The Fight of the Century"—the 1971 showdown of unbeaten heavyweights that somehow exceeded its hype and confirmed Joe Frazier as the undisputed champion by unanimous decision—so was his veneer of invulnerability.

Even in the fights Ali won, he absorbed some vicious beatings. In the 1974 "Rumble in the Jungle" against George Foreman, the massive puncher who'd wrenched the title from Frazier with six knockdowns inside two rounds, Ali lay on the ropes, his forearms raised to shield his face like a turtle in a shell, and let the younger, stronger champ bang away with sledgehammers to the body and head. Only after Foreman had punched himself into exhaustion did Ali spring from his "rope-a-dope" shell to shock everyone with an eighth-round knockout and reclaim the championship.

Defending that title the next year against Frazier in the epic "Thrilla in Manila," Ali would have to survive a grueling war of attrition that tested each man's will, courage, and resilience. With Frazier relentlessly and remorselessly pounding thunderous hooks to the body and head, Ali slumped on his stool after the tenth round and gasped, "I think this is what dying is like." Just when all hope seemed lost, Ali summoned strength from somewhere deep down inside and rallied like a wounded lion ferociously fighting off a fierce enemy. He punched Frazier's legs to rubber and eyes to slits, but spent the last of his own reserve and resolve doing so. At the end of a fourteenth round savage enough to make even bloodthirsty fight fans feel guilt over their voyeuristic bloodlust, Ali dragged himself to his corner, wearily held out his gloves, and told his trainer, "Cut 'em off." Before Ali had a chance to quit, Frazier's trainer, Eddie Futch, beat him to it, placing his hands firmly on his own protesting fighter's shoulders and commanding, "Sit down, son. It's over." By not letting his defenseless charge answer the bell for the fifteenth and final round, Futch had mercifully stopped history's best and most brutal bout because he "didn't want Joe's brains scrambled."

Given all the damage that Ali and Frazier inflicted on one another through the forty-one rounds of their three-fight blood feud, their heroic rubber match should have put an exclamation point on both of their storied careers. "What you saw," Ali said slowly an hour afterward when he'd finally summoned enough strength to face the press, "was next to death. Closest thing to dyin' that I know of." His eyes vacant and his voice a halting raspy whisper, he would later confide to a reporter, "Why I do this? It was insane in there. Couple of times, [it felt] like I was leaving my body. I must be crazy. For what? This is it for me. It's over."

If only Ali had indeed walked away then. If only he'd had an Eddie Futch in his corner to save him from himself. The closest thing to that in his own entourage was Dr. Ferdie Pacheco, the physician who'd been in his corner since the night a young Cassius Clay shockingly beat the fearsome ex-con Sonny Liston into submission to win the title in 1964. Now, eleven years later, as Pacheco performed his customary postfight checkup back at the Manila Hilton, he examined Ali's puffy face—forehead ridged with bony lumps, eyes swollen half shut above angry purple welts, lips scraped raw as if sandpapered—and envisioned a brain that must likewise have become "a swollen, scar-filled mess." Pacheco, haunted by the specter of someday seeing "the most joyful, talented guy in the world stumbling around and mumbling to himself," decided the time had come to advise Ali to retire. Ali nodded knowingly, then ignored doctor's orders.

A year later, minutes after barely retaining the title with a controversial decision over Ken Norton, Ali lay flat on his back, exhausted and strangely silent, in an eerily quiet Yankee Stadium dressing room as Pacheco examined him. "I don't have it anymore, Doc," Ali said softly, breaking the silence. "I see the things to do, but I can't do them. I've got to get out of this before I get hurt. Am I through, Doc? Should I quit?"

"Yeah, Champ, I wish you would," Pacheco sighed, "but you won't."

Pacheco knew better. Pacheco knew all about the ego that had stoked Ali's competitive fire and the vanity that now threatened his well-being. Pacheco knew all about Ali's mounting financial worries due to lavish spending, alimony payments, and the responsibility of providing for eight children. More than that, Pacheco knew all about what he diagnosed as Ali's susceptibility to "the most virulent infection in the human race: the standing ovation." For the self-proclaimed "People's Champion," his own personal siren call became the rhythmic chants that echoed loudly through arenas the world over: "Ah-lee! Ah-lee! Ah-lee!"

Pacheco's intensifying crisis of conscience reached a tipping point a year later after Ali barely retained his title by decision over the hardest puncher he ever faced, Earnie Shavers. At a press conference the next day, Madison Square Garden's matchmaker, Teddy Brenner, privately urged Ali to announce his retirement and then publicly made a startling announcement of his own: the mecca of boxing would never again host an Ali fight, Brenner declared, because "I don't want him to come over to me someday and say, 'What's your name?'" The very same day, a New York State Athletic Commission doctor handed Pacheco a lab report revealing that Ali had serious kidney damage as well as neurological deterioration. Pacheco immediately wrote Ali a letter begging him to retire and sent copies of it along with the lab report to his wife, trainer, and manager by certified mail. When the letter elicited no responses, Pacheco did what Ali wouldn't—he quit. Pacheco, whose work in Ali's corner had made him a celebrity in his own right known internationally as "The Fight Doctor," left the famous entourage and the fight game itself.

Ali kept right on fighting for another year, losing the title to the inexperienced Leon Spinks and then regaining it for an unprecedented third time, before announcing his retirement at thirty-seven. As it turned out, though, Ali was no more immune than Sugar Ray Robinson, Joe Louis, and Jerry Quarry to the prizefighter's curse. Ignoring the pleas of his wife and his mother, Ali decided two years later to challenge for the title he'd vacated by retiring.

Because of mounting controversy over his slurred speech and slowed reflexes, he had to pass a neurological exam at the Mayo Clinic as a precondition for a Nevada boxing license. Though medically cleared for a 1980 title challenge in Las Vegas, he proved no match for the unbeaten Larry Holmes, his onetime sparring partner who'd succeeded him as champion in his absence. Holmes pulled his punches throughout the first ten rounds, continually imploring the referee to mercifully stop the beating before his idol got seriously hurt or worse. The slaughter finally ended with Ali slumped on his stool, unable to answer the bell for the eleventh round. By then so impaired that no U.S. site would sanction a farewell fight, Ali ignominiously ended his career in the Bahamas a year later with a dismal, defenseless defeat against an artless, awkward trivia answer named Trevor Berbick.

When Ali finally hung up the gloves for good, he looked and felt much older than his thirty-nine years. Although the head blows had stopped once and for all, the troubling symptoms—slurred speech, slowed movement, crushing fatigue, sluggish reflexes, hand tremors—were getting progressively worse.

Just seven months into his hard-earned retirement, Ali was hospitalized at UCLA Medical Center with those telltale signs of parkinsonism. He complained to doctors there that he was "walking like an old man," slurring his speech with low volume, drooling on occasion. A year later, he was back at the UCLA hospital, complaining that he was "moving like a mummy" and that his speech was becoming unintelligible. This time, CAT scans and neuropsychological tests revealed signs of brain damage significant enough for doctors to prescribe L-dopa, the drug of choice for treating parkinsonian symptoms. The meds helped ease the symptoms b' replacing the dopamine his brain was no longer able to produce in sufficient amounts, but when the condition kept worsening over the next year, Ali became more worried. No longer in denial, he resolved to get to the bottom of whatever was causing these problems. Which is what brought him to Columbia-Presbyterian Medical Center in 1984 for eight days of extensive testing at its Neurological Institute.

The neurologist he had been referred to was Dr. Stanley Fahn, director of the hospital's center for movement disorders, who'd built a reputation as the Muhammad Ali of Parkinson's experts. During their intake consultation, Fahn could sense how much the tremors and sluggishness troubled the once-graceful athlete celebrated as the fastest and smoothest heavyweight of all time. More than that, Fahn could sense how much the slurred and mumbled speech distressed the voluble firebrand notorious for taunting his foes in verse and for sparring verbally with reporters. "People say to me, 'What did you say? I can't understand you,'" Ali reported. "I'm not scared, but my family and friends are scared to death."

Upon examination, Fahn found such telltale signs of parkinsonism as stiffness, slowed movement, and decreased facial expression. A CAT scan showed atrophy of the cortex and a hole in the septum, and an MRI revealed damage to the brainstem. Neuropsychological testing uncovered slowed reflexes and response times, but there was no evidence of memory loss or declining intelligence.

At the time of Ali's discharge, Fahn issued a brief public statement explaining that his famous patient was exhibiting "some mild symptoms of Parkinson's syndrome"—not punch-drunk syndrome, not dementia pugilistica—and that he didn't appear to have a progressive degenerative condition. At Ali's request, Fahn did not disclose what he believed to be the cause of the parkinsonism.

Not until several years later did Fahn, at Ali's behest for an authorized biography, reveal that he had indeed linked Ali's condition directly to boxing. His actual diagnosis, Fahn disclosed in the 1991 Ali biography, "was a post-traumatic Parkinsonism due to injuries from fighting." In Parkinson's disease, he explained, the cells that produce dopamine in the substantia nigra of the brainstem progressively degenerate and die, depriving the central nervous system of a neurotransmitter essential for motor control. "In Muhammad's case, there's damage to these cells from physical trauma," Fahn told biographer Thomas Hauser in *Muhammad Ali: His Life and Times*. "Muhammad himself told me he thinks that most of the damage came from the third Frazier fight, the one in Manila. That may be where he started to get his damage, but it's highly unlikely that it all came from one fight. My assumption is that his physical condition resulted from repeated blows to the head over time."

The manifestation of that damage was evident even before Ali's 1980 comeback fight against Holmes, when reporters accustomed to interviewing a loquacious loudmouth had to lean in close to hear his mumbled, slurred words. Noting how Ali had shown clear parkinsonian symptoms since that time, Fahn told Hauser, "One might argue that his Parkinsonism could and should have been recognized earlier from the changes in his speech. That's speculative. But had that been the case, it would have kept him out of his last few fights and saved him from later damage. It was bad enough to have some damage, but getting hit in the head those last few years might have made his injuries worse. Also, since Parkinsonism causes, among other things, slowness of movement, one can question whether the beating Muhammad took in his last few fights was because he was suffering from Parkinsonism and couldn't move as quickly as before in the ring, and thus was more susceptible to being hit."

Certain symptoms led Fahn to diagnose what had long been described in the medical literature as "pugilistic parkinsonism." Numbness in the face and lips, rendering Ali unaware of when food needed to be wiped away, indicated damage to the brainstem due to boxing. So did his sleep disturbances. The early onset of his speech problems, like that of the sleep problems, provided more evidence that the cause was brain trauma.

Over the decade following the diagnosis, Ali receded from the spotlight, becoming as conspicuous by his silence as he had been by his booming presence. Of all the names speculated as candidates to light the Olympic cauldron at the 1996 Summer Games in Atlanta, no one thought to mention the ailing legend who had stamped himself the world's most famous athlete after bursting into the public consciousness as a brash eighteen-year-old gold medalist at the 1960 Games. But then suddenly there he was, at the climactic moment on the grandest stage in the world, materializing high on the platform at the far end of Atlanta's Olympic Stadium, greeted by an astonished gasp that built into a reverential roar.

It was an unforgettable sight: Muhammad Ali, a six-foot-three specter dressed head to toe in white, standing larger than life on the pedestal, his left arm performing an involuntary dance at his side, his empty left hand trembling, while his right arm held the flaming Olympic torch aloft. It would remain an indelible image: Muhammad Ali, expressionless behind a parkinsonian mask, emerging as the public face of a disease many sufferers prefer to keep private and the public face of traumatic brain injury from the sport that had brought him to this Olympic peak before billions of viewers.

Paradoxically, the more Parkinson's slowed his movements, the more mobile he became after his Olympic rebirth, traveling the globe in his role as cultural icon and goodwill ambassador. With Parkinson's continuing its relentless march through his central nervous system, however, Ali became more and more a shadow of the glib and graceful figure remembered for promising to "shock the world" and then delivering on that boast time after time. The most recognizable face on the planet, once so animated and stunningly handsome that he never missed a chance to remind everyone how "pretty" he was, had become a lifemask. The familiar voice, once so strident that it inspired his original Louisville Lip nickname, was stilled. The fancy footwork, once so quick that the "Ali Shuffle" could be appreciated only in slow-motion replays, had given way to the Parkinson's shuffle.

Although Fahn hadn't treated him since the 1984 evaluation, the neurologist tracked the inexorable worsening of Ali's symptoms over the following two decades. The pattern led Fahn to believe that the Parkinson's syndrome had progressed into full-blown Parkinson's disease, the traumatic blows having kicked off an irreversible sequence of destruction in Ali's brain.

What made Ali's case unusual among boxers was that the parkinsonian symptoms predominated to the apparent exclusion of dementia symptoms. Pugilistic parkinsonism, as first described in the medical literature by Harrison Martland back in 1928, is relatively rare. Dementia pugilistica is not. It could ravage whole weight classes—and whole families.

Jerry Quarry was not the only one of Jack Quarry's sons to go into the risky family business. Jack, a onetime fighter of sorts with the letters

H-A-R-D tattooed across the knuckles of his left hand and L-U-C-K across his right fist, schooled all four Quarry boys on boxing technique and toughness as a rite of passage. By the age of five, when they were required to step into the ring for real bouts against real opponents, they already had their father's family motto tattooed into their brains: "There's no quit in a Quarry." The oldest, Jimmy, did manage to quit before he could turn pro and before boxing could do too much damage to his brain. Jerry and his two kid brothers weren't so lucky.

Mike, younger by six years, idolized Jerry but wanted desperately to emerge from his shadow, their sparring sessions degenerating into brawls in which both would fling off their headgear to see who could withstand the hardest punches. A jab-and-move stylist who lacked the punching power that made Jerry a top heavyweight contender, Mike ran off thirty-five straight wins to earn a shot at the world light-heavyweight championship. In that 1972 title fight, on the undercard of Jerry's rematch with Ali, Mike was knocked out in the fourth round by a left hook so devastating that the champion, Bob Foster, was sure he'd killed his unconscious challenger. Mike would never be the same after that, but, like Jerry, he had too much heart and not enough quit in him.

Five years later, Mike was taking a bloody beating when Jerry, working his corner, stopped the fight after the sixth round. In the locker room afterward, Jerry caressed Mike's swollen face and declared, "I'll never let him fight again, not if I can help it. He's gonna quit. I will make him quit." Then he turned to Mike and said firmly, "Say it."

Mike countered, "I'm gonna fight one more to go out a winner—"

"Say it!" Jerry shot back, his voice rising.

Mike nodded in resignation as Jerry leaned over and kissed him on the neck. But Mike didn't say it, and he didn't do it. He fought nine more times over the next five years, finally retiring after his eighty-second pro bout ended in a dismal loss. Within a few years, he was forgetful and disoriented, walking on his heels, losing his balance, punching holes in walls. He spent the next decade bouncing from job to job—construction worker, insurance salesman, hairdresser, landscaper's assistant, church janitor—only to get fired over and over because he couldn't remember what he was supposed to do. In time, his wife became his round-the-clock caregiver, feeding him, bathing him, sitting him down on the toilet while she showered so he wouldn't wander off. Finally, she had no choice but to move him into a full-care facility, where he gradually lost the ability to walk and to talk.

Mike Quarry's descent into dementia pugilistica paralleled that of the famous big brother he echoed both in life and in death. Despite his own deteriorating condition, Jerry had the presence of mind late in his life to apologize to his little brother for hitting him so hard and so often. By the time Mike died at age fifty-five in 2006 from the same dementing disease that had killed Jerry seven years earlier, their brother Bobby, the youngest by twelve years, was battling pugilistic parkinsonism following a short, mediocre heavyweight career.

If boxing was the family legacy, brain damage was the family curse. To be sure, the Quarry brothers had inherited a lot from their father: the toughness, the passion for the fight game, the motto that kept them from quitting before it was too late. But they also may have inherited something worse: genes that made them more susceptible than other boxers to punch-drunk syndrome.

Dr. Barry Jordan didn't need to see dementia pugilistica racing through families for him to wonder whether there was a genetic predisposition. All he had to do was glance up from his ringside seat at boxing matches everywhere from Madison Square Garden to small clubs in upstate New York.

As chief medical officer for the New York State Athletic Commission since 1987, Jordan was the physician responsible for clearing all boxers to fight professionally anywhere in his jurisdiction. A neurologist at the Hospital for Special Surgery in Manhattan, he had gravitated to boxing only because he was interested in brain injuries and knew he would see a lot of them as a ringside doctor for fights featuring George Foreman, Mike Tyson, Sugar Ray Leonard, and numerous lesser lights. Even he was surprised when he became a fan of a sport that the American Academy of Neurology and the American Medical Association condemned and pushed to have banned. Believing that such a prohibition would send boxing underground and lead to more injuries and deaths in bootleg bouts, he resolved to make the sport safer through stricter regulations, closer medical supervision, and further scientific research.

Through the years, Jordan observed many boxers with brain damage and, in his research, tried to figure out why some were more prone to dementia pugilistica. No single factor could completely explain why some became punch-drunk and others didn't. He would see two boxers with identical exposure to the sport and wonder why one appeared healthy while the other was walking on his heels. He began to suspect there might be some sort of genetic predisposition. Then in the early '90s, when scientists discovered a genetic mutation that predisposed people to typical late-onset Alzheimer's, a bell went off in his head. Recalling earlier studies that showed head trauma raised the risk for the disease, he started thinking about his punch-drunk boxers. The dementia they suffered seemed very similar to Alzheimer's, from the debilitating symptoms right down the plaques and tangles in their brains. Maybe, he thought, the boxers who developed dementia pugilistica possessed the recently discovered genetic mutation.

To test his hypothesis, he recruited twenty-seven retired boxers and three active ones for a study he led with Dr. Norman Relkin, director of the Memory Disorders Program at Cornell Medical Center in Manhattan. The two neurologists and their colleagues conducted detailed examinations of the thirty boxers and found nineteen had symptoms of chronic traumatic encephalopathy. At the same time, DNA samples were analyzed to determine whether the boxers possessed the genetic mutation implicated in Alzheimer's. The mutation, an allele of the apolipoprotein E gene dubbed apoE ε4, was found to significantly increase the risk for Alzheimer's in people who had at least one copy; the risk rose as much as tenfold in those who inherited copies of it from both parents. What was more, a subsequent study showed that people with the allele who had suffered a traumatic brain injury were five times more likely to develop Alzheimer's compared to those who possessed the allele but no history of TBI.

When Jordan and his colleagues analyzed the boxing data, they determined that fighters who had the mutation were far likelier to get dementia pugilistica and to get it more severely and at a younger age. Among the boxers showing obvious symptoms, 50 percent had at least one copy of the mutation, as compared to 11 percent of the others. All three of the boxers with severe symptoms had at least one copy. Boxers who had fought more than twelve pro bouts suffered worse symptoms if they possessed the allele.

With its 1997 publication in the *Journal of the American Medical As-*

sociation, the study raised an ethical question that extended far beyond the confines of the ring. The hypothesis that apoE ε4 conveys a genetic predisposition to chronic traumatic encephalopathy, the authors wrote, "potentially has extraordinary ramifications for the regulation of health and safety in boxing and other high-risk sports including American football, soccer, and ice hockey."

As it turned out, apoE ε4 wasn't a strong enough predictor for anyone to revoke even a boxing license. But Jordan, now director of the Brain Injury Program at Burke Rehabilitation Center, is still hunting for a better biomarker. Sitting in his cluttered office in White Plains, New York, surrounded by photos from his days as a ringside doctor, Jordan mulls over the conundrum presented by a disease you don't see until it's too late. By the time boxers develop symptoms of dementia pugilistica, he points out, "the horse is already out of the barn," so you need to find a way to identify which ones are genetically at risk before they even start to fight. That at least would enable you to advise susceptible boxers on their risks, to follow them more closely with mandatory exams and scans, and to alert their doctors about the need for heightened vigilance.

If scientists ever discover a biomarker that could predict with absolute certainty which athletes would develop trauma-induced dementia, it will create an ethical dilemma: Do officials have the right to stop them from participating in contact sports? Until medical science can offer a solution, everyone must continue grappling with the real dilemma that has predominated the century and a half since the Marquess of Queensberry rules reformed boxing into its modern era: How do you make the most brain-damaging sport safer?

Hours after retaining the world welterweight title with a left hook that knocked Jimmy Doyle into a coma from which he never awoke, Sugar Ray Robinson was summoned to the Cleveland morgue to testify at a coroner's inquest.

"Did you intend to get Doyle in trouble?" the coroner asked the champion.

"Mister," Robinson replied deliberately, "it's my *business* to get him in trouble."

Thus did Robinson speak for all the boxers who have unintentionally killed or maimed men in a legally sanctioned sport where the goal is to injure an opponent's brain by inflicting damaging blows to the head. Each high-profile ring death from acute brain trauma, like Doyle's in 1947, would invariably spur a new round of calls for the abolition of a sport that killed an average of ten boxers a year. Sweden outlawed boxing in 1969 and Norway in 1981, but the United States did little to discourage it since the late teens when brief bans in some American locales succeeded only in driving fights underground into backrooms and onto barges.

The medical community had a stronger case than politicians, on moral and ethical grounds. In 1984, the American Medical Association formally called for the elimination of both amateur and professional boxing. Dr. George Lundberg, editor of the *Journal of the American Medical Association*, had fired the first shot in the AMA's crusade with a 1983 editorial demanding that boxing be banned, calling it an "obscenity [that is] less sport than is cockfighting" and "a throwback to uncivilized man [that] should not be sanctioned by any civilized society."

The AMA offered a smoking gun the following spring when its prestigious journal published a study that evaluated eighteen retired and active boxers with neurological exams, EEGs, CAT scans, and neuropsychological tests. Thirteen of the fifteen professional boxers in the study— a staggering 87 percent—showed definite evidence of brain damage on at least two of the four measures. Eight of the eighteen professionals and amateurs had abnormal CAT scans, including 75 percent of those with more than twenty pro bouts. All eighteen had abnormal neuropsych test results. "Existing medical controls and safety measures did not prevent chronic brain damage in this group of boxers," Ira Casson, the neurologist who had recently found Jerry Quarry's brain damage, and his co-authors concluded. "There is no reason to believe that future generations of boxers will be any more fortunate."

The AMA was hardly alone in its campaign against boxing. The World Medical Association started waging its own fight to ban what it called a "barbaric" sport, as did the national medical associations of Britain, Australia, Canada, and other countries. All cited the alarming incidence of not only acute brain injury from a knockout punch but also chronic brain damage from repeated head blows.

Until the fall of 1984, the American Academy of Neurology held out hope that its seven thousand member neurologists could help find ways to make the sport safer. But its president, Dr. Nelson Richards, changed his mind after hearing Muhammad Ali give an unintelligible TV interview and then hearing colleague Stanley Fahn's diagnosis of the ex-champion's parkinsonism. With Richards joining the fight against "a so-called sport that defines itself by having one man try to destroy another," his organization formally called for a ban, as did the American Neurological Association.

Even if there were a ban, of course, the odds of ever stopping people from boxing are about as good as changing what fighting reflects in human nature. With no realistic hope of outlawing the sport or even banishing head blows from it, the medical community found at least one thing that boxing officials couldn't fight them on: the need for safety reform. Unfortunately, the federal government's attempt at reform, the Professional Boxing Safety Act of 1996, was like putting a Band-Aid on a bleeder, failing even to set up a national regulatory body to oversee the health and safety of fighters. That left licensing decisions up to the individual state commissions, many of which would clear boxers to fight based on the most cursory of physicals by any kind of doctor.

New York proved an exception. During Jordan's fifteen-year tenure as chief medical officer, the New York State Athletic Commission enacted the strictest medical code of any state in the nation: all boxers had to pass annual neurological exams, CAT scans, and EEGs before they could be licensed to fight professionally, with MRIs required every three years. Revoking licenses and denying applications in as many as 5 percent of cases, Jordan noted, "We saved a few lives."

It wasn't just about saving lives, but also about preserving quality of life for the countless survivors like the protagonist in Simon and Garfunkel's 1969 hit—"The Boxer"—who "squandered [his] resistance for a pocketful of mumbles." The concern extended beyond the short-term effects of acute TBI to the long-term effects of chronic TBI. For every boxer who becomes symptomatic while still active, countless more develop deficits years after retirement. So insidious is the disease that brain damage inflicted during their glory days may not manifest itself until their golden years.

That's how it caught up with Floyd Patterson. The youngest world champion ever when he won the heavyweight crown at twenty-one in 1956, Patterson had gone on to distinguish himself in many ways throughout a twenty-year pro career. He was an anomaly—too slender, too insecure, too mild-mannered to survive without a killer punch and a killer instinct. He was the sensitive soul who, after becoming the first man ever to regain the heavyweight title, delayed his own celebration to cradle his knocked-out opponent in his arms before helping him off the canvas. He was the tortured soul who would pack a fake beard and mustache in his equipment bag as a disguise so he could slip out of arenas incognito should he suffer a humiliating defeat.

Patterson found more and more use for the disguise after being separated from his senses and his crown with seven knockdowns in the third round of his 1959 title defense against Ingemar Johansson. Though Patterson avenged that knockout a year later by rendering Johansson unconscious for eight minutes to regain the title, the humiliating losses would come as furious and fast as the fists of Sonny Liston and Muhammad Ali. Liston needed just two minutes to knock out Patterson and take away the title in 1962, and just two minutes to embarrass him again in their 1963 rematch. Two years later, Patterson challenged Ali, who'd taken the title from Liston, in a grudge match fueled by the ugly barbs they had traded over which one would be the better role model for black America. Throughout their 1965 title bout, Ali taunted, teased, and toyed with Patterson, continually pummeling him to the point of collapse only to back off as if to deliberately extend the torture. The mortifying punishment went on for twelve rounds until the ref stopped it with the challenger out on his feet. Patterson fought for another eight years until a knockout loss in his 1973 rematch with Ali convinced him to finally leave the ring at age thirty-seven.

In retirement, Patterson was often asked about the most dubious of all his feats: being knocked down more than any other heavyweight champion. "Yes," he'd reply with a proud smile, "but I also got up more than anyone." Maybe he shouldn't have. His weakness—the glass jaw that signaled his inability to take a punch—wouldn't have been such a health liability if not for his determination to keep getting up only to absorb more punishment. Beyond all the knockdowns and knockouts, there were all the punches that the aging Patterson had absorbed over twenty-two rounds in two bouts against a young up-and-comer named Jerry Quarry, the first a draw and the second a loss by split decision. The impact of all the punches a boxer like Patterson took over the course of his career—from the hardest hooks to the softest jabs—could add up to more brain damage than the knockout blows.

Patterson was maybe fifty when the cumulative effect of sixty-four professional bouts and countless sparring sessions caught up with him. In the mid-'80s, he began showing signs of dementia, often forgetting the names of people he'd known for years. Within a few years, it was clear that his affliction was more than mere forgetfulness. Even when he was appointed chairman of the New York State Athletic Commission in 1995, it was already an open secret among boxing insiders that he was no longer capable of handling a job whose duties were anything but demanding.

Three years later, the secret became public during a deposition Patterson gave for a civil suit brought by a promoter challenging the commission's ban on "ultimate fighting." Although he still appeared to be in fighting trim at sixty-three, there was a confused look behind his pleading hangdog eyes. Under questioning from a lawyer, Patterson couldn't remember the name of the heavyweight champion he dethroned to first win the world title. He couldn't remember the site or the year of that career-making title fight. He couldn't remember the names of his other opponents. He couldn't remember the names of his closest aides, his secretary, the commission's lawyer. He couldn't remember the name of his predecessor as chairman of the commission. He couldn't remember the names of his two fellow commissioners. "One's a lady and one's a man," he said finally.

This went on for three hours with no referee to step in and stop it. He seemed as dazed and bewildered as a boxer stumbling around the ring. He was confused about the most basic rules of boxing, unable to recall the size of the ring or the number of ringside judges; he didn't remember that the length of title fights had been cut to twelve rounds over a decade earlier in the wake of a nationally televised ring death. At one point, he said, "What are we talking about? I'm lost. Who's the plaintiff?" Over and over, he tried attributing his memory lapses to lack of sleep. "It's hard for me to think when I'm tired," he explained. "Sometimes, I can't even remember my wife's name, and I've been married thirty-two, thirty-three years. Sometimes, I can't even remember my own name."

Floyd Patterson, as gallant and gracious an ambassador as the savage sport had ever known, immediately resigned his position. When he died eight years later, Patterson was remembered for his familiar storybook rise, from the mean slums of Bedford-Stuyvesant to the heavyweight championship of the world, and for his all-too-familiar descent into the depths of Alzheimer's dementia—the latest in a long line of ring legends to succumb to the occupational hazard of their chosen profession.

Chapter 10

Ticking Time Bombs

On a cool fall Saturday in 2002, Dr. Bennet Omalu sat with his first cup of coffee in his Pittsburgh apartment, flipping through the channels catching bits and pieces of the morning news. One story grabbed his attention and made him set down the remote: Football Hall of Famer Mike Webster had died at the age of fifty after years of bizarre behavior and homelessness. What intrigued Omalu was not the replays of Webster's career highlights, but rather the description of the man's decade-long descent into mental illness after retiring from the NFL.

With bulging biceps and steely tenacity that won over every lunch-pail football fan in Pittsburgh, Iron Mike Webster had spent seventeen savage seasons forging a reputation as the best center in NFL history and powering a Steelers dynasty to four Super Bowl titles. Toward the end of his career, the warrior hailed for his iron will as much as his physical toughness started to come apart. By the time Webster retired at thirty-eight, his behavior had already become so odd that his wife and four kids were scared. He'd fly into rages, smashing his cherished football memorabilia, once even demolishing a porcelain sink. More disturbing were episodes like the time he got up from the dinner table, walked over to the stove, opened the oven, urinated into it, and then casually returned to the table as if he'd just used the bathroom. Webster was unable to hold down a job and squandered the family's savings through bad business investments. When the same ex-teammates who'd once voted him Steelers captain offered to help, he pushed them away. Soon he was wandering the streets homeless, sleeping some nights slumped in his dilapidated pickup truck in deserted parking lots, other nights huddled in the downtown

Pittsburgh train station near the stadium where he'd once basked in the cheers of sixty thousand Steelers fans. He spent his final years drifting in and out of lucidity, overwhelmed by dread, depression, and paranoia.

As Omalu drove to work that gray Saturday morning, still mulling over the story he'd just seen on TV, he wondered how this could have happened to such a tough, hulking, seemingly indestructible athlete. The radio droned on with talk show hosts and callers slamming Webster— once a beloved Steel City icon—as yet another sports hero who couldn't make the transition from ballfield to real life. All the talk made Omalu angry. He was sure something must have happened to Webster's brain that would explain his behavior. Omalu thought about how violent football was and how he avoided watching it for that very reason. He wondered whether the hits that linemen like Webster sustained on every play might somehow be comparable to the blows absorbed by boxers: Was it possible that football players were susceptible to something like dementia pugilistica? Omalu shook his head and thought, "It doesn't matter anyway. I'm just an insignificant doctor with no clout. What can I do?" He parked his car and, as he opened the door to his building, resolved not to spend any more time dwelling on something he could do nothing about.

Omalu walked into the coroner's office, wondering what he would find today on his autopsy table, and instantly recognized the embalmed body from what he'd just been watching on TV. It was Mike Webster.

Omalu stepped out of the autopsy suite to ask why Webster was there, since initial news reports had attributed the death to a heart attack. He was told that Webster's physician had written "chronic concussive brain injury" on the death certificate, implying that an element of trauma had contributed to the player's demise. Because that meant the death might not be due to natural causes, it fell to the coroner's office to perform an autopsy. As the forensic pathologist on duty, Omalu was responsible for determining cause of death. He cracked open Webster's chest, removed the heart, and examined it. He quickly determined that Webster had indeed died as a result of a heart attack.

Omalu, however, wasn't ready to finish the autopsy. The neuropathologist in him was sure that if he examined the brain, he could find answers to his questions about Webster's descent into depression and dementia. He carefully cut an incision from ear to ear over the crown of

Webster's head and then peeled the scalp away from the skull. After saw-
ing through the bone, he removed a cap-shaped piece of skull, revealing
the pink, corrugated lump of tissue that was Webster's brain. He carefully
slid his gloved hands under the brain and gently lifted it from the skull.
He stared at it from every angle, looking for imperfections among all the
ridges and crevices, but there were none. It looked perfectly normal. He
ran his fingers over the bumpy surface, feeling for soft spots, but there
were none. He was disappointed. With the degree of mental deterioration that Webster had exhibited in the twelve years since his retirement,
Omalu had expected to find visible signs of brain damage.

Instinctively, he started to do what he normally would when finishing
up an autopsy. He scooped up the brain and started to put it back into
Webster's skull to prepare the body for burial. But then suddenly, Omalu
heard a voice in his head whispering, "Bennet, save this brain." Omalu
paused and wondered if this was Mike Webster's soul trying to speak to
him, telling him to keep searching for the answer. Omalu knew that people could have significant symptoms with only microscopic brain damage.
If he had a chance to cut up the brain and make slides to examine under
his microscope, he might find some clues. As a rookie pathologist with
just two months on the job, he would need permission from the coroner
as well as from Webster's family to perform a more extensive examination
of the brain. In the meantime, he tucked it in a jar of preservative solution. Then he called Webster's lawyer to get permission from the family
to examine it in more detail. He explained to the lawyer that this was a
chance for Mike Webster to tell the world in death what he was unable to
say in life. It didn't take long for Omalu to get his answer—and the brain.

Omalu went to work thin-slicing the brain. He sent some of the slices
off to the University of Pittsburgh for mounting on slides and staining
with dyes that would highlight the two telltale proteins suffusing the
brains of Alzheimer's patients and of boxers suffering from dementia
pugilistica. Sure enough, when the slides came back and he put them
under his microscope, he saw clear proof of brain damage. On the slides
stained to highlight tau, he saw dark brown bloated neurons, indicating
cells stuffed with tangles of twisted protein threads. On the slides stained
to highlight amyloid beta, he saw irregular smudges of reddish brown in
between neurons, indicating clumps of the sticky protein.

Omalu wasn't sure what it all meant, so he took his slides over to the University of Pittsburgh to consult with one of the nation's leading Alzheimer's experts. Dr. Steven DeKosky pored over the slides and said, "Bennet, this is not Alzheimer's." DeKosky explained that Alzheimer's disease always starts in the hippocampus and then, over the years, wreaks havoc on that deep brain region. Omalu's slides showed no traces of damage to the hippocampus. Omalu suggested that perhaps what they were seeing was the same disease that led to dementia in boxers. Since much of the damage appeared in Webster's cortex, that made sense to DeKosky. He and Omalu both recognized the significance of the finding: the first autopsy-confirmed case of a football player found to have the same dementing brain disease previously thought to strike only punch-drunk boxers who'd taken countless blows to the head.

Omalu, who regarded pathologists like himself as advocates defending and speaking for the dead, raced off to tell Mike Webster's children and ex-wife what the brain had told him. Now he could assure them that all of the odd and inexplicable symptoms—the memory loss, the emotional swings, the behavioral problems—were not Mike's fault but rather the fault of twenty thousand hits to his helmet. It explained how the loving, caring, funny father they once knew came to be begging them to zap him into unconsciousness with a Taser gun in a desperate attempt to escape his back pain and get some sleep. It explained how he came to be squeezing Super Glue onto his gums in a confused attempt to reattach rotted teeth to his jaw. The forensic findings finally gave the family some peace and some closure—as well as some more ammunition in their ongoing battle with the NFL.

Webster had spent the last three years of his life fighting the league and its players' union for disability benefits based on his traumatic brain injury. After his claim was filed in 1999, the NFL's pension plan awarded him only partial benefits, a fraction of what he would have received for a full disability related directly to playing football. His lawyer promptly filed an appeal that included medical reports from a psychiatrist, a psychologist, and a neurologist who was handpicked by the NFL. The doctors all agreed on the diagnosis: a dementing disorder that resulted from multiple head injuries sustained playing football and that had left him disabled since his retirement in 1990. Following his death, the NFL pension board denied the appeal for retroactive benefits, holding that his disability did not show up until long after his retirement.

Now, with Omalu's autopsy, a neuropathologist had provided hard scientific evidence of the same diagnosis that the psychiatrist had made three years earlier based on symptoms: chronic traumatic encephalopathy caused by repeated head trauma sustained while playing on the offensive line. The courts would find all the medical evidence overwhelming. A federal judge ruled in favor of Webster's claim in 2005, and when the NFL challenged that, a federal appeals court unanimously upheld the ruling and awarded more than $1.5 million to the estate in retroactive benefits. Everyone seemed to agree that Iron Mike Webster had been completely and permanently disabled as a result of brain injuries from playing pro football. Everyone, that is, except the NFL.

Omalu would discover just how deep the league was digging in its cleats when he submitted his groundbreaking case study to *Neurosurgery*, the same medical journal that was in the midst of publishing a series of papers written by the NFL's Mild Traumatic Brain Injury Committee. The publication of Omalu's article in the July 2005 issue of *Neurosurgery* rocked the football establishment, coming as it did just six months after the journal had printed a study by the NFL committee concluding that multiple concussions were benign, transient events with no long-term consequences. Dr. Elliot Pellman, the NFL committee's chairman and the lead author on its controversial study, joined with his co-author Ira Casson, an expert on dementia pugilistica, in trashing Omalu's article in a long letter to the editor. They attacked everything about Omalu's paper, starting with the title—"Chronic Traumatic Encephalopathy in a National Football League Player"—because they claimed there was no evidence that Webster's condition was chronic or traumatically induced or, for that matter, even encephalopathy. They claimed the article had "serious flaws," specifically a "serious misinterpretation" of its own neuropathological findings, a "complete misunderstanding" of the condition that afflicts boxers, and a failure to show causation through an adequate clinical case history. They demanded that Omalu and DeKosky "retract their paper or sufficiently revise it and its title after more detailed investigation of this case."

Not only did Omalu refuse to retract or revise it, but by now he had another case study to back it up.

As luck would have it, Omalu had shown up for work one spring day in 2005 to find the body of another former Steelers lineman on his autopsy table. Terry Long had played eight seasons for the Steelers, the first five right alongside Webster on the offensive line. After Long retired in 1991, having already attempted suicide once with sleeping pills and rat poison, he plunged into a mental decline that paralleled Webster's. Long became volatile, irrational, impulsive, and paranoid. A tempest of bad business decisions left him deep in debt and under indictment for felony fraud. Clinical depression led to more suicide attempts and three hospitalizations for psychiatric treatment. He was just forty-five when he died after drinking antifreeze. Because suicide was suspected as the cause of death, his body wound up on Omalu's table at the Allegheny County coroner's office in Pittsburgh.

Omalu, struck by the parallel to the Webster case, jumped at the fortuitous opportunity to examine the brain of another former NFL player. To the pathologist's naked eye, Long's brain looked as normal as Webster's had. As with Webster's, Omalu stored Long's brain in preservative solution for slicing, staining, and examination. As with Webster's, Omalu peered through his microscope at Long's slides and saw clear evidence of brain damage. The dark brown blotches riddling Long's brain reminded Omalu of the bloated neurons that he'd seen on Webster's slides. Their appearance signaled the presence of tau tangles, the true telltale sign of chronic traumatic encephalopathy. With Long's slides showing none of the amyloid beta plaques found in Webster's, the tau was all Omalu needed to confirm the second case of a middle-aged football player whose brain resembled that of a demented old man twice his age.

Omalu's boss, Cyril Wecht, the controversial coroner notorious for offering expert commentary on high-profile deaths, immediately saw another chance to jump into the fray. To the lengthy list of cases he'd made news consulting on and commenting on over the years—John F. Kennedy, Elvis Presley, Sunny von Bülow, JonBenét Ramsey—Wecht added the name Terry Long. Wecht, the forensic pathologist who'd been a lightning rod since he challenged the single-bullet theory in JFK's assassination, released his office's autopsy report attributing Long's death to inflammation of the brain lining from repeated head injuries on the gridiron. "This is analogous to what is colloquially known as being punch-drunk," Wecht declared. "We believe the microscopic changes in the brain are consistent with chronic traumatic encephalopathy or a degeneration over time that set the stage for the final result. You don't have to be a doctor or an engineer or even a football player to realize that the helmet does not block out all the measured force produced when some three-hundred-pound player with a hand the size of a Christmas ham whacks you in the head dozens of times a game, season after season."

The team neurosurgeon for the Steelers, Dr. Joseph Maroon, responded quickly by attacking Wecht's statements and Omalu's findings. "I think the conclusions drawn here are preposterous and a misinterpretation of facts," Maroon told reporters. "I think it's fallacious reasoning, and I don't think it's plausible at all. Given Mister Long's history of drug abuse and suicide attempts or whatever altercations may have contributed to his demise, I think it's just bad science to conclude that football caused his death. To go back and say that he was depressed from playing in the NFL and that led to his death fourteen years later I think is purely speculative. I think it's not appropriate science when you have a history of no significant head injuries. I was the team neurosurgeon during his entire tenure with the Steelers. I rechecked my records. There was not one cerebral concussion documented in him during those entire seven years. Not one."

The fact was, Long had indeed once sustained a documented concussion severe enough that Maroon recommended he sit out at least one week. How many more went unreported was anyone's guess. That was even truer with Iron Mike Webster, a warrior revered for playing through all manner of pain for 177 consecutive games. Since neither Webster nor Long had a significant history of diagnosed concussions, alarms should have sounded as soon as chronic traumatic encephalopathy was found on autopsy. Playing on the line of scrimmage, where the collisions aren't nearly as spectacular as the full-speed crashes in the open field, Webster and Long absorbed hits to the helmet from defensive linemen launching at them every time the ball was snapped. Omalu's autopsy findings raised questions about the cumulative effect of these countless blows—the same formula implicated in the boxing epidemic known as dementia pugilistica.

Although Long's death certificate would later be amended after toxicology tests linked his fatal brain swelling directly to the antifreeze he drank, Omalu maintained that the football-induced chronic traumatic encephalopathy was a contributing factor by causing the depression that led to the suicide. By the time Omalu's second case study was published in the November 2006 issue of *Neurosurgery*, the acronym CTE had entered the football lexicon and a new variant of dementia pugilistica had crept from the ring to the gridiron.

The NFL responded by slamming Omalu in the newspapers and on television. NFL doctors attacked the science, and then the scientist. They said he was too young and too inexperienced, just a rookie pathologist in his mid-thirties who was out of his depth. They insinuated, he'd later recall with a shake of his head, that he was practicing "voodoo medicine." They questioned his motives and his ethics, denigrating him as some for-eigner—a Nigerian—out to destroy America's game and, by extension, the American way of life.

Omalu was stunned by the personal attacks. He had written his pa-pers to share what he'd learned with the world, not as an assault on the sport. He understood the appeal of sports, even if he wasn't a fan of foot-ball. While growing up in Nigeria, where he'd been born a refugee in the jungles of secessionist Biafra during a civil war air raid, he'd played the popular sport that most of the world calls football: soccer. His only exposure to American football then was through highlights glimpsed on CNN. He didn't see the appeal of American football, and didn't under-stand the game. He thought the players looked like extraterrestrials in their helmets and shoulder pads, and he found the tackling too ferocious. That opinion didn't change when he immigrated to the United States in his mid-twenties to attend college and then medical school. He was sure he was the only man in Pittsburgh who didn't spend Sunday afternoons rooting religiously for the Steelers.

Omalu, who hadn't heard of either Mike Webster or Terry Long until the day of their autopsies, would eventually come to wish he had never heard their names or looked at their brains. He hated picking up the newspaper and seeing his own name dragged through the mud by the NFL doctors trying to discredit and dismiss his findings. He felt threatened by the NFL; he was just a little doctor going up against a multibillion-dollar goliath. Next time an ex-player died, he wouldn't be so anxious to perform the autopsy.

On a cold winter night late in 2006, Omalu had just settled onto his living room couch to watch the evening news when the phone rang. Annoyed that the phone was intruding at dinnertime, he decided to ignore it. His wife quietly got up from the couch and answered it. She didn't recognize the name of the caller and was about to hang up on him. Then she paused and decided to ask her husband if he knew someone named Chris Nowinski. The name rang a bell with Omalu. Mildly curious what it was about, Omalu nodded to his wife and took the phone.

Chris Nowinski had called Omalu with an unusual, albeit simple, proposition: If Nowinski could get another football player's brain, would Omalu be willing to perform the autopsy? Nowinski had seen an obituary of a former NFL player as he was reading his morning newspaper and something had sparked in his brain. He wondered if Philadelphia Eagles star Andre Waters might have been suffering from the same concussion-related problems as Mike Webster and Terry Long. Now, Nowinski was offering to call Waters's family to ask if they would allow Omalu to examine the player's brain; Nowinski would tell the family that an autopsy might help not only answer their questions surrounding Waters's odd behavior and suicide, but also shed more light on the possible connection between football and dementia.

Nowinski had a personal stake in the answer to that question. Over the years, he'd experienced many hits to the head as a college football player and a pro wrestler, and he was currently suffering from post-concussion syndrome. He wanted to know if he was at greater risk of developing early-onset dementia.

A big, athletic kid, Nowinski had always been drawn to football, but his mom had vetoed his participation until high school. She was aware of all the injuries in younger kids and she didn't want her son hurt. Once he reached high school and went out for the team, it was clear that he was made for the sport. He had the hundred-page playbook memorized in a single afternoon and was voted captain the third day of practice. Nowinski played hard, and by the time he was a sophomore, he'd injured both his shoulders. That didn't slow the enterprising linebacker down a bit. He just switched from battering with his shoulders to hammering with his head.

He quickly realized that this was actually an improvement since it was an even more effective means of thrusting opposing players out of the way. It never once occurred to him that the technique could hurt his brain—he figured that he was big and tough and that his head was protected by a helmet.

By the time he was a junior, a host of colleges, including Harvard and Princeton, were courting the student with exceptional SAT scores, an excellent grade point average, and prodigious football talent. Nowinski chose Harvard on the advice of his high school coach and was soon using the head-as-battering-ram technique to bowl over players in college games as an All–Ivy League defensive lineman. He still wasn't worried about his brain, even after one concussion left him calling friends by the wrong names at dinner and another turned the sky a strange orange hue.

When graduation time rolled around in the spring of 2000, Nowinski was at a loss to figure out what to do with his life. In college, he'd developed an interest in acting and he was hoping to find some sort of career that would allow him to explore that further. He had also become a big fan of professional wrestling, often crowding around the TV with his roommates and hailing each rousing bodyslam with a shout and a high-five. He thought it looked like fun, and as a lark, he checked to see what was involved in becoming a pro wrestler. The more he learned, the more it sounded like a real option to him. Here was a chance to have a job that would be an outlet for both his love of theater and his penchant for the physical. The promoters at World Wrestling Entertainment welcomed his acting talents, his sculpted six-foot-five physique, and the cachet of having a Harvard-educated star to hype.

Always with a flair for the dramatic, he enjoyed strutting out into the ring with his varsity letterman jacket and assuming the character of "Chris Harvard" before huge crowds of screaming fans. Though the beginning and ending moves were choreographed ahead of time, much of the rest was improvised. It reminded him of plays and drama classes he'd enjoyed in college. He had a lot of fun playing the vilified Ivy League snob—until the concussions started piling up.

Over the course of three years, he had four major concussions, each one worse than the last. Still, he managed to bounce back from the headaches, the blackouts, and the temporary blindness after the first three concussions without giving a thought to long-term consequences. Then, during a tag-team match in 2003, Nowinski got kicked in the chin by an opponent. As the boot made contact, it seemed as if everything around him exploded. He lay on his back staring up at the lights wondering why they were so fuzzy, wondering where he was and what he was doing there. Then he turned his head to the side, saw the screaming crowd and the referee, and suddenly remembered the match. He thought about getting up, but his head felt like it was in a vise. Before he could even register what was happening, another wrestler appeared seemingly out of nowhere and leapt through the air, landing his full three hundred pounds on Nowinski. The pain in Nowinski's head was now excruciating. Somehow he made it through the rest of the match, but when it was over, he went to the locker room and stretched out on the cold cement floor without pausing to put on a shirt. His head hurt too much for him to move.

This time the concussion symptoms hung on tenaciously, even after weeks of rest. His head would throb for days on end. Each night he'd lay his head on the pillow, hoping that the ache would be gone in the morning. His memory, which had been almost photographic, was now spotty at best. He couldn't recall anyone's names; he'd forget important appointments; he couldn't even summon his password when he sat down at the computer.

Nowinski went to doctor after doctor only to receive the same response every time: Just be patient, you'll be better in a couple of weeks. After several months had passed, he realized that his doctors didn't understand what had happened to him any better than he did. Resolving to find out more on his own, he became a regular at Harvard's medical school library, pulling and photocopying every study that said anything about concussions, and about brain injury in general. The research came naturally to him. Since college he'd been working part-time as an analyst for a Boston-area biotech firm that did consulting work for pharmaceutical companies. It didn't take long to dig up all the studies—there just wasn't that much information out there.

Some of what he read made him shake his head in disbelief. Study after study found concussions to be relatively rare in athletes. Nowinski knew from personal experience that that couldn't be right, but he understood how the researchers might have gotten it so wrong. He thought,

"OK, I've had six concussions that I know of. I told zero people about them. That must be what everyone else is doing, too." Nowinski dug deeper and eventually found studies showing that up to half of football players were being concussed every season. That made a lot more sense. So did the studies showing that concussions seemed to add up, with increasing numbers of jolts to the head leading to longer recovery times and a heightened risk of sustaining more concussions. Nowinski saw references to something called post-concussion syndrome and figured that might explain the symptoms that had been dogging him for the past year. What worried him was that nobody seemed to be able to predict how long the syndrome might last. It was at about this time that a friend referred Nowinski to Dr. Robert Cantu, one of the nation's leading concussion experts.

Cantu did a series of tests and confirmed that Nowinski did indeed have post-concussion syndrome. The neurosurgeon explained that concussions could signal actual damage to the brain and that the damage could result in permanent deficits. Cantu couldn't tell Nowinski exactly when—or if—all the concussion symptoms would resolve. What Cantu could say was that another concussion would lead to worse symptoms, a longer recovery time, and maybe permanent brain damage. That was enough to convince Nowinski to retire, at twenty-four.

Though he now had his diagnosis, Nowinski continued to scour the scientific literature for information on concussions. Some of what he found was downright scary. He read the studies showing that traumatic brain injury increased the risk of developing Alzheimer's disease. Then he saw population studies suggesting that the risks of depression and dementia were higher among pro football players than the general population. Each time Nowinski found some new and startling result, he'd e-mail the researchers to get more information.

All the while, he was thinking about the significance of what he was learning. He started to wonder about all the other players who assumed, just as he had, that concussions were benign and transient. More important, he started thinking about the millions of kids playing football. In the back of his mind were the words his mother spoke as he was heading off to college. "You were born with gifts," she'd said, "and you have an obligation to use those gifts to help people." He decided it was his responsibility to sound an alarm. When he talked things over with Cantu, the neurosurgeon suggested that Nowinski write a book that would expose football's threat to the brain.

As Nowinski continued to dig through the scientific literature, he stumbled upon Omalu's first paper. He was stunned, and a little frightened, to see that a pathologist had found concrete evidence of chronic traumatic encephalopathy in a football player. After reading the paper, Nowinski wanted to know more. He shot off an e-mail to Omalu explaining his interest in long-term damage from concussions and asking if the neuropathologist would consent to an interview for a book. During the hour they spoke, Omalu told Nowinski about the Webster and Long cases, about the symptoms the players had exhibited after their retirements, and about the pathology he had found in their brains. He explained what was known about CTE from studies of boxers. Nowinski put it all down in a chapter in his book and then moved on to other topics.

He didn't think about Omalu again until the day he opened the newspaper and saw Andre Waters's obituary. Nowinski remembered Waters as an aggressive defensive back for the Eagles, one of the hardest hitters in the NFL. The safety's fierce tackles and ferocious hits had earned him the nickname Dirty Waters and had led to a rule banning defensive players from hitting quarterbacks below the waist while still in the pocket. That hard-hitting reputation got Nowinski wondering about Waters's concussion history. Sure enough, the more Nowinski searched the web for clues, the more concussions he uncovered. He found one newspaper clip in which Waters was asked in the midst of his twelve-year career how many concussions he'd sustained. Waters had replied simply, "I think I lost count at fifteen." Another clip told about the time Waters was hospitalized following a seizure on the team plane after a game in which he'd suffered a concussion.

What happened to Waters after his 1995 retirement reminded Nowinski of Webster and Long. As Waters drifted from job to job as an assistant college football coach, he fell into a frighteningly familiar pattern of mental deterioration: memory loss, paranoia, depression, suicide attempts. A few days before Thanksgiving of 2006, Waters shot himself in the head at his Florida home. The report of his death at the age of forty-four made Nowinski think immediately of Long's descent into suicidal depression. Nowinski thought that two former NFL players committing suicide in their mid-forties couldn't just be a coincidence. So he called the pathologist who had examined Long's brain as well as Webster's.

Omalu listened to Nowinski's proposition and then said he'd be willing to examine Waters's brain. But Nowinski would have to be the one to convince Waters's family that the autopsy could answer important questions—both for them and for others. Once Omalu was on board, Nowinski realized the enormity of what he'd volunteered to do. He was nervous about making what he recognized would be the hardest cold call he'd ever made. He sat down and typed out a script so he'd get the words right on the first try. He would explain that he, too, had suffered damage from repeated concussions and that he believed that Waters's brain might help prove dementia could result from them.

He went to his office at the consulting firm and shut the door so he wouldn't be disturbed. He took a deep breath and picked up the phone and rang Waters's mother. There was no answer and no message machine. Over the next few days, he tried a few more times. Then he found a phone number for Waters's sister Tracy Lane. After several attempts, he was finally able to get her on the phone.

He looked down at his script and began: "Hi, I'm Chris Nowinski. I used to play football and I used to be a professional wrestler. I had a lot of concussions, and that's why I care about this and why I'm calling." Lane listened quietly as he went on. "I was hoping you might allow your brother's brain to be examined by a pathologist to see if he had brain damage from all those concussions," Nowinski said. "I think your brother's brain could help future generations because it could help us confirm a link between concussions and depression and maybe dementia."

Lane told Nowinski that the family did want to know what had gone wrong with Andre, why he had transformed from gregarious and giving to depressed and paranoid. Most of all, they wanted to understand why he had killed himself. Nowinski told Lane that a brain autopsy might give them the answers they needed. She said she'd talk to the rest of the family and get back to him.

Nowinski waited impatiently—until one day the phone rang with Waters's niece on the other end. Kwana Pittman told him that the family had designated her as their representative. She asked him to again explain why he needed her Uncle Andre's brain. Nowinski pulled out the script again and started at the top. When he was done, Pittman told him that the family had researched his background and checked out his just-published book, *Head Games: Football's Concussion Crisis*. She told him that she trusted that his heart was in the right place and that she thought his experience with concussions would give him empathy. "OK," she said finally, "let's do this." They talked for a few minutes longer, and as Pittman was about to hang up, she said, "You know, the only reason I'm doing this is because you were a victim."

The next step was to get the brain from the Tampa coroner's of-fice. The medical examiner there told Nowinski that only a few scraps of brain tissue remained, adding up to less than one-tenth of the original brain. When the package arrived in the mail, Omalu tore it open and was shocked to find how little of Waters's brain remained. The five pieces fit easily in the palm of Omalu's hand. He worried that there might not be enough brain tissue for an accurate analysis. As it turned out, there was more than enough to prove that Waters had developed CTE.

Once Omulu had the diagnosis, he arranged to meet Nowinski down in Tampa, where they could present their findings to Waters's family and get a history of the former player's symptoms. When Nowinski and Omalu arrived, the family couldn't help but be struck by the appearance of this odd couple at the door: the trim, six-foot-five former lineman towering over the stubby, round-faced scientist. The family would come away from the meeting relieved to have an explanation for Waters's tragic decline. Nowinski and Omalu came away with a partnership.

They were now in the business of brain hunting, Nowinski surfing the web each day to find brains for Omalu to slice up. Since the work had nothing to do with his day job, Omalu had to take it home. That's how he had done it with Waters's brain. He had set up an impromptu lab in his garage, where he could slice the brain into sections to be sent off for staining and mounting on slides.

When the Waters story broke on the front page of *The New York Times*, it focused public attention on the possibility that America's most popular sport might be destroying the brains of its own stars. This was the third case of CTE that Omalu had documented in middle-aged NFL re-tirees. It was becoming harder and harder to argue that his findings were just anomalies. The partnership with Nowinski gave Omalu some much-needed moral support. He didn't feel so alone anymore. He and Nowinski earned a reputation as muckrakers confronting the NFL's concussion deniers. The story began to take on a life of its own. Nowinski became a go-to guy for interviews on the concussion controversy, popping up on national TV shows and all over talk radio. He was clean-cut, soft-spoken, and articulate, the voice of the odd couple both in public and in private. He was still the one who took on the responsibility of calling the grieving relatives to ask for the brain of a recently deceased loved one.

Early in 2007, Nowinski and Omalu heard that a coroner's office in upstate New York might have some brain tissue from another former NFL player. Justin Strzelczyk, a Steelers offensive lineman like Webster and Long, was only thirty-six when he died in a fiery wreck after a high-speed police chase in 2004. In the six years since a knee injury ended his nine-season NFL career, Strzelczyk had spiraled into depression and paranoia. Friends and family no longer recognized the mountain of a man who looked like a grizzly but acted more like a teddy bear off the field. His behavior became erratic, his moods mercurial. He was sure his phone was tapped by the devil, and he complained of hearing voices from "the evil ones." One morning, after his pickup truck brushed a car on the New York State Thruway while speeding at 100 mph, Strzelczyk caught the attention of some highway patrolmen, who gave chase. Forty miles later, when he failed to even slow down, the police threw spikes onto the road. With one tire blown out, he continued to fly down the highway, crossing over the median into oncoming traffic and, after another four harrowing miles, smashed into a tanker truck head-on. The autopsy showed no drugs or alcohol in his system. Strzelczyk's friends and family were at a loss to explain what had happened to him.

Three years after the wreck, Nowinski called Strzelczyk's mother and told her that he might be able to find some answers and give the family some closure. All he would need was her permission for Omalu to examine Strzelczyk's brain for signs of CTE. Omalu received the brain early in the spring and began the process of slicing it up, sometimes moving his operation from his garage out to the balcony when the weather was warm and sunny. Once again, he sent the tissue samples out for staining and mounting. Once again, they came back with clear signs of CTE, this time verified by two independent neuropathologists. What was particularly striking about Strzelczyk's case was that he was just in his mid-thirties and he had no reported concussions playing football at any level. That was the fourth case of CTE that Omalu had found out of the five brains he'd examined. The one brain with no abnormal proteins came from an active player who was just twenty-four when he died, which wasn't surprising because CTE is a progressive disease that takes years to develop. Omalu began to lobby to have football-induced CTE recognized as a distinct condition. "Gridiron dementia," he dubbed it.

Nowinski wasn't limiting his investigations to football players. In the summer of 2007, when he read the shocking news that pro wrestler Chris Benoit had murdered his wife and his seven-year-old son before hanging himself, Nowinski wondered whether CTE had played any role in the tragedy. Nowinski knew Benoit from their WWE days and felt comfortable approaching the family to ask for the wrestler's brain. When the stained slides came back, Omalu saw in a forty-year-old brain the worst case of CTE he'd observed up to that point. The findings made sense to Nowinski because Benoit had once admitted to having more concussions than he could count.

Benoit was the first athlete examined under the auspices of a newly formed organization called the Sports Legacy Institute. Nowinski, Omalu, Cantu, and another neurosurgeon, Dr. Julian Bailes, had founded the institute to formalize research into CTE. From the beginning, the group planned to affiliate with a major university. As it turned out, there was one right in Nowinski's backyard. He learned of it fortuitously: one of his friends had been impressed with a presentation by a Boston University neuropsychologist, Robert Stern, on the link between head trauma and Alzheimer's disease. The friend immediately called Nowinski suggesting he contact Stern, co-director of the Alzheimer's Disease Clinical and Research Program at BU.

Stern and the Alzheimer's program seemed to be exactly what Nowinski wanted for the Sports Legacy Institute. What made BU even more enticing was its connection with the Brain Bank at the Bedford VA Medical Center. Better still, the connection would offer a neuropathologist with decades of experience. Dr. Ann McKee had the kind of expertise that Nowinski was looking for. She was not only the neuropathologist for the Bedford VA, but she was also director for several brain banks housed there: the BU Alzheimer's Disease Center, the Framingham Heart Study, and the Centenarian Study.

Not long afterward, the Sports Legacy Institute joined with the BU Alzheimer's Disease Center to form the Center for the Study of Traumatic Encephalopathy. The new center would go a long way toward legitimizing research that had previously been in danger of being dismissed as sloppy and seat-of-the-pants. With her extensive experience examining both healthy and diseased brains, McKee would give the new center the credibility it needed.

Taped to the door of Ann McKee's office is a broad black banner asking everyone who enters a whimsical question in white block letters: "got brains?"

The sign gives visitors their first sense of the scientist who works in the small, tightly packed office on the first floor of a nondescript brick building at the Bedford VA in eastern Massachusetts. Step inside and there are plenty of other clues to who she is. McKee's desk is surrounded by curiosities that echo the whimsical note sounded on her door. Huddled atop one filing cabinet, Mr. Potato Head shares space with a skull and a bobblehead doll of New England Patriots quarterback Tom Brady. A statuette of another superstar quarterback, Brett Favre in his Green Bay Packers uniform, stands alongside medical texts on a bookshelf as a nod to the storied hometown franchise she's rooted for since she was a little girl back in Wisconsin. A tomboy who grew up playing backyard football every summer, she would have followed her two older brothers onto the gridiron—"if," she quips, "I hadn't had the misfortune of being born a girl."

The walls of the office are papered with photos of family and friends—and poster-sized images displaying the brains of people she's become close to only after their deaths. Stacked in a small wooden filing cabinet beside McKee's cluttered desk are sliding shelves containing stained slices from brains she's already examined. McKee refers to each glass shelf by the name of the brain's former owner—unless she's been asked by family members not to divulge the identity of the person to whom the tissue belonged. In those cases, she simply refers to the shelf by some other identifying detail: the boxer, the football player, the eighteen-year-old.

She grabs one of the glass shelves and lays it on her desk to point out the differences between CTE and Alzheimer's disease. Early on you can distinguish the two by their symptoms, she explains. Alzheimer's patients exhibit memory problems right from the start. Those who suffer from CTE are more likely to demonstrate personality changes, like moodiness or anger. Late in the course of the two diseases, it can be impossible to tell them apart if you're going only on symptoms. But when you look at the brains, the differences are unmistakable. Pointing to the brain tissue under glass, McKee says, "This was a man with Alzheimer's disease. You can see how evenly distributed and regular the tau is." The slice isn't even magnified and still it's impossible to miss the brownish tinge that signifies the presence of tau tangles in a multitude of neurons. Then she pulls out a second glass shelf and lays it next to the first one. "And this is a football player," she says. "You can see how much more selective and patchy the tau deposits are." What's even more telling, she says, is that the brain of this football player, like many others with CTE, has no amyloid beta deposits. Though CTE sometimes comes with amyloid beta, the deposits are generally small.

Next, McKee points to a brain image from a boxer—her first case of CTE, back in 2003. She got the boxer's brain shortly after he died. When the brain arrived, she didn't know that it had come from a boxer, or even that he was old when he died. Whenever McKee first meets a new brain, she makes sure she has no background information on the person who originally owned it. She doesn't want to know anything about the former owner's death, or any diagnosed diseases. That kind of information would only serve to bias her first impression. She wants to make sure her judgments of this new acquaintance will be based solely on the brain tissue before her.

When she started to examine the boxer's brain slices, she was puzzled. She had never seen anything like this before: there was no amyloid beta, and the tau was distributed in an odd, patchy fashion. She could tell that this person had suffered from some sort of neurodegenerative disease, but she didn't recognize which one it was. The one thing she did know for sure was that it wasn't Alzheimer's because there was no amyloid beta.

As the weeks passed, McKee continued to puzzle over the brain. She had her staff slice and prepare additional sections, but the more closely she examined the damage, the less it looked like anything she'd ever seen. There was one clue, though. Some of the slides suggested that the brain's former owner had suffered from some sort of head trauma because the heaviest damage was in regions that are often harmed when the head is hit. But she couldn't explain what that had to do with all the deterioration she was seeing. She pored through neuropathology texts, until one day she finally saw illustrations showing brain tissue from some ex-boxers. They looked so much like her guy that she was sure she was looking at someone who had been punch-drunk when he was alive.

As it turned out, the man had been living at the VA for years before his death at age seventy-two and his doctors had diagnosed him with Alzheimer's disease. When McKee went to them with her findings, they told her that the man had been a professional boxer, a world champion in fact. They had assumed that the boxing had nothing to do with his dementia because he'd retired more than two decades before he started showing symptoms. They had assumed that if his dementia arose out of blows to the head while boxing, there would have been signs much sooner. McKee told the doctors what she had only recently learned herself: the neurodegenerative process that is kicked off by boxing usually doesn't manifest itself with clear symptoms until many years after a fighter has quit the ring.

As far as the outside world was concerned, Paul Pender had died with Alzheimer's disease. That's what the obituaries all reported, quoting a Bedford VA spokeswoman who had gotten the diagnosis from his doctors. And that's what the public perception would remain, since McKee and others have never revealed the identity of the CTE patient. Pender, a skinny Brookline firefighter-turned-prizefighter, was an unknown when he challenged Sugar Ray Robinson for the world middleweight championship in 1960. "Paul who?" the aging champ had deadpanned. Pender wrested the title from Robinson in a stunning upset, then proved that it wasn't a fluke five months later by winning their rematch with another fifteen-round split decision. Pender went on to lose and regain the title over the next two years, then retired at age thirty-two after forty-eight pro bouts.

Eventually McKee put the intriguing case aside and didn't think much about it until three years later, when another brain showed up with the same type of pathology. She quickly concluded that this was another boxer with CTE. Just as in the first case, the man had been living at the VA for years before he died. But when McKee went back to his doctors with her diagnosis, they told her that she must be wrong: the patient had no history of head trauma. They were convinced this was a case of Alzheimer's, based on his symptoms. McKee was so sure her diagnosis was right that she called the man's family to ask about his life and whether he'd had any history of head trauma. A little surprised, the family said that the man had indeed boxed in his twenties.

Two years later, when Chris Nowinski contacted her about examining brain tissue for the Center for the Study of Traumatic Encephalopathy, McKee was excited and enthusiastic. Here was a group offering to bring her more brains with possible CTE. She signed on right away. What made the partnership even more interesting to her was the promise of brains from athletes other than boxers. This was a chance to begin to answer questions about CTE, like how much head trauma it took to spark the development of the neurodegenerative disease.

The first of the football player brains arrived in fairly short order. It belonged to John Grimsley, a former Houston Oilers linebacker who had accidentally shot himself to death while cleaning a pistol early in 2008. During the years after his retirement, Grimsley had begun to show symptoms that worried his wife, Virginia. He had always been an easygoing guy, but now he was short-tempered and snappish. His memory problems were impossible to ignore. Over and over, she'd tell him something and it just wouldn't stick in his brain. He'd go to the video rental store and bring back movies they'd just watched. On top of that, he was having regular headaches and problems sleeping. Virginia couldn't figure out what was going on with her husband—until she saw a TV program that featured Chris Nowinski's crusade to make football safer. The report included the stories of football players like Mike Webster and Terry Long, and their descent into dementia. Not long after that, John Grimsley shot himself. Virginia was sure the accident was the result of his deteriorating memory, that he had just forgotten there was a bullet in the chamber.

She was making arrangements for his funeral when the phone call came. A friend in the next room picked up and then called out to Virginia, "It's someone named Chris Nowinski. He—"

Virginia interrupted and said, "Tell him I know who he is, and I know what he wants. Tell him he can have it."

John Grimsley's brain came to McKee from the coroner sliced and ready to be stained. Once she had the slides in front of her, McKee couldn't help but be struck by how similar this brain looked to those of the boxers. Here again was the dark brown ribbon of tau tracing the outer rim of the brain. As with the boxers, there was so much tau that she could easily see the clumps with the naked eye. When she looked at the slices under the microscope, she could see that neurons had died in several regions of the brain, including the hippocampus—which might explain Grimsley's problems with memory. She could also see dense patches of tau tangles scattered throughout a number of brain regions. Like the first boxer's, this brain had not even a trace of amyloid beta. McKee was convinced: this was another case of CTE.

When asked how she knew that the pathology she was seeing in the forty-five-year-old football player was due to head trauma and not something that normally occurs in the general population, McKee had a ready answer. "I've looked at thousands of brains," she said. "I have examined the brains of lots of eighty-year-olds from the Framingham study and it's not normal to have this much tau. There are eighty-year-olds with nothing. In fact, I've examined the brain of a one-hundred-and-ten-year-old and it was pristine. I can tell you, this is not a normal part of aging."

McKee wrote up a scholarly review of all known cases of CTE that had been confirmed by a neuropathologist and included her two boxers and the football player. The article was published in the *Journal of Neuropathology & Experimental Neurology* in July 2009. Meanwhile, athletes' brains were showing up at a rate of one a month. By spring of 2010, McKee had examined the brains of twelve football players whose ages when they died ranged from eighteen to over eighty. All twelve had pathology consistent with CTE, varying from mild to severe. By this time McKee had also examined the brains of twelve other athletes in high-contact sports—boxers, wrestlers, and hockey players—and found CTE in all of them. Not all of the athletes had shown symptoms before they died. But in general, the more severe the pathology, the more likely it was that an athlete would have been showing clear signs of the disease.

McKee wasn't the only neuropathologist busily autopsying athletes' brains in search of CTE and other traumatically induced diseases. Bennet Omalu was also still on the trail of "gridiron dementia." Following an acrimonious split with Nowinski, Omalu had teamed up with another disgruntled Sports Legacy Institute co-founder, the neurosurgeon Julian Bailes. The two doctors had become close after Bailes publicly defended Omalu's groundbreaking postmortem studies in the face of the NFL's harsh criticism. Bailes had a personal connection with the former players Omalu had autopsied, having gotten to know Mike Webster, Terry Long, and Justin Strzelczyk during a ten-year stint as a Steelers team physician. In 2009, Bailes launched his own CTE lab at West Virginia University, where he'd long served as chairman of neurosurgery, and tapped Omalu to help build a brain bank similar to the one Nowinski and McKee ran. In short order, a heated rivalry sprang up between the two labs. They would compete for the brains of recently deceased players, once asking a family to split the brain 50-50 and sometimes publicly squabbling over which group deserved credit for a particular CTE diagnosis. Bailes and Omalu found themselves having to play catch-up with the well-oiled assembly line and publicity machine that Nowinski had built at BU with McKee and Cantu.

Nowinski, in the meantime, was innovating another strategy to build his brain bank: he had begun to solicit living players for brain donations. Instead of getting easier, it was getting harder to make cold calls to grieving relatives to ask for the brains of their just-deceased loved ones. He decided it would be a lot less daunting to ask the living to agree to donate their own brains upon death. By spring of 2010, he had commitments from more than three hundred athletes to donate their brains to his brain bank. "Some of the guys are doing it to protect their sons," Nowinski says. "They recognize this is a problem, and they think if they can be part of the solution, they want to do it." Included among athletes who agreed to donate their own brains is Nowinski himself. On the list of donation agreements gathered by Nowinski are some that had to be signed by wives rather than the athletes themselves. Though the players are still alive, they are too debilitated by dementia to make the decision. Among them are two former NFL teammates, John Mackey and Ralph Wenzel.

• • •

The reception for former NFL players was getting noisy and Sylvia Mackey decided to retreat to an empty conference room to get her husband away from the din. As they sat quietly at a conference table, she noticed another couple coming through the door, the wife tightly grasping her husband's hand. Sylvia didn't recognize the hulking sixty-three-year-old former player or his wife, but she did recognize the signs of the disease that was ravaging his brain.

Sylvia got up, walked across the room, and introduced herself. Then she looked directly into Eleanor Perfetto's eyes and said gently, "Your husband has dementia."

Eleanor nodded and replied softly, "Yours does, too."

Even though she hadn't spotted John Mackey's symptoms from across the room, Eleanor recognized the name. Like most everyone else in Baltimore, she knew that John Mackey had been diagnosed with dementia, just as she knew that he had been a superstar for the team that once enthralled the city, the Colts. Now she finally had the chance to bond with another wife who was going through the same ordeal that she was with her husband, Ralph Wenzel. Sitting at the conference table, the two women shared experiences as their husbands stared blankly off into space.

They started with day-to-day caregiving challenges, but soon moved on to the topic that was threatening to make their lives impossible: finances. Sylvia said she'd had to go back to work several years earlier at the age of fifty-six, taking a job as a flight attendant. The Mackeys needed the money as well as the health insurance the job afforded. They never had much of a nest egg—John had earned less than $50,000 per season during a ten-year Hall of Fame career that ended in 1972—and his pension of $1,950 a month wasn't enough to cover their living expenses, let alone the escalating cost of his care. For her part, Eleanor was afraid that Ralph's worsening dementia might send them into bankruptcy. Though she had a good job as a senior director at a major pharmaceutical company, she knew it wouldn't be enough as Ralph's disease progressed. Ralph, who had made so little during his seven-year career as a backup lineman that he depended on offseason jobs to make ends meet, was receiving only $925 a month from his NFL pension. Eleanor was already searching for an assisted-living facility because she knew she wouldn't be able to care for him at home much longer. Good ones were expensive, and she didn't know where the money was going to come from.

Sylvia nodded reassuringly and told Eleanor that help might be on the way. She'd been lobbying the NFL to create a program that would help families take care of former players who had developed dementia. A few months earlier, in the spring of 2006, Sylvia had written a three-page letter to the NFL commissioner, Paul Tagliabue, in which she described her husband's decline and explained how it was going to ruin her family financially. She told him that dementia was "a slow, deteriorating, ugly, caregiver-killing, degenerative, brain-destroying, tragic horror." She pleaded with him to help her family and all the others struggling to care for retired players with disabilities like her husband's.

When it came to dealing with the NFL, Sylvia had learned the art of negotiation by borrowing a page from her husband's playbook. A soft-spoken leader by example on the playing field, John Mackey had emerged as the outspoken ringleader of the fledgling players' union at the bargaining table. Elected the first president of the modern NFL Players Association in 1970, he organized a strike and led the union through bitter negotiations to win an improved pension and benefits package, then sued the NFL for the right of players to bargain with any team and become true free agents once their contracts expired. By taking on the NFL's imperious owners and beating them at their own game, he cleared the way for the players who followed him to become rich. Unfortunately, Mackey and his peers never got to reap the rewards of the multibillion-dollar monopoly they helped build. Salaries were low—players earned less in a full season than today's stars can make in a single series of downs—and careers short. Even today, the average NFL career lasts barely three years; football remains the only major sport that does not have guaranteed contracts that pay off in the event of career-ending injury; and an alarming number of players limp away with physical infirmities and with cognitive impairments that might not show up until years later. For retirees from Mackey's generation, those consequences were here now.

Sylvia Mackey knew better than to apply for disability benefits from a league notoriously stingy with pensions related to football's occupational hazards. She considered filing a worker's compensation claim, but the futility of that was clear to anyone following Mike Webster's tortuous case. Now that her husband could no longer advocate for himself, Sylvia found another way to appeal to the NFL for help on his behalf. She took her case to Tagliabue and then to his successor as NFL commissioner, Roger Goodell, to win support from the owners her husband once battled. Then she pressed the Players Association for months until the union her husband once led finally acquiesced.

The night they met, Sylvia told Eleanor that the details were currently being worked out on a program to help take care of retirees suffering from dementia. She said she was pretty sure that the NFL would do the right thing and put it in place soon. In the meantime, the women exchanged phone numbers and e-mail addresses, and soon became a support group of two.

A few months later, the league adopted the 88 Plan, named for the number John Mackey had worn on his jersey. The program would provide up to $88,000 per year for institutional care and up to $50,000 per year for home care. Sylvia and Eleanor were among the first to apply, and their husbands became the first two recipients.

The NFL made it clear that the 88 Plan was in no way an admission that concussions sustained on the football field were linked to dementia. Rather, the program was promoted as simply an effort to help care for the growing population of aging retirees suffering from dementia. Sylvia had never pressed the NFL to admit to a link, though she certainly had reason to suspect that football was the likely cause. All she had to do was think back to those fall Sunday afternoons she spent watching the Colts and remember the way her husband played the game.

The NFL had never seen a receiver quite like John Mackey. He possessed the strength of a lineman, the speed of a sprinter, the hands of a surgeon. Whenever he caught a pass, defensive backs would cringe at the sight of this six-foot-two, 225-pound locomotive, ball cradled under one of his massive arms, rumbling toward them like a runaway train. Rampaging around, over, and through would-be tacklers, Mackey revolutionized the position of tight end. To a position previously reserved for lumbering blockers, he brought the electrifying ability to break open a game with a single rousing play—like the pass he grabbed, after it tipped off two sets of fingertips, and then converted into a record seventy-five-yard touchdown to help lead the Baltimore Colts to their first Super Bowl title in 1971. The same breakneck style that made him history's greatest tight end may also have made him football's most famous dementia victim. In Sylvia's mind, the touchdown that stuck out most did not occur in the 1971 Super Bowl, but rather in a meaningless exhibition game six years earlier. She was haunted by the frightening image of him galloping across the goal line, crashing headfirst at full speed into an unforgiving goalpost, then staggering in dazed confusion to the opposing team's huddle and then over to a seat on the opposing team's bench. That concussion was so spectacular that it led the NFL to move the goalposts back off the goal line deep into the end zone. Whether it also led to her husband's early onset of dementia is something Sylvia could only suspect.

John was barely into his fifties when Sylvia began to notice signs that something was wrong with him. His memory was becoming spotty, his judgment impaired, his moods volatile. Always a tireless ball of energy who inspired teammates with his work ethic, he was now lying in bed for hours on end just staring at the Weather Channel. Once so articulate a union leader that he could go jaw to jaw with arrogant NFL owners and rally striking players with spellbinding speeches, he was now often at a loss for words.

By the time he was sixty, his symptoms had intensified to the point where Sylvia was worried enough to take him to a neurologist. The doctor diagnosed frontotemporal dementia, a rare degenerative brain disease that starts in the frontal lobes. The diagnosis could explain his behavioral and personality changes as well as his lapses in judgment, especially when it came to business decisions. That was small consolation to Sylvia, who now realized that nobody could help her husband and that his condition was just going to deteriorate. The only saving grace was that John seemed completely oblivious to his fate.

He still loved being John Mackey, football hero. He still loved going out in public and signing autographs for adoring fans. He would proudly flash his oversized Super Bowl ring and Hall of Fame ring. And he would proudly tell his favorite story—about his record seventy-five-yard touchdown in the Super Bowl—over and over again to the same fan without realizing he'd already told it. He could remember the 1971 Super Bowl like it was yesterday, but he couldn't remember what he did yesterday. He could pick out old teammates from highlight reels, but he couldn't recognize them when he ran into them at alumni events. He could spend hours playing with his grandchildren, but he couldn't remember their visit minutes after they'd left.

Even more troubling than the memory problems were the personality and behavioral changes. Once calm, measured, and mild-mannered, he now had a hair-trigger temper and would sometimes scream and curse at his wife in public. At times he was so explosive that he scared even Sylvia. This wasn't the man she had married four decades before. They had made the perfect All-American couple—the handsome football star and the beautiful fashion model—always the envy of the eyes watching them dance at galas as if they were Fred and Ginger. The advent of John's symptoms changed all that. At first, they irritated his wife and strained relationships with his grown children. When the diagnosis came, it brought understanding and compassion. Sylvia missed the man she married, but she stuck by the man he'd become. She didn't blame him for the outbursts, the insensitivity, the ugly words—she blamed the disease.

Getting others to understand was another matter. John's paranoia made him suspicious of people, sure that they were trying to steal his possessions. A few years after the diagnosis, John and Sylvia were traveling to an autograph-signing event when his Super Bowl and Hall of Fame rings set off an airport metal detector. He refused to remove the rings, his most prized possessions. When two armed security guards moved in and grabbed him by the arms, he elbowed his way past them and marched toward the gate. It took four guards to wrestle him to the ground while Sylvia screamed, "Don't kill him! Please don't kill him!" The sight of her husband handcuffed, confused, and agitated, coupled with the realization that he could very well have been shot to death, left Sylvia shaken. Life would never be the same. John already needed round-the-clock monitoring, the family's only respite coming when he was at an adult daycare center. Soon he would require full care in a nursing home.

Sylvia glimpsed that sad future on the winter day in 2007 when she brought John to visit Ralph Wenzel at the Annapolis assisted-living facility that Eleanor had recently moved her husband into. The two men had played together on the same offensive line with the 1972 San Diego Chargers late in their careers, but the onetime teammates now had no memory of that or of each other. Even after they were reintroduced to one another several times, neither could remember the other's name.

"Do you remember playing with Ralph at all, John?" Mackey was asked.

"Who's Ralph?" Mackey replied.

"The guy sitting to your left," he was told.

Turning toward Wenzel, he said, "You're Ralph?"

"Yes."

"I'm John Mackey," he declared, staring blankly ahead.

Sylvia and Eleanor looked at each other and smiled sadly. They would exchange a lot of knowing glances throughout the visit. During lunch, John used a spoon to drink his coffee, thinking it was soup, while Ralph had to be fork-fed by Eleanor. John uttered non sequiturs like "I got in the end zone," while Ralph could only mumble a few nonsensical syllables. Ralph, his head drooping, was unresponsive for much of the visit. Eleanor tried to jog his memory by pointing to a black-and-white photo of the Steelers teammate who had been his best friend. Ralph couldn't remember the man, and Eleanor couldn't help feeling she was losing a little more of her own best friend.

When Ralph's symptoms had first begun to appear, Eleanor hadn't realized that this was a sign that her husband was slowly slipping away. She put his bout of depression down to a job loss. She teased him when he misplaced his wallet or forgot to transfer money from the couple's savings account to cover checks he'd written—he was in his early fifties and she figured the memory lapses were just a sign that he was hitting middle age. She did think it was a little strange when he began to have problems making simple decisions without her help, like picking something to order at restaurants. But all the changes were too subtle to set off any alarm bells.

Though he never said anything to Eleanor, Ralph knew there was more to those subtle changes than she suspected. The short-term memory lapses had been worrying, but then he had an experience that convinced him that something was going very wrong with his brain. As football coach for a private school in Washington, D.C., he would start each practice by describing the play his kids would be working on. One day, as he started to explain what they would be doing, one of the players stopped him and said, "We did that yesterday, Coach." At first Ralph didn't believe them. But when they repeated, almost verbatim, what he was planning on saying this day, Ralph was shocked. He knew they were right. But he still couldn't remember anything from the day before. He never told Eleanor. But as time went on, his memory lapses became more frequent and profound, and she realized that it was time to take him for an evaluation.

They sat across from the neurologist as he questioned Ralph about his symptoms. The doctor quickly zeroed in on the memory problems and asked how long Ralph had been experiencing them. Ralph told him about the episode with the high school kids, which had happened almost five years earlier. Eleanor was stunned. She couldn't believe that Ralph had been able to compensate and to cover everything up for so long. Then the doctor moved on to Ralph's concussion history.

"Have you ever had a concussion?" the neurologist asked.

Ralph laughed and then responded, "More than I can count."

"Were you ever completely knocked out?"

"Oh, yeah."

"How many times?"

"I really don't remember how many times. But it was a few."

"Were you ever knocked out and, when you came to, you really didn't know where you were or what you were supposed to be doing or what had happened?"

"Oh, yeah. I remember a game where I got knocked out. When I came to, I got up and I got back on the line. I was in the next play, and when I was supposed to run, I ran in the wrong direction. After that they pulled me off the field."

Ralph was diagnosed with mild cognitive impairment and the couple was warned that there was a good chance it could progress to Alzheimer's disease as time went on. Eleanor was surprised that someone as young as Ralph could be in the early stages of a disease that had struck no one else in his family. Both his parents, who were in their eighties, were still mentally sharp, as was his older brother. The neurologist suggested that the cognitive impairment might be related to Ralph's years playing football: "It seems to me that we're dealing with some damage that happened as a result of the head injuries you had in your life."

As the neurologist was finishing up, he asked Ralph, "Do you understand what is happening to you?"

"I sort of do," Ralph replied.

"What's it like?"

"I feel like there's a door in my head that closes. And it closes when it wants and it opens when it wants. And I can't control that."

As time went on, Eleanor saw that the door in Ralph's head was closing more and more often. When it was open, she'd see glimpses of the man she'd fallen in love with two decades before, the shy, quiet guy with the dry sense of humor who would casually drop a one-liner in the middle of a conversation that would send everyone into fits of laughter. She'd been captivated by that sense of humor from the first night she met the big, burly bear of a man at a Halloween party at the Indian reservation where they'd both been working, he as a thirty-something coach and teacher, she as a pharmacist just out of college.

They'd connected instantly and soon became inseparable. Over the years they zigzagged around the country, moving any time either of them got a particularly good job offer. Though they socialized, they were happiest when they could spend time alone together working on some domestic task. Cooking was something they both especially enjoyed sharing, and Ralph was always happy when he could create a new culinary masterpiece.

Ralph's decline was mirrored in the meals he cooked. Often when Eleanor was working late, he'd have a sumptuous repast ready when she walked in the door. But as his cognitive skills declined, he started to have problems figuring out meal plans. He'd greet her enthusiastically with some steaks he grilled, but there'd be nothing to eat with them. He'd gotten so absorbed cooking the meat that he'd just forgotten to make anything else. Eventually Eleanor took over all the cooking. She felt a sadness descend each time she walked into the kitchen to cook a meal, remembering that this was something that she and Ralph had delighted in and now she was preparing food just to keep them fed.

Within a few years, Eleanor had to hire a "housekeeper" to look out for her husband when she wasn't around. Over the course of seven years, the housekeeper went from a few hours a day to full-time. It was hard, but they seemed to be managing—until late in 2006 when the couple took a trip to the West Coast to visit relatives. Out of the familiar surroundings of home, Ralph seemed to deteriorate overnight. He became obsessive and paranoid and started having frightening delusions. When he became violent, threatening to hurt both Eleanor and his father, the family took him to a local hospital where doctors worked to calm him down enough to allow the couple to fly back home. One day, while Eleanor was waiting for Ralph to stabilize, a friend brought over a newspaper story that had appeared on the front page of *The New York Times* describing football-related dementia and a crusader who was trying to bring the issue to the public's attention. Eleanor made a mental note that she would contact both the crusader, Chris Nowinski, and the *Times* reporter, Alan Schwarz, when she and Ralph got home.

Eventually, with the help of two hulking male nurses, Eleanor was able get Ralph on a plane and back to Maryland, where he was admitted to a hospital with a dementia unit. Eleanor started to look for an assisted-living facility since she'd realized she wasn't going to be able to take care of him at home anymore. It wasn't easy. Many facilities told her they weren't set up to care for a patient like Ralph. They were used to getting dementia patients who were much older—and frail. Though Ralph had declined mentally, he was still in fairly good health. The facilities didn't want to deal with a big, and potentially dangerous, patient.

Once Eleanor did find a place for Ralph, she dug out the names of the crusader and the reporter. She'd decided she needed to find a way to let the world know about the wreckage football could create. When she connected with Nowinski and Schwarz, they suggested that the best way to tell Ralph's story might be to go to his new home and describe for the world what concussions had wrought. Eleanor wasn't sure whether it would be fair to expose Ralph to this kind of publicity. And she wasn't sure she'd even be able to get him to comprehend what was being asked of him. But when she explained to Ralph that it might help everyone understand the dangers of football, it seemed that the door had once again opened, if only for a few brief moments. "Yes," he said. "It's for the kids."

Eleanor and Sylvia discussed the issue and agreed that they would bring their husbands together for stories that would run on the front page of *The New York Times* and on an HBO special report spotlighting football's connection with dementia. Those stories were just the beginning. Both women continued their fight to make football safer, though they chose very different strategies.

Sylvia worked from the inside to advocate for health benefits for retired players. She had a close relationship with Goodell, watching the 2009 Super Bowl with him in the commissioner's box. She was happy with the fruits of her quiet diplomacy and proud that her husband's bittersweet legacy—the 88 Plan—was already providing nearly a hundred former players with benefits. "I feel I get more with sugar than with vinegar," she said, explaining the difference between her and Eleanor. "But we need Eleanor's personality on our side. When you're fighting a fight, or you're trying to win fair benefits or recognition, you need different types of people on different roads going for the same thing."

Eleanor took on the NFL establishment head-on as an outsider who never liked football, and she didn't care if the commissioner himself was mad at her. When Goodell organized an NFL meeting to examine the later-life care of retirees, Eleanor showed up, insisting that she needed to be there to speak for Ralph and all the others who could not speak for themselves. As she tried to enter the room, Goodell barred the door and told her that the meeting was for players only. Eleanor publicly criticized her exclusion and continued to ratchet up her activism, testifying before Congress and filing a worker's compensation claim. She described herself as "one very pushy broad" advocating for her husband both as a caregiver and as a crusader.

It would take just that kind of pushiness on the part of all the reformers if anything was ever going to change.

Chapter 11

Seeds of Change

For years, the entire sports world had been flicking off the periodic warnings from scientists as if their dire-sounding concussion studies were just pesky flies. The spate of retirements due to post-concussion syndrome was dismissed as casually as the bumps on the head that caused them. Not even the deaths from second-impact syndrome could change the reckless way we played our games—that tragic specter could be rationalized away as too rare to worry about. But dementia was something else entirely.

Although no one knew how common it was, the very idea that playing sports could result in early-onset dementia gave everyone pause. Some tried to suggest that it was just as rare as second-impact syndrome. But ultimately, no one could guarantee that it wasn't a time bomb ticking away in every player's brain. The more cases that turned up, the more worried everyone got. Everyone, it seemed, except for the National Football League.

In the spring of 2007, the NFL convened a summit meeting that would bring the opposing sides of the concussion controversy face to face. The league summoned team physicians and trainers from its thirty-two franchises to what figured to be a heated debate: the NFL's doctors stubbornly defending their dangerous concussion policies against brain injury experts relentlessly criticizing such a head-in-the-sand approach. For months, the two sides had been on a collision course, exchanging harsh words and harsher critiques of each other's opinions on both the short-term and the long-term effects of concussions. Now, finally, the opposing voices would clash jaw to jaw at the daylong summit behind the closed doors of a conference room in a hotel near Chicago's O'Hare Airport.

The NFL's doctors came armed with the fourteen studies conducted by its Mild Traumatic Brain Injury Committee and published over the previous four years. Those studies, which affirmed NFL medical practices that returned fully half of concussed players to the same game in which they were injured, suggested that concussions were benign and concluded that multiple concussions did not lead to long-term consequences. The outside experts, dismissing the NFL's studies as "industry-funded research," came armed with a raft of independent studies as evidence to the contrary.

Dr. Julian Bailes, a former team neurosurgeon for the Pittsburgh Steelers, stood up at the lectern and presented findings that debunked the NFL's position and policy on concussion management. He talked about a survey of 2,552 retired NFL players that correlated concussions with increasingly higher incidences of depression and dementia, and about two resulting journal articles he'd co-authored with that study's principal investigator, University of North Carolina concussion expert Kevin Guskiewicz. One showed that retirees with at least three concussions were three times more likely to be diagnosed with depression than those with no history of head injury; the other showed that retirees with at least three concussions were three times more likely to suffer significant memory problems and five times more likely to be diagnosed with the pre-Alzheimer's condition called mild cognitive impairment. Though the NFL had dismissed those survey findings as "virtually worthless," Bailes could turn to harder scientific evidence.

His PowerPoint presentation was loaded with slides from the brains in which Dr. Bennet Omalu had recently found chronic traumatic encephalopathy. Up came the slides from Mike Webster and Terry Long and Justin Strzelczyk, three Steelers Bailes had gotten to know personally as a team physician, as well as the slides from Andre Waters. The slides from all four middle-aged brains showed splotches the color of a football—clear evidence of the CTE that had manifested in depression and dementia shortly after the players retired from the NFL. As soon as Bailes concluded his presentation, the league's doctors went on the offensive. Suddenly Bailes found himself trading barbs with the NFL's new concussion czar, Dr. Ira Casson.

Casson had replaced Dr. Elliot Pellman as chairman of the NFL's Mild Traumatic Brain Injury Committee just four months earlier. The league had hoped that Casson would be less of a lightning rod than Pellman, a rheumatologist whose lack of concussion knowledge had infuriated brain injury experts. Casson, at least, was a neurologist, and the experts hoped his background would lead to a more enlightened discussion about the long-term impact of concussions. It quickly became apparent, however, that Casson was going to pick up right where Pellman left off as a pugnacious protector of the status quo. Just like Pellman, Casson attacked the brain injury experts whose research contradicted the league's position, downplayed the accumulating evidence on the risks of concussions, and defended NFL policies that critics said set a dangerous precedent for millions of kids playing football.

In an HBO interview shortly after replacing Pellman, Casson had fielded pointed questions about the mounting evidence on the dangers of concussions. He parried them all without missing a beat.

"Is there any evidence, as far as you're concerned, that links multiple head injuries among pro football players with depression?"

"No."

". . . with dementia?"

"No."

". . . with early onset of Alzheimer's?"

"No."

"Is there any evidence, as of today, that links multiple head injuries with *any* long-term problem like that?"

"In NFL players? No."

"So you don't think they're rolling the dice, really?"

"As far as chronic brain damage is concerned? No, I don't."

In a word, Casson had neatly summed up the NFL's position going into the summit. So when Bailes finished presenting the CTE slides there, it wasn't surprising that Casson immediately argued that there was no evidence that any of the four former players sustained brain damage from football. "The only scientifically valid evidence of chronic encephalopathy in athletes is in boxers and in some steeplechase jockeys," said Casson, who two decades earlier had conducted seminal scanning studies that showed CTE in active and retired boxers. "It's never been scientifically, validly documented in any other athletes." Bailes countered that the slides spoke for themselves. "We can't be sure, but football is by far at the top of the list for me," he said, "and I don't see many other clear candidates for how that damage got there." And so it went.

The summit may not have settled any scientific arguments, but its mere existence signaled the willingness of the NFL's rookie commissioner, Roger Goodell, to at least listen to the critics beseeching him to tear down the Berlin Wall of concussion denial. Goodell, who had learned about leadership growing up the son of a principled U.S. senator respected for denouncing the Vietnam War in the late '60s as a liberal Republican, had barely settled into the commissioner's office the previous fall when he found himself confronted with a heap of inherited crises. Naturally assuming that the NFL's most urgent problem was the spate of headline-grabbing scandals involving players' off-the-field misconduct, he may have underestimated the silent concussion epidemic that his predecessor had allowed to fester untreated for years. It was a growing abscess that would explode into his most consuming problem, what *The Washington Post* proclaimed "the biggest crisis the sport has ever faced." To tackle it, Goodell would need to first play catch-up on the fast-evolving scientific research, then admit there was indeed a serious problem, and then finally figure out a way to fix it.

As if to show he wasn't just paying lip service to reform, Goodell announced new NFL standards for concussion management on the same day he called for the summit conference. He mandated neuropsychological baseline testing for all players before each season, adopting an objective tool that had been required by the National Hockey League for a decade already. He stipulated that players knocked unconscious could no longer be returned to action the same day. He announced that return-to-play decisions had to be based on health rather than competitive considerations and had to be made solely by team medical personnel without pressure from players, coaches, or executives. To help ensure that, he instituted a "whistleblower" hotline enabling anyone to anonymously report an incident in which a concussed player was pressed back into action before the injury could heal.

The whistleblower edict resulted from a recent allegation by retired linebacker Ted Johnson that he had been pressured to return too soon after a concussion. The story Johnson revealed to reporters was a warning about the danger not only of concussions but also of the culture that fostered them.

Back in 2002, Johnson had been knocked out of a preseason game by a concussion sustained in a head-on collision. Four days later, at the New England Patriots' next full-contact practice, the head trainer issued him a red jersey as a signal to teammates that the linebacker was not supposed to be hit. Johnson told reporters that, just before a high-impact running drill, an assistant trainer raced over with a standard blue jersey to replace the red one. Johnson was sure that the order to change jerseys came from head coach Bill Belichick. Worried about losing his roster spot along with his nonguaranteed contract, Johnson pulled on the blue jersey and lined up for the drill. On the first play, he collided with a running back and instantly felt dazed and disoriented. He continued on in a fog, not mentioning his symptoms to anyone. It wasn't until after practice that he angrily strode up to the head trainer and growled, "Just so you know, I got another concussion." The trainer paled and sent Johnson to the hospital, where a neurologist confirmed that the player had sustained another concussion and sidelined him for the next two weeks. Upon his return to practice, Johnson confronted Belichick about pressuring him back too soon after the first concussion. "You played God with my health," Johnson told the coach. "You knew I shouldn't have been cleared to play, and you gave me that blue jersey anyway." Belichick would later tell reporters, "If Ted felt so strongly that he didn't feel he was ready to practice with us, he should have told me."

Johnson played through that season and the next two without reporting symptoms from at least half a dozen concussions, fearing he'd be branded as an injury-prone player. But with his symptoms of fatigue, depression, and cognitive impairment taking on a frightening permanence, he shocked fans by retiring at age thirty-two in 2005, mere months after winning his third Super Bowl ring in four years. When he went public with his cautionary tale two years later, it made front-page news not because of what it said about Belichick, the acerbic coaching genius who denied pressuring Johnson, but because of what it revealed about football's concussion culture.

In 2009, Johnson returned to the Super Bowl, this time to publicize his story as part of a growing crusade lobbying the NFL to change its culture of concussions. In the two years since the concussion summit, even as the mounting scientific evidence continued to pour in, the safety reforms had slowed to a drip. As a sign of its continuing denial, the NFL was still distributing an informational pamphlet to all players and their families that minimized the consequences of multiple concussions: "Current research with professional athletes has not shown that having more than one or two concussions leads to permanent problems if each injury is managed properly."

Throughout the week leading up to the 2009 Super Bowl in Tampa, the concussion crusaders, led by Chris Nowinski, raised the pressure on the NFL by taking the fight to its biggest stage, exploiting the event's attendant media circus. Five days before Super Sunday, Nowinski's Center for the Study of Traumatic Encephalopathy held a press conference at a Tampa hotel to announce the sixth autopsy-confirmed case of CTE in a former NFL player between the ages of thirty-six and fifty. The center's neuropathologist, Ann McKee, presented findings that showed the condition in a forty-five-year-old former lineman for the hometown Tampa Bay Bucaneers, Tom McHale. More shockingly, she presented the youngest known case of CTE: an eighteen-year-old boy who had sustained multiple concussions playing high school football. Pointing at a slide that showed brown specks of abnormal tau, she declared, "This is something you *never* should see in an eighteen-year-old brain. This is something that's highly alarming."

To McKee, it was more than that—it was downright "chilling." When she first saw the brown specks on the eighteen-year-old's slide, she froze and thought, "That could just as easily be my son." Her son was also eighteen and an athlete, a goalie on his high school soccer team. The concussion crisis that she had coolly and clinically played a key role in uncovering suddenly hit home in a way that any other soccer mom could empathize with.

The revelation of CTE in an eighteen-year-old—expanding the issue of long-term brain damage to youth sports—should have fueled the urgency of dealing with this burgeoning public health crisis. Instead, the Tampa press conference drew fewer than two dozen reporters from among the thousands in town for the Super Bowl. It was clear that changing the culture would not be easy.

That left the crusaders with no choice but to try to beat the NFL at its own masterful PR game. Taking to the airwaves on everything from National Public Radio to *Nightline* and *60 Minutes*, they kept the pressure on the league like linebackers blitzing a quarterback. Nowinski may have been the most visible provocateur, slamming the NFL goliath with his slingshot every chance he got, but he was hardly alone: brain-injured ex-players advocated for changing the just-rub-dirt-on-it culture; wives begged for help on behalf of retirees too demented to do so themselves; parents of children maimed or killed by second-impact syndrome pleaded for safety reform; and, all the while, *New York Times* reporter Alan Schwarz kept the unfolding story on the front burner and the front page with a series of muckraking exposés. In the end, the most effective argument would come from the scientists.

In the spring of 2009, barely three months after McKee had crashed the Super Bowl party with her scary slides, the NFL invited her and other leading researchers to New York City to meet with its Mild Traumatic Brain Injury Committee at the league's plush Park Avenue headquarters. As she stepped into the huge mahogany boardroom plastered with posters of Vince Lombardi exhorting the Green Bay Packers dynasty she'd grown up rooting for, McKee couldn't help feeling that she was entering the lion's den. It didn't help that she was the only woman in a room designed to celebrate the most testosterone-fueled team sport. She took a deep breath and calmly presented her CTE findings to all the male doctors arrayed around the large conference table. The reaction of the NFL doctors, predictably, was skepticism. One of them, she later told reporters, actually accused her of making up the disease.

It was a clear sign of just how entrenched the NFL was. Changing the culture was a game not of yards, but of inches. Every once in a while, the NFL would indeed capitulate with a concussion concession, like adopting a rule that banned certain types of deliberate helmet-to-helmet hits. But when it came to the long-term ramifications of repeat concussions, the NFL's position remained immovable: no admission of any problem, pending the findings in a few years of its own ongoing research study of 120 retirees.

While the NFL's internal research continued to limp through its fifteenth year, another independent study pushed the issue toward a tipping point. For that study, which had been commissioned by the NFL itself, University of Michigan researchers asked 1,063 retired players if they had ever been diagnosed with "dementia, Alzheimer's disease, or other memory-related disease." The phone survey found that ex-players over forty-nine years old were five times more likely to receive such a diagnosis than men of the same age in the general population. More alarming, retirees aged thirty to forty-nine were nineteen times likelier to be diagnosed with a memory-related disease than men of the same age in the general population. Two days after *The New York Times* broke the story on its front page, the House Judiciary Committee announced that it would hold congressional hearings to look into the impact of head injuries on football players and on society in general.

On October 28, 2009, before a standing-room-only crowd in the Rayburn House Office Building on Capitol Hill, the NFL absorbed a barrage of hits during a hearing that left Roger Goodell sputtering like a battered quarterback. Defending the league's policies in the face of heated criticism from a steady stream of lawmakers, doctors, safety advocates, and ex-players, the NFL commissioner repeatedly refused to acknowledge a direct link between football and brain injury, between football and cognitive impairment, between football and dementia. This time, however, he was facing foes more formidable than the critics the NFL had been stiff-arming for years. Two California congresswomen, in particular, took turns expressing exasperation with his evasiveness under the tough questioning about the long-term impact of concussions.

At one point, Representative Linda Sánchez asked Goodell to read aloud from the NFL's educational pamphlet informing its players that concussions hadn't been proven to cause permanent problems, and then rebuked him. "The NFL has this blanket denial or minimizing of the fact that there may be this link," she said. "And it reminds me of the tobacco companies, pre-nineties, when they kept saying, 'Oh, there's no link between smoking and damage to your health.'"

At another point, Representative Maxine Waters, whose husband had played linebacker for six NFL seasons, became so irritated that she interrupted Goodell to deliver a finger-jabbing accusation. "I think you're an eight-billion-dollar organization that has not taken seriously your responsibility to the players," she scolded. "I know you do everything you possibly can to hold on to those profits, but I think the responsibility of this Congress is to take a look at the antitrust exemption you have and take it away."

The threat to revoke an antitrust exemption worth billions to the league in TV revenue wasn't just about doing right by the two thousand active NFL players and the sixteen thousand retirees. It was also about the millions of amateur players on every level from the colleges to the high schools to the peewee leagues. Panelist after panelist testified about the impact of the concussion culture trickling down to the kids emulating their NFL heroes. That's why it was so important for McKee to present evidence of CTE not only in seven middle-aged NFL retirees, but also in the eighteen-year-old high school player and four former collegians who had never played pro football. And that's why the most moving testimony was delivered not by any doctor or player or executive, but by a burly, bearded father who spoke for all the parents and for all the kids.

Dick Benson told the story of his son Will, a seventeen-year-old quarterback who had collapsed during a high school game two weeks after suffering a concussion and died from second-impact syndrome. He chronicled how he'd spent the next five years lobbying Texas state legislators to pass a high school safety bill in his son's memory. Periodically dabbing a tissue to his face as photos flashed on screens showing Will from baby swing to football field, Dick Benson concluded his testimony with a plea to the NFL and to Congress. "My one request is," he said, pausing several times to fight back tears, "don't . . . let it . . . happen . . . again." He composed himself just long enough to add, "Please."

When the daylong hearing was finally over, the NFL and Goodell had been beaten into submission. In the end, the chastened commissioner insisted, "We are changing the culture of our game for the better." While the words sounded the right note, no one seemed convinced that they would translate into action anytime soon given the NFL's long history of recalcitrance.

The fallout from the hearing, however, would be stunning in its speed and its breadth. Almost overnight, the NFL did a complete reversal: the most public voice opposing concussion reform was now suddenly supporting it.

Just a month after the hearing, Goodell announced a series of changes that signaled a stricter policy designed to "protect the health and safety of our players, and set the best possible example for players at all levels and in all sports." The NFL would now require that outside neurologists and neurosurgeons independently clear concussed players, taking return-to-play decisions out of the sole control of team physicians who were vulnerable to conflict-of-interest pressures from their employers. What's more, the NFL would now require players with any significant sign of concussion to be removed from a game or practice and be barred from returning the same day. The ruling meant that concussed players, who as recently as 2007 could still return to games even if they had been knocked unconscious, would now be automatically sidelined for the day if they experienced such signs of concussion as confusion, disorientation, amnesia, and memory loss, whether or not those symptoms quickly subsided; players could still return to the field the same day they experienced headache and dizziness, but only if those symptoms did not persist. In a league that had long maintained it was safe for players to return to action as soon as their symptoms cleared, such a major policy shift would take time to permeate the play-through-pain mindset.

The week Goodell announced the stricter concussion policies, the increased focus was as conspicuous on the field as the absence that Sunday of Ben Roethlisberger and Kurt Warner, the two starting quarterbacks in the 2009 Super Bowl. Each had suffered a concussion the previous Sunday and then had been cleared to return after passing neurological exams and neuropsychological tests, but their teams decided to err on the side of caution. Even though Roethlisberger lobbied Steelers coach Mike Tomlin to play despite the headaches that returned at a midweek practice, the team neurosurgeon, Dr. Joseph Maroon, recommended that he sit out the next game. In the locker room after the Steelers lost in overtime, wide receiver Hines Ward questioned Roethlisberger's toughness and said the team was split 50–50 on whether their star quarterback should have played despite the concussion. "We needed him out there, we wanted him out there," said Ward, noting that he had lied to doctors many times in the past and played despite concussions. "This is the biggest game of the year. Me being a competitor, I just wish we would've had all our weapons out there. It's frustrating." By challenging his team's enlightened handling of Roethlisberger's fourth diagnosed concussion, Ward underscored what an uphill battle it would be to change attitudes so ingrained in the culture.

Goodell's reforms weren't limited to policy changes. He also accepted the resignations of Casson, the chief critic of the evidence linking football to cognitive decline, and Dr. David Viano as co-chairmen of the NFL's concussion committee. Casson and Viano had joined Pellman in authoring the controversial 2005 study that concluded "it might be safe" for high schools and colleges to adopt the NFL's practice of allowing concussed players to return to play the same day they were injured. In the wake of Casson's resignation, the NFL suspended the study he was conducting into the impact of concussions on retired players. As Linda Sánchez had quipped on the eve of the congressional hearings in ridiculing that study, "Hey, why don't we let tobacco companies determine whether smoking is bad for your health or not?"

To avoid any perceived conflict of interest, the NFL decided to fund outside research. The league even teamed up with its biggest nemesis: Chris Nowinski and his Center for the Study of Traumatic Encephalopathy. For so long, Nowinski, McKee, and their colleagues had been accused of trying to kill the American institution known as football. When Nowinski began his crusade four years earlier, Gene Upshaw, the hard-nosed Hall of Fame lineman then running the NFL Players Association, had dismissed him as a greedy author just trying to sell books. When McKee showed her CTE slides to her big brother Charles, a family physician in Wisconsin who had been an All-American quarterback at Lawrence University, he had warned her, "You're going to ruin football." For their part, McKee and Nowinski were rabid football fans who saw themselves not as a game wreckers, but as game changers. They considered it vindication that the NFL was now donating $1 million toward their center's ongoing research into CTE, no strings attached.

By the end of the 2009 season, the NFL, the same league that used to promote head-rattling hits in commercials, was airing a public service announcement to warn kids, parents, and youth coaches about the dangers of concussions. The thirty-second message, created in conjunction with the CDC at the behest of Congress, featured the NFL logo and an announcer's authoritative voiceover: "Concussions and other head injuries must be taken seriously. If you're a player, protect yourself and your teammates. If you think you're hurt, don't hide it. Report it, and take time to recover. If you're a coach or parent, know concussion symptoms and warning signs, and never let athletes return to action before a health professional says it's OK. Help take head injuries out of play."

To ensure that its own players got the message, the NFL produced a poster warning them about the dangers of concussions and admitting that multiple head injuries could indeed lead to permanent brain damage as well as depression and dementia. In the wake of the NFL's stubborn denial of such long-term consequences, this signaled a reversal of position that was as astounding as it was overdue. By the opening kickoff of the 2010 season, the poster—headlined CONCUSSION in big block letters—hung in every locker room throughout the league. Subtitled "A Must Read for NFL Players," it was the football equivalent of the Surgeon General's Warning on every pack of cigarettes that smoking can kill you: "[Traumatic brain injury] may lead to problems with memory and communication, personality changes, as well as depression and the early onset of dementia. Concussions and conditions resulting from repeated brain injury can change your life and your family's life forever." That warning was also handed to every player, replacing the brochure that since 2007 had insisted there was no evidence of any long-term effects.

Stripped across the bottom of the NFL poster, a string of photos showed boys and girls playing soccer, hockey, baseball, and lacrosse, as well as football. The accompanying text offered a reminder in bold letters to the players that they were role models for kids across America: "Other athletes are watching . . ."

The posters had been up for barely a month when Roger Goodell journeyed to Seattle on a mission to spread his newfound gospel beyond the NFL's locker rooms. "We know, in the NFL, that we set a standard in sports," he declared at a conference on concussions in youth sports. "When we change our approach, others take notice. And they will follow." Leading by example, however, was no longer enough for the newly converted commissioner. He was unveiling a new poster, patterned on the NFL's, designed to hang in school locker rooms across the nation—"so that every girl who plays soccer, basketball, or field hockey and every boy who wrestles or plays football or competes in lacrosse [will] be aware of the symptoms of concussions."

Goodell was just getting started. He introduced the former middle school football player whose debilitating brain injury had inspired Washington's landmark state concussion law. With Zackery Lystedt by his side, Goodell vowed to lobby aggressively for similar safety laws in other states. "This must become the standard for how youth concussions are treated," Goodell said. "I have made it a league priority to keep this going until all fifty states have passed Zackery's law or found a way do something that is just as significant."

Goodell had already sent a letter to the governors of the forty-four states without concussion laws, urging them to push for similar legislation to protect young athletes from head injuries. From the moment it was enacted in May 2009, the Zackery Lystedt Law had become the template for every state formulating legislation on concussion safety: it required that any youth athlete suspected of sustaining a concussion be immediately removed from play and then prohibited from returning without written clearance from a licensed healthcare provider trained in concussion management. Because provisions varied widely in the six states that had already adopted concussion laws, federal bills were introduced in both the Senate and House of Representatives to try to bring some uniformity to concussion policies. The crisis was escalating too fast, however, for Goodell to wait for legislative initiatives to take their course.

That's why he had resolved months earlier to seek help from the dean of concussion specialists, Dr. Robert Cantu. No one could provide the commissioner a broader perspective on the problem than the Massachusetts neurosurgeon, whose pioneering work ranged from authoring the first concussion guidelines in 1986 to teaming with McKee at the vanguard of today's CTE breakthroughs. So when Goodell was in Boston for the NFL's 2009 fall owners meeting a couple of weeks before the congressional hearings that would spur its stunning reversal on the concussion issue, he asked Cantu to swing by his hotel for a private one-on-one discussion. For ninety minutes, Goodell sounded out Cantu on ways to move the league forward on the concussion problem. Cantu urged him to strengthen the league's return-to-play guidelines and player education efforts—two initiatives that could immediately benefit the pros and that would invariably trickle down to college, high school, and youth athletes. What Cantu couldn't stress enough was the responsibility of the NFL to attack the problem from the grassroots up and the importance of better concussion education on the youth and high school levels. He suggested that the NFL already had the ideal vehicle to accomplish this: its partnership with USA Football, the national governing body on the youth and amateur levels. Two months after the meeting, USA Football integrated concussion awareness into its flagship program that trains and certifies thousands of youth league coaches throughout the nation.

The urgency of dealing with the concussion crisis was growing with each succeeding diagnosis of CTE in younger players. In the summer of 2010, two cases in particular made it painfully clear that CTE was not just a phenomenon striking retired pros in middle age and later—it was developing in the younger brains of players who were still active. The football world was shaken when Dr. Bennet Omalu uncovered the first case of CTE in an active NFL player: Chris Henry, a notoriously troubled wide receiver who was just twenty-six when he fell or jumped to his death from the back of a speeding pickup truck during a frenzied domestic dispute. Then came the even more shocking news that Dr. Ann McKee had uncovered the first case of CTE in an active college football player: Owen Thomas, a junior lineman at the University of Pennsylvania who was just twenty-one when he committed suicide with no previous history of depression. More to the point, he also had no previous history of concussion. Because he'd never been diagnosed with one, McKee suspected that the CTE was caused by concussions Thomas had never reported, the "subconcussive" hits linemen absorb on every down, or a combination of both factors. Unlike the eighteen-year-old brain in which she'd found only incipient traces of disease, this twenty-one-year-old brain was by far the youngest to merit a firm diagnosis of CTE—mild, but definite.

When McKee showed her colleagues the Thomas slides, they were shaken—especially Cantu. Peering at the now-familiar brown splotches, Cantu shook his head and resolved to ratchet up his longtime crusade for concussion safety. "We can, and we must, develop brain trauma guidelines similar to the 'pitch count' regulations now used in Little League baseball," he declared. "We count the pitches of every baseball player to ensure a small number do not develop shoulder and elbow problems—and yet we don't count how often children get hit in the head playing football, even though it can lead to early dementia or possibly depression and suicide years later. We have pitch counts for pitchers from Little League to the Major Leagues who want to limit the number of pitches they throw and protect their arms; we're probably going to have to go to hit counts to the head in our football players to protect the brain."

The inspiration for Cantu's "hit count" proposal came from research conducted by his colleague Kevin Guskiewicz. As director of the University of North Carolina research center poignantly named after a local teen who died from a traumatic brain injury suffered in his very first high school football game, Guskiewicz had been studying the effects of head impacts to analyze just how much punishment players' brains sustain on a daily basis. Since 2004 he had monitored the impact of every hit at every UNC football game and practice with a new technology known as HITS, shorthand for Head Impact Telemetry System. Small sensors placed inside the players' helmets measured the force and location of each hit, then transmitted the data in real time to a laptop computer on the sideline.

What Guskiewicz saw on his computer screen would shock him: players were routinely absorbing multiple impacts in practice exceeding what most scientists theorized was the concussion-causing threshold of seventy to seventy-five times the force of gravity. Players were averaging a thousand to twelve hundred head hits per season, with some linemen estimated to log up to eighteen hundred of them. Perhaps most troubling, fully 20 percent of hits were located at the top of the helmet, meaning that far too many players were leading with their heads as a battering ram or lowering their heads dangerously just before impact. A 2010 study of three NCAA football teams raised the alarm: each team averaged three thousand hard hits to the head during one full season of practices—three hundred of which fell in the concussion-causing range of 80 to 119 g's and two hundred of which exceeded 120 g's.

Even more alarming was a study that extended those results to younger athletes. That study also monitored head impacts, this time on a high school football team through the entire 2009 season. What stunned the researchers wasn't what they found in the concussed players, but rather what they found in a control group of eight teammates with no reported concussions or observable symptoms. Four of the eight controls surprisingly demonstrated cognitive deficits (on neuropsych tests) and neurophysiological impairments (on functional MRI scans); what's more, the most impairment was found not in the three concussed players, but rather in nonconcussed linemen who'd absorbed numerous hits below the concussion-causing threshold of 80 g's. By designating a new category of athletes who are functionally but not observably impaired, the researchers from Purdue University underscored the value of monitoring the number of hits sustained by players at every level.

With 58 percent of all documented college football concussions occurring on the practice field, Guskiewicz began spending his weekday afternoons using the HITS technology to monitor severe impacts that might otherwise go unnoticed as well as unreported. He used it to identify dangerous techniques and then teach at-risk players safer ones to protect their brains; like a coach breaking down games films, he would show a player 3-D computer images diagramming hits to the top of the head and correlate them with replays of the perilous plays in question. Based on Guskiewicz's research, UNC head coach Butch Davis cut back on full-contact practices, hoping to reduce the toll on players' brains.

UNC was not alone. At Virginia Tech, which pioneered the HITS technology in 2003, the team physician, Dr. Gunnar Brolinson, had long turned the practice field into a virtual lab. His head-impact data convinced the coaching staff to do away with the universal training camp ritual of two-a-day practices and to limit the time spent on certain drills that HITS showed to be most dangerous to the brain.

In theory as well as in practice, the impact-sensing helmets made perfect sense. In reality, the cost—up to $1,000 per helmet—proved prohibitive for most colleges and virtually all high schools. If high schools couldn't afford to hire a certified athletic trainer—only 42 percent of them have access to one—and if they wouldn't invest $500 for neuropsychological testing software like ImPACT, then they certainly weren't about to pony up $60,000 to buy helmets with sensors.

Even among those schools that did employ such software, a recent study showed that an alarming number of athletic trainers were administering the tests incorrectly, misinterpreting the results, or flat-out ignoring them. The 2009 study of ImPACT usage found that only half of high school and college trainers bothered to make sure that athletes hadn't purposely scored low on baseline tests; those skewed results would make it impossible to accurately interpret cognitive status after a concussion and evaluate when it might be safe to return an athlete to play. Most troubling, 10 percent of trainers reported that they would clear a concussed athlete who scored below baseline, and another 4 percent said they might return such a player if the game was really important. While nearly all of the trainers administered baseline tests to football teams, only two-thirds did so for soccer and basketball.

Some school districts were using the potential misuse of neuropsychological tests as an excuse for not including them as part of a comprehensive concussion-management protocol. Even in the state of Washington, where the adoption of the Zackery Lystedt Law set the standard of care for the rest of the nation, at least one school district rebuffed calls to implement neuropsych tests in large part because its insurance provider did not recommend them, citing the liability opened up by the potential for improper or inconsistent use.

Another loophole in the Lystedt Law was that it did not require emergency or medical personnel to be at games. With only 34 percent of Washington high schools having access to a certified athletic trainer—less even than the national average of 42 percent—it's clear that cost considerations could trump safety concerns even in the state deemed the most enlightened on the concussion issue. "The best advice I can give is to have appropriate medical personnel in place," says Guskiewicz, the leading concussion expert among certified athletic trainers. "Trust me, this is not self-serving; it's just what we know. If you have a certified athletic trainer who understands the signs and symptoms, that person can help the team—from the coaches to the players to the parents—better understand brain trauma. If you can't have that, then you might want to give strong consideration as to whether or not your school should offer contact sports."

Of course, not even the presence of trainers can assure safe management when so few of them follow proper procedures. Guskiewicz, the lead author of the National Athletic Trainers' Association position statement on concussion management, had been dismayed to discover that only 3 percent of the certified athletic trainers he surveyed for a 2005 study were complying with the organization's guidelines advocating the use of symptom checklists, neuropsych tests, and balance exams for managing sports-related concussions.

After the NFL reversed field and became a leading voice on the issue of concussion management, the lower levels did exactly what Cantu and Goodell had predicted—they followed suit. The NCAA, the National Federation of State High School Associations, and USA Football all beefed up their return-to-play guidelines. The NCAA and the NFHS, for example, each instituted a new policy mandating that players with any concussion symptoms be held out for the remainder of the game.

Unfortunately, the new policies, like the emerging science, remained way ahead of the culture. No sooner had the 2010 college football season kicked off than fans were treated to this nationally televised spectacle: a head coach berating his team physician on the sideline for refusing to let a star player return to the same game in which he'd been knocked unconscious. As soon as Dr. Sam Haraldson diagnosed a concussion based on loss of consciousness as well as problems with balance and memory, Texas Christian University running back Ed Wesley should have been sidelined automatically per the new NCAA policy. But Haraldson found himself debating the return-to-play issue with TCU coach Gary Patterson in full view of ESPN's cameras. "I was literally verbally accosted by the coach, screaming at me insanely at the top of his lungs that he doesn't think [Wesley] has a concussion and what right do I have to hold him out," Haraldson said later.

Such inconsistent use of mandated policies and management protocols meant that the quickest fix to the urgent concussion crisis remained the most fundamental: changing the way the game was played. USA Football did just that in 2010 by toughening its rules against head hits, penalizing the use of the shoulder or forearm—not just the helmet—to make contact with an opposing player above the shoulder. And in the other collision sport where hits were intrinsic to the game and concussions long ago reached epidemic proportions, USA Hockey continued to set a standard for vigilance.

At a Mayo Clinic concussion conference in the fall of 2010, a group of 250 doctors, researchers, and hockey officials formally recommended that head contact be banned at every level, urging the NHL and its minor leagues to follow the example set by all the amateur organizations that had already done so. The NHL was not ready to sign on for such revolutionary change. Having just instituted a rule penalizing blindside hits to the head and bodychecks targeting the head, the league immediately

dismissed any suggestion of penalizing head-on checks and even distributed an explanatory video showing what it termed "an example of a legal
shoulder check to the head"—the very type of jarring hit responsible for
60 percent of its seventy-five concussions per season. Kerry Fraser, who
had just retired after refereeing an NHL-record 2,165 games over thirty
years, responded to the league's recalcitrance by calling for a complete ban
on head hits. "Really, what it takes is *this*," he said as he brandished a silver
referee's whistle. "You need to blow the whistle, call the penalties, and get
everybody on the same page. The culture will change very quickly."

In the meantime, since the pros seemed too deeply entrenched to
accept a leadership role that would filter down to all the amateur levels,
the Mayo Clinic conference focused on youth hockey, where the rate of
concussion was surprisingly only slightly lower than in the NHL. The
group of experts strongly urged hockey officials to delay the age at which
bodychecking is introduced to thirteen, two years older than what the
rules currently allow. They cited a new Canadian study showing that the
concussion rate among eleven- and twelve-year-olds in Alberta, where
bodychecking was allowed, to be four times higher than in Quebec, where
it was prohibited. The study's authors concluded that moving back the
age in Alberta would reduce concussions among the nine thousand kids
playing hockey there from seven hundred to three hundred per season.

As the conference came to a close, the concussion experts left hockey-
crazed Minnesota determined to spread their message at other conferences and to other sports. "You can hear the sounds of change," James
Whitehead, executive vice president of the American College of Sports
Medicine, observed. "Historic, game-changing, breakthrough change."

Nowhere, of course, was that sound more audible than in the NFL.
Sixteen years after forming its Mild Traumatic Brain Injury Committee
to study concussions, the league had finally realized that there was no
such thing as a "mild" traumatic brain injury and renamed it the Head,
Neck and Spine Medical Committee. More significant, the NFL completely overhauled the committee, replacing the doctors who had been
impediments to change from the inside with those who had been agents
of change from the outside. The league even brought in as adviser one of
the harshest and longest-standing critics of its concussion policies, Dr.
Robert Cantu, a quarter century after he began preaching what eventually

became a mantra throughout the medical community: "When in doubt, sit them out."

The opening of the 2010 NFL season brought the promise of a new era of enlightenment. Posters papering locker room walls preached the league's newfound gospel warning players about the dangers of concussions. Players had been drilled on the recent policy changes designed to treat concussions more seriously than ever before. And now, all eyes were watching the NFL to see how the sea change would play out on the field. They didn't have to wait long.

On the very first Sunday of the season, Philadelphia Eagles linebacker Stewart Bradley was attempting to make a diving headfirst tackle when his helmet slammed directly into a teammate's hip. He woozily tried to rise, stumbled to his feet, staggered a few steps on rubbery legs, and then collapsed back to the turf. His teammates frantically waved for medical assistance and then watched in concerned silence as he was being attended to and helped off the field.

More than twenty-eight million viewers across America saw all this live on TV. More than sixty-nine thousand Eagles fans witnessed it in person at Lincoln Financial Field. The only people who didn't see it, apparently, were the medical personnel on the Eagles sideline.

As a national TV audience watched slow-motion and real-time replays of the episode, the Fox broadcasters narrated the scene with concern in their voices. "Clearly confused and dazed," observed the color commentator, Troy Aikman. "It's hard to imagine him coming back into the game, with all the attention paid to head injuries."

Less than four minutes later, Bradley was sent back onto the field. "That surprises me," Aikman told viewers. His play-by-play partner, Joe Buck, agreed and added that Bradley must have passed the standard sideline assessment tests so he was "OK to return." Neither Buck nor Aikman, the Hall of Fame quarterback whose own concussion history had prematurely ended his career and brought the problem to fans' attention a decade earlier, raised the question of how it was possible that an obviously concussed player had been cleared to return to play and put back into the game with just three minutes left in the first half.

At halftime, Bradley was examined, diagnosed with a concussion, and pulled from the rest of the game. For all the NFL's strong words about how far the league had come on concussion safety, the incident spoke volumes about how much farther it still had to go. The Eagles tried to rationalize away their failure to adhere to new, stricter concussion policies prohibiting any player from being returned to the very game in which he was concussed. They insisted that none of their medical personnel had seen the collision or the subsequent collapse. And more importantly, they said their three-minute sideline exam revealed no concussion—an explanation that boggled the minds of brain injury experts across the nation, and in the NFL itself.

"I doubt they did any kind of neurologic, thorough assessment," Cantu declared, noting that sideline evaluations require at least fifteen minutes. "You just can't do it that fast. You need to assess the player both at rest and then after exertion." Cantu shook his head. "It's a shame it was seen on national TV," he said, "but it points out needed work to be done."

It also raised frightening questions for every parent of a sports-playing child: If a concussion this obvious could be missed by the well-trained medical staffs that populate NFL sidelines, what about high school and youth league games where there are no team physicians or athletic trainers? And if a concussion this glaring could go unnoticed under the NFL's spotlight and microscope, how many go unnoticed on high school fields, youth league fields, and playgrounds across America?

Epilogue

Seven years after post-concussion syndrome forced him to drop out of Rutgers, Dave Showalter went back to college. He was tentative at first, signing up for just one course to see if he could handle the work. But by fall of 2008, he was back at Rutgers full-time, enthusiastically pursuing a degree in anthropology. School was different this time. Some of the concussion damage had been permanent, and learning didn't come as easily as it once had. Before the brain injuries, he had needed only to attend lectures to get a good grade, often skipping reading and homework assignments. Now if he wanted to do well, he needed to read every word from the assigned books, sometimes more than once, and could never skip a homework assignment. This time, though, he was excited about his major and happy to put in all the extra work, maintaining nearly a 4.0 GPA in the classes he took since his return. By the spring of 2010, he had a diploma in hand and an open door to new dreams that included graduate school, perhaps even a career as a professor.

Showalter was philosophical about the years he took off from school. He wasn't sure he would have been as motivated if he had tried to come back sooner. One thing he was sure of was that he had spent too long assuming that his cognitive abilities would never return. No one had told him that he could retrain his brain by plugging away at the tasks that had become so difficult for him. Among the most important lessons he learned from his first class back was that the brain could be rehabbed just like any muscle in the body. The more he read, the easier it got. The more he expressed himself, the more fluidly he wrote and spoke. He still read more slowly than he did when he started college back in 1998 and occasionally found himself fumbling for words, but he learned that he could still excel in the classroom. He accepted the fact that his brain didn't work as well as it once had. He was happy that it seemed to be working well enough to take him where he wanted to go. He started rewriting his old concussion speeches in his head. Now he wanted to tell all the high school and college students whose lives had been derailed by concussions that they needed to keep at it and push themselves to reclaim the skills stolen by brain injury. He hoped that nowadays fewer kids would need to hear this advice, that the sports world had finally gotten the message that concussions were serious injuries.

As he watched games during the first few weeks of the 2010 NFL season, Showalter was amazed to see what Roger Goodell had managed in just a few short months. Players were actually being pulled from games because of concussions. Though the changes meant the sport might have fewer of the exhilarating big hits, he figured a little less excitement was a small price to pay to protect players' brains.

Not everyone felt the same way.

As the 2010 season swung into high gear, so did the violence. Despite warnings from league officials that certain types of brain-rattling head hits would be harshly punished, playing styles hadn't changed one bit. In fact, it seemed like this season was even more brutal than previous ones. By mid-October, there had already been at least fifty-three concussions. And then came a Sunday that instantly became famous for its level of brutality: violent head hits sent one player to the hospital on a backboard and knocked four others out of games. Overnight, Goodell upped the ante, threatening suspensions in addition to fines for offenders. Ultimately, the commissioner decided to mete out only fines this time, but he sent a memo to every team warning that there would be an immediate crackdown and that from now on players who delivered illegal blows to the head and neck would receive suspensions as well as hefty fines.

The crackdown wasn't popular with the players or their union. The most notorious of the three fined players, James Harrison of the Pittsburgh Steelers, threatened to pick up his football and go home. "How can I continue to play this game the way that I've been taught to play this game since I was ten years old?" said the hard-hitting All-Pro linebacker. "And now you're telling me that everything they've taught me from that time on for the last twenty-plus years is not the way you're supposed to play the game anymore. If that's the case, I can't play by those rules. You're handicapping me."

Many other players insisted that they couldn't learn a new style of play, one that didn't include using the head and body as a battering ram. The league decided to show them that they could. That week in the film rooms of all thirty-two NFL teams, players were forced to watch a league-produced video showing examples of flagrant hits that would no longer be tolerated—a highlight reel of helmet-to-helmet hits and of shots to the heads of "defenseless" receivers. The players' response was similar to what you'd expect from a roomful of junior-high boys forced to watch *Reefer Madness* as a drug-education video. There were catcalls and wads of paper hurled at the screen. All that was missing were spitballs. As the video's narrator warned that they'd now be disciplined for these kinds of hits, the players provided their own commentary, making cracks like "Did this guy ever play?!"

All-Pro linebacker Brian Urlacher of the Chicago Bears spoke for many of them when he scoffed that the NFL should just issue flags instead of protective pads and rename itself "the NFFL—the National Flag Football League." The union president, former All-Pro center Kevin Mawae, ridiculed the crackdown, saying, "The skirts need to be taken off in the NFL offices."

Perhaps more surprising was the response from sportswriters who were concerned that all the new rules were going to ruin the game they loved to watch and write about. William Rhoden, a columnist at *The New York Times*, the very newspaper that ran dozens of front-page stories alerting the public to the dangers of concussions, wrote, "A number of parents with young children are wringing their hands and saying they would never allow their children to play football. That's precisely why there is a premium on those who do play football: it takes a rare breed to play this violent game at any level. Football has always been dangerous— and that's why we like it, for the vicarious thrill of watching someone do something we would never or could never do."

There were some who saw it differently, who recognized the value of protecting players from themselves. Brad Wilson, a columnist for a small paper in Pennsylvania's Lehigh Valley, put it this way: "There are a few fans, one would like to think a minority, who view football as a bloodsport and will decry the new rules and changes they cause as wimpy and only good for sissies. These are the same people who didn't like it when Rome stopped feeding its criminals to the lions because it spoiled their day out at the Colosseum. These people can go watch 'Saw' movies and leave football for everyone else."

After the NFL's fall 2010 crackdown in the wake of what became instantly infamous as Black-and-Blue Sunday, concussions increasingly seeped into the public consciousness and conversation. No matter where people sided on the concussion debate—whether with the reformers striving to make contact sports safer or the traditionalists fighting to preserve the fabric of rough-and-tumble games—it was getting harder and harder to ignore the impact that head injuries have on our brains and our favorite pastimes.

Concussions had entered the vernacular everywhere from the sportscasts that entertain us to the video games that enchant our children. It was indeed a sign of the changing times when *Madden NFL*, which through its first two decades as America's hottest-selling video game wowed nearly a hundred million kids with head-rattling hits even more exaggerated than anything seen in real-life games, announced in the spring of 2011 that its next version was being redesigned to stress the seriousness of head injuries, the urgency of sidelining concussed players, and the responsibility of teaching safer tackling techniques.

Although the public hadn't fully absorbed the message about the menace of head injuries, at least Americans were finally starting to recognize that concussions are indeed injuries to the brain.

All the concussion talk certainly was weighing heavily on Dave Duerson's mind that February night when he penned a chilling suicide note in block letters: PLEASE, SEE THAT MY BRAIN IS GIVEN TO THE NFL'S BRAIN BANK. He proceeded to aim a revolver at his chest rather than his head and shoot himself through the heart so that his brain could be preserved for science. Duerson had suspected that all the head blows he'd absorbed through his eleven-year NFL career as a hard-hitting safety were responsible for his downward spiral from a two-time Super Bowl champion and successful businessman to a bankrupt fifty-year-old battling memory loss, impulse control issues, and mood volatility. It surprised no one three months later when BU's Center for the Study of Traumatic Encephalopathy revealed that Duerson's brain evidenced the same trauma-induced disease previously found in the autopsies of more than twenty former NFL players. In becoming what *Time* magazine called "football's first martyr," he left this legacy for all those suffering in silence: a sword of Damocles that must now haunt everyone who's ever sustained repeated concussions or absorbed multiple head jolts, from the Dave Duersons to the Dave Showalters.

And it wasn't just America's most popular sport being threatened by the ticking time bomb of head injuries. Less than three months after the NFL's Black-and-Blue Sunday, the NHL found itself facing a concussion flashpoint of its own.

At the epicenter was hockey's supreme superstar: Sidney Crosby, the sublimely skilled center hailed as the second coming of Wayne Gretzky himself. Whether leading the Pittsburgh Penguins to the Stanley Cup or Team Canada to the Olympic gold medal, Crosby has been the face of hockey ever since his 2005 NHL debut. By missing the entire second half of the 2010–11 season due to concussion symptoms, he would also become the face of an injury that threatens anybody who plays contact sports.

It is a cautionary tale that highlights the consequences of failing to take head injuries seriously. During the NHL's annual New Year's Day spectacle on a makeshift outdoor rink built over the very Heinz Field gridiron where the Pittsburgh Steelers illuminated football's concussion crisis, sixty-eight thousand spectators and millions of TV viewers watched Crosby get flattened by a blindside shoulder to the head, struggle to his feet, and then skate slowly, dazed and doubled over, off the ice. That wooziness should have been enough of a red flag to automatically sideline him for the remaining twenty minutes of play. Instead, shaking off what he dismissed as just common neck soreness, he played on without missing a shift and started the Penguins' next game four nights later despite a feeling of fogginess that sneaked up on him gradually. His brain was still foggy late in the second period when he was rammed into the boards by an illegal blindside check, slamming his head against the glass. It wasn't until he reported feeling headachy and sick after finishing the game that he was finally sent to the University of Pittsburgh's renowned concussion clinic for evaluation.

Even then, the diagnosis, "mild concussion," and the prognosis for his return to play, "about a week," minimized the seriousness of the head injury. With Crosby's headaches and other symptoms persisting much

longer than expected, doctors waited ten weeks before clearing him to
resume even light skating; and when his noncontact workouts triggered
a recurrence of the concussion symptoms five weeks later, they ordered
him to stop all physical activity. The Penguins' medical personnel, still
stinging from widespread criticism over not taking the New Year's Day
hit more seriously, were now taking no chances in the aftermath of their
team captain's first diagnosed concussion. By season's end, Crosby had
been disabled for four months and had resigned himself to the specter of
a long roller coaster of recovery and rehab from a scary injury that was
threatening his brilliant career at the age of just twenty-three.

It took the loss of hockey's transcendent star to spur the NHL into
taking action. Late in the season, the league toughened its head injury
protocol to require that any player who shows signs of concussion be removed from the bench and examined by a team doctor for fifteen minutes
in a quiet room away from the ice. At the same time, the Crosby controversy—coupled with the finding of CTE in two NHL retirees notorious
for their aggressive style—poured gasoline on the smoldering debate over
whether all head hits should be banned. Crosby himself joined the growing chorus of prominent voices criticizing the NHL when it failed to
discipline either player who'd blindsided him and calling for a prohibition
on all head hits once and for all.

"How much damage is it going to take before we finally wake up and
we make those changes?" wondered Pat LaFontaine, the Hall of Famer
whose forced retirement had inspired him to become a vocal advocate for
concussion awareness. "I pray it doesn't mean somebody doesn't get up off
the ice to realize this is a serious problem."

As important as those types of changes would be for the pros, they are
all the more imperative for the kids.

The YouTube video got hundreds of thousands of views: Two eight-year-
old boys are charging toward one another in a tackling drill as a female
voice yells "Go! Go!" They lower their heads and ram into each other,
helmet to helmet, with a sickening crack. The boy carrying the ball is
knocked flat on his back and begins to cry and writhe in pain as a coach
casually walks over.

The video encapsulated everything that is wrong with the way we play sports in America. We glorify the big brain-rattling hits, cheering the players who deliver them and rewarding the coaches who teach them. We entrust our children to coaches who would blithely unleash two eight-year-old heads on one another without a thought to the vulnerability of the developing brains inside the helmets.

Inevitably, people who want to keep the game the same will suggest that the problem can be solved with better helmets. But that's just wishful thinking. Helmets can't protect a brain during a collision any better than a shell can protect an egg yolk if the egg is shaken back and forth. Like the yolk, the brain slams around in its "shell" when the head suddenly accelerates or decelerates. No matter how sophisticated the design of a football helmet, nothing can prevent the brain from being damaged by the shaking. The only way to protect athletes' brains is by changing our culture of concussions on every level from the pros all the way down to the peewees.

We need to educate not just the athletes—millions of whom aren't old enough yet to make informed decisions—but also the parents, the coaches, and everyone else involved with youth and school sports. Only through education and information will Americans come to accept the reality that concussions are indeed traumatic brain injuries.

America needs a hero, a celebrity willing to step forward and speak for all the millions suffering in silence with brain injuries that they prefer to keep hidden for fear of being stigmatized.

Troy Aikman, America's Quarterback himself, would have made an ideal spokesman after multiple concussions forced him to retire at age thirty-four. To the millions of kids looking up to him as a role model, he could have told a cautionary tale about the dangers of playing through concussions and offered a heads-up about the urgency of managing them safely. Instead, as a leading broadcaster on the NFL's network telecasts, he chose to send a different message—by minimizing them and insisting that they must be accepted as a risk inherent in the sport. Even after the NFL finally accepted the need for safety reforms under withering media and political pressure in 2009, Aikman seemed less concerned with the long-term effects of concussions on the players' brains than with the long-term impact of the increased awareness on "the game of football as we know it." In the face of the mounting scientific evidence exposing football-related dementia among NFL retirees, he pointed out that he has no cognitive deficits in his forties and focused not on that vulnerability but on the trickle-down effect on the sport. "I wonder what the impact of the concussion studies will have at the grassroots level," he wrote in his *Sporting News* magazine column. "If you're a parent and you hear repetitive contact in football could cause long-term health issues, are you inclined to let your 10-year-old son participate? And if fewer kids are allowed to play, what effect will that have on the NFL 10 or 15 years from now?"

Troy Aikman, bemoaning how he and fellow Hall of Fame quarterback Steve Young had become "the poster boys for concussions," wasn't about to become a crusader for concussion safety. If only some marquee superstar like Aikman could have followed the example set by Harry Carson.

During his thirteen seasons as one of the NFL's hardest-hitting linebackers, Carson had caused countless concussions and sustained at least fifteen himself without ever reporting them to a trainer. He never connected them with the odd symptoms that dogged him through much of his Hall of Fame career—not even the depression so profound that once, while driving across the Tappan Zee Bridge on his way to Giants Stadium for practice, he had to resist the strong impulse to steer his car through the guardrail and into the Hudson River. It wasn't until Carson began his second career as a TV commentator that the symptoms he'd played through became too noticeable to ignore: migraines, blurred vision, sensitivity to light and noises, short-term memory loss, concentration problems. He would be on air, live, and he'd lose his train of thought in mid-sentence. He found himself misidentifying players and teams, blanking on the names of interviewees in mid-question, mispronouncing words, stammering as he fumbled to retrieve them from his thesauruslike vocabulary. Sure that he had a brain tumor, he finally consulted a neurologist two years after he'd retired from the NFL. The belated diagnosis of post-concussion syndrome explained the symptoms that cost him his broadcasting career and his first marriage.

It also led to a new calling. In 1994, four years after he was diagnosed with a syndrome that was then just starting to force other NFL stars into early retirement, Carson was asked by the Brain Injury Association of America to promote concussion awareness. At a time when the concussion controversy was first emerging, Carson started by trying to educate former teammates and opponents. "Once I went public with this concussion thing, they were looking at me as being sort of brain-damaged, drooling and all this stuff," he recalls, "but it is an injury just like one to your knee or hip." That's the message he delivers, passionately and eloquently, whenever he speaks to athletes, parents, and coaches at educational conferences.

With a sensitive and soft-spoken manner belying the ferocity he brought to the football field, Carson makes just as effective a leader in the fight for retiree disability benefits as he had been as captain of the New York Giants' first Super Bowl championship team. Still suffering post-concussion symptoms fully two decades after retirement, he worries about the future implications for his own brain and regrets whatever role the hits he delivered may have had in the dementia suffered by too many of his teammates and opponents. If he had known then what he does now about the long-term consequences of concussion, Carson doubts he ever would have played in the first place. When medical conditions forced his older son to give up football before an NFL tryout and his younger son to give it up before a major-college tryout, Carson was relieved rather than disappointed. "Every parent should sit up and pay attention," he says. "When you look at the players who have played the game and are now dealing with serious neurological issues, you have to ask yourself, 'Is it worth the risk to allow my child to play the game?'"

America needs more Harry Carsons, sports stars willing to talk publicly about brain injuries that most sufferers strive to keep private. The famous among us need to be just as courageous as the everyday people who made this book possible by sharing their lives and struggles. If the most visible among us won't talk about their invisible wounds, traumatic brain injury is fated to remain silent and hidden.

Appendix I

Concussion Symptoms

All head injuries should be taken seriously. A concussion may be an invisible injury, but its symptoms and signs can often be spotted by parents, friends, coaches, athletic trainers, and others who know the head-injured individual. The following symptoms or signs of concussion may occur after a bump, blow, or jolt to the head:

Observed Symptoms

- Appears dazed or stunned
- Vomiting or complaining of nausea
- Confusion
- Memory problems (difficulty learning new information)
- Amnesia (loss of memories from before and/or after the injury)
- Any loss of consciousness
- Difficulty with coordination or balance
- Behavior or personality changes
- Slowed thinking, reaction, speaking, or reading
- Slurred or nonsensical speech
- Seizures

Reported Symptoms

- Feeling dizzy, dazed, or lightheaded
- Headache, neck pain, or a sensation of pressure in the head
- Increased sensitivity to light or sounds
- Feeling hazy, foggy, or groggy
- Feeling sluggish, fatigued, or unusually tired
- "Seeing stars"

- Blurred vision or double vision
- Ringing in ears
- Mood changes (e.g., sadness, listlessness, irritability, anxiety, loss of motivation)
- Difficulty concentrating, thinking, or making decisions
- Sleeping longer than usual or having trouble sleeping
- Loss of sense of taste or smell

Sources: Adapted from the Centers for Disease Control and Prevention's "Heads Up Toolkit for Youth Sports," the "Sport Concussion Assessment Tool 2" developed and adopted in 2008 by the Third International Conference on Concussion in Sport, and concussion education articles published online by the University of Pittsburgh Medical Center and the University of California–Los Angeles Health System.

Appendix II

Resources for Patients and Families

The following are some useful resources for information on traumatic brain injuries in general and concussions in particular:

Brain Injury Association of America
1608 Spring Hill Road, Suite 110
Vienna, VA 22182
Phone: 800-444-6443
Website: www.biausa.org

The nation's oldest and largest brain injury organization offers education, research, and advocacy for individuals with brain injury, their families and friends, and healthcare professionals. The BIAA offers a nationwide network of more than forty chartered state affiliates and hundreds of local chapters and support groups. Its National Directory of Brain Injury Services offers a comprehensive online directory of TBI providers.

CDC's National Center for Injury Prevention & Control
4770 Buford Highway, NE
Mail Stop F-63
Atlanta, GA 30341
Phone: 800-232-4636 (800-CDC-INFO)
Website: www.cdc.gov/injury

This CDC website provides comprehensive information on brain injury in general and concussion in particular. Access its "Concussion and

Mild TBI" homepage directly through www.cdc.gov/concussion. The homepage offers links to separate sections on sports concussions and on clinical diagnosis and management, as well as links to tools and resources for downloading and mail-ordering educational materials. There are links to download its "Heads Up on Concussion" toolkits, a series of free guides, and other educational materials for coaches, parents, athletes, and health-care professionals that provide information on preventing, recognizing, and responding to concussions. They include "Heads Up: Concussion in Youth Sports," "Heads Up: Concussion in High School Sports," "Heads Up to Schools: Know Your Concussion ABCs," and "Heads Up: Brain Injury in Your Practice."

National Library of Medicine's Medline Plus
Website: www.nlm.nih.gov/medlineplus

This government site provides comprehensive information and links. Type "concussion" into the search engine for the latest news and a host of external links.

Traumatic Brain Injury National Data and Statistical Center
Website: www.tbindsc.org

For information on the sixteen federally funded centers that pro-vide comprehensive systems of TBI care and rehabilitation, click on the "TBIMS CENTERS" homepage link or go directly to the address www.tbindsc.org/Centers.aspx.

Acknowledgments

In the five years since we first stumbled upon this hidden epidemic and realized how little was known about it, we've had to rely on countless people to help us comprehend the impact of the invisible injury and to bring an emerging public health crisis out of the shadows.

First and foremost, we'd like to thank all the TBI sufferers who've courageously shared the stories of their struggles to overcome an injury that most prefer to keep private. Chief among them are those you've met in these pages: Dave Showalter, Willie Baun, Melissa Inzitari, Katrina Majewski, Brian Radke, Chari Abb, Anne Forrest, Mike Zacchea, Mark Lenkiewicz, and Angelica Kruth. We'd also like to thank their family members for opening lives and hearts to us: Whitey and Becky Baun, Nova Radke, Diane Lenkiewicz, Doreen Kruth, Eleanor Perfetto, Jovita Bollig, and Chari Stoesser, among others. We owe a debt of gratitude to all those whose stories have played out in the media—from the teenage athletes struck by second-impact syndrome to the professional stars who've battled post-concussion syndrome and early-onset dementia. Thanks to all who have shared their compelling stories in an effort to help and to inspire the countless TBI survivors who suffer in silence.

We'd like to acknowledge all the doctors who have devoted their careers to treating patients with brain injuries and who graciously took time out of their tight schedules to talk with us. Among them, we'd especially like to thank Bob Cantu and Mark Lovell—pioneers in the diagnosis and treatment of concussions. Other clinicians who were generous with their time, insight, and experience include Jill Brooks, Richard Saunders, Robert Harbaugh, Mark Sementilli, Tom Thompson, Wayne Gordon, Tamar Martin, James Hill, Warren Lux, Joe Maroon, and Barry Jordan.

Without the help of the scientists who took many hours of their time to explain very complicated research to us, we wouldn't have been able to describe what goes on in the brains of TBI sufferers. Dave Hovda and Doug Smith welcomed us into their state-of-the-art labs and were always available to patiently explain difficult concepts, occasionally many times over. We also relied on many other researchers to help us put the emerging science in perspective: Ann McKee, Bob Stern, Bennet Omalu, Julian Bailes, Kevin Guskiewicz, Fred Mueller, John Povlishock, Ed Hall, Jon Lifshitz, Michael Lipton.

We all owe a debt of gratitude to those who struggled early on to educate the public about the dangers of concussions. In particular, we'd like to thank Leigh Steinberg for sharing the story of his drive to change football's concussion culture and for providing insights on the evolution of concussion awareness. We'd also like to thank Chris Nowinski for providing us with an inside look at the crusade he's led to force safety reforms in football as well as other contact sports.

We'd like to acknowledge our fellow journalists for writing the first draft of history on this emerging story. We are particularly indebted to Alan Schwarz for the relentless reporting that put concussions on the front page of *The New York Times* and helped raise the nation's awareness about this growing public health crisis.

This book could not have happened without Jane Dystel, literary agent extraordinaire. Jane believed in the project right from the start, and whenever the going got tough and we got discouraged, she was always there to remind us that this was an important issue that needed to be written about. She tenaciously sought a publishing house that would agree and, eventually, found just the right home for the book.

We couldn't have anticipated the enthusiasm with which Simon & Schuster embraced the project, from its publisher on down. We were heartened by Jonathan Karp's suggestion that this book could change the way America looks at concussions. We are indebted to our editor, Roger Labrie, for helping mold the manuscript. He saw what needed to be pruned and where we needed reorganization to make the book's message more powerful. His guidance made our manuscript into a much better book.

We are fortunate to have friends who were willing to read multiple drafts and to offer specific suggestions for improvement. We're especially grateful to Peggy Loper, Michael Keller, and Diane Nafis, the one person who may have read the manuscript more times than we did. Thanks, as always, to Dale Maharidge for the wisdom of his experience—starting with the warning that writing a book is "like climbing a ten-thousand-foot wall of ice, carving one new handhold at a time"—and the encouraging advice on how to scale that ice cliff.

Finally, we'd like to thank our families for living with this project for the past five years—especially Mariela, who only rarely complained that Mommy was often too busy working on the book to come out and play.

Source Notes

Introduction

Parents' concussion knowledge: Survey data came from 2010 University of Michigan report titled "C. S. Mott Children's Hospital National Poll on Children's Health."

Hospitalization statistics: Data came from Lisa L. Bakhos et al., "Emergency Department Visits for Concussion in Young Child Athletes," *Pediatrics* 126:e550–56, 2010.

Concussion incidence: CDC estimates for sports-related concussions came from Jean A. Langlois et al., "The Epidemiology and Impact of Traumatic Brain Injury," *Journal of Head Trauma Rehabilitation* 21:375–78, 2006.

Long-term deficits: Statistic came from David F. Meaney and Douglas H. Smith, "Biomechanics of Concussion," *Clinics in Sports Medicine* 30:33–48, 2011.

Chapter 1: Just a Bump on the Head

Dave Showalter's story: Narrative based on interviews with Dave Showalter and Jill Brooks, Ph.D.

Chapter 2: The Emerging Epidemic

Concussion incidence: CDC estimates for sports-related concussions came from Jean A. Langlois et al., "The Epidemiology and Impact of Traumatic Brain Injury," *Journal of Head Trauma Rehabilitation* 21:375–78, 2006.

Participation statistic: Estimate by the National Council of Youth Sports came from its 2008 market research membership study titled "Report on Trends and Participation in Organized Youth Sports."

Cantu guidelines: Narrative based on interviews with Robert Cantu, M.D. Details on his guidelines came from Robert C. Cantu, "Guidelines for Return to Contact Sports after a Cerebral Concussion," *Physician and Sports Medicine* 14:75–83, 1986.

Second-impact syndrome discovery: Narrative based on interviews with Richard Saunders, M.D., and Robert Harbaugh, M.D. Details on their findings came from Richard L. Saunders and Robert E. Harbaugh, "The Second Impact in Catastrophic Contact-

Sports Head Trauma," *Journal of the American Medical Association* 252:538–39, 1984. Works cited for influencing their research include the seminal textbook describing catastrophic injuries, Richard C. Schneider, *Head and Neck Injuries in Football: Mechanisms, Treatment, and Prevention* (Baltimore: Williams & Wilkins, 1973); and an animal study, Robert A. Moody et al., "An Evaluation of Decompression in Experimental Head Injury," *Journal of Neurosurgery* 29:586–90, 1968.

Enzo Montemurro's story: Frederick Mueller, Ph.D., director of the National Center for Catastrophic Sports Injury Research at the University of North Carolina–Chapel Hill, and the public affairs office at Dartmouth College helped identify the Cornell student who succumbed to second-impact syndrome. Details on the injury and its aftermath came from articles reported by the Associated Press and several newspapers. Particularly helpful were stories on his treatment ("Gridder Remains Critical; Doctor Explains Condition," *Cornell Daily Sun*, October 27, 1981) and his death ("Cornell Gridder Dies of Injuries," *Ithaca Journal*, October 30, 1981).

Second-impact deaths: Invaluable assistance in identifying college and high school athletes killed by second-impact syndrome was provided by Frederick Mueller. Details on the deaths of the high school football players cited came from their local newspapers. Particularly helpful were articles on Billy Rideout ("Football Player, 17, Dies after Injury," *New York Times*, November 10, 1986) and on Freddy Mendoza ("Prep Player Dies After Collapsing," *Los Angeles Times*, October 8, 1991).

Second-impact syndrome statistics: The CDC provided the number of known second-impact deaths in a report titled "Sports-Related Recurrent Brain Injuries—United States" in its *Morbidity and Mortality Weekly Report* of March 14, 1997.

Brandon Schultz's story: Narrative constructed from "Playing Hard," *PBS NewsHour with Jim Lehrer*, January 26, 2000, along with information from the law firm that represented Schultz in his landmark suit, Nelson Langer Engle.

Steinberg-Aikman-Young concussion awakening: Interviews with Leigh Steinberg formed the basis of the narrative. His quote on role models came from "Playing Hard," *PBS NewsHour with Jim Lehrer*, January 26, 2000. Background on the multiple concussions leading to the retirements of Troy Aikman and Steve Young came from various periodicals. Details on Young's retirement came from Dave Kindred, "In the End, Young Had No Choice," *Sporting News*, June 19, 2000. Details on the concussion that hospitalized Aikman came from "A Common N.F.L. Question: How Many Fingers Do You See?" *New York Times*, January 26, 1994. The Concussion Bowl reference came from Mark Starr, "Arms Like Lead! Hit 'Em in the Head!" *Newsweek*, December 1, 1997. Details on Aikman's conversations with Young came from "Giants Want Aikman Stopped but Conscious," *New York Times*, October 13, 2000. Background on Al Toon's post-concussion syndrome and retirement came from multiple *New York Times* news stories.

Guskiewicz research: Narrative based on interviews with Kevin Guskiewicz, Ph.D. Description of his findings came from Kevin M. Guskiewicz et al., "Cumulative Effects

Associated with Recurrent Concussion in Collegiate Football Players: The NCAA Concussion Study," *Journal of the American Medical Association* 290:2549–55, 2003, and Michael McCrea et al., "Acute Effects and Recovery Time Following Concussions in Collegiate Football Players: The NCAA Concussion Study," *Journal of the American Medical Association* 290:2556–63, 2003.

Studies illuminating dangers of multiple concussions: Details of the college and high school football study showing that risk of concussion goes up with each head jolt came from Eric D. Zemper, "Two-Year Prospective Study of Relative Risk of a Second Cerebral Concussion," *American Journal of Physical Medicine & Rehabilitation* 82:653–59, 2003. Information on the link between cognitive deficits and multiple concussions came from Michael W. Collins et al., "Relationship between Concussion and Neuropsychological Performance in College Football Players," *Journal of the American Medical Association* 282:964–70, 1999, and Grant L. Iverson et al., "Cumulative Effects of Concussion in Amateur Athletes," *Brain Injury* 18:433–43, 2004.

Incidence of sports concussions: Statistics on high school football came from Wayne Langburt et al., "Incidence of Concussion in High School Football Players of Ohio and Pennsylvania," *Journal of Child Neurology* 16:83–85, 2001. Statistics comparing college and high school basketball, soccer, and football came from Luke M. Gessell et al., "Concussions among United States High School and Collegiate Athletes," *Journal of Athletic Training* 42:495–503, 2007.

Jamie Carey's story: Narrative constructed from multiple newspaper stories, including "The Science of Hard Knocks," *Chronicle of Higher Education*, June 15, 2007; "Concussions Knock Out Stanford Star's Dream," *San Jose Mercury News*, November 8, 2000; "Concussion Aside, Jamie Carey Tries to Resume Career at Texas," *Dallas Morning News*, July 26, 2002; "Texas Women's Hoops Transfer Brings Issue of Concussions to Forefront," *Kansas City Star*, August 24, 2002; "Concussions Are Just Part of Game for Longhorns' Carey," *New York Times*, April 6, 2003; and "Her Courage Is Untouchable," *Hartford Courant*, May 20, 2005. NBA-WNBA concussion rates came from John R. Deitch et al., "Injury Risk in Professional Basketball Players: A Comparison of Women's National Basketball Association and National Basketball Association Athletes," *American Journal of Sports Medicine* 34:1077–83, 2006.

Zack Lystedt's story: Narrative constructed from published and televised reports. Most helpful was "Knocking Heads," *Dan Rather Reports*, HDNet, March 3, 2009. Some details of the injury and its aftermath were drawn from newspaper stories, notably "Special Report: The Dangers of Adolescents Playing Football with Concussions," *Seattle Times*, November 4, 2008. Research showing that athletes returned to play too soon came from Ellen E. Yard and R. Dawn Comstock, "Compliance with Return to Play Guidelines Following Concussion in U.S. High School Athletes, 2005–2008," *Brain Injury* 23:888–98, 2009.

Chapter 3: Head Games

The Bauns' story: Narrative based on interviews with Willie, Whitey, and Becky Baun. Background came from Christopher Nowinski, *Head Games: Football's Concussion Crisis* (East Bridgewater, Mass.: Drummond, 2007).

NFL violence: Details on Fox commercial, TNT ad, and ESPN highlights came from "Scorecard," *Sports Illustrated*, October 16, 1995, and "NFL Is Playing Head Games," *New York Post*, September 6, 1995. Vince Lombardi's philosophy came from multiple sources, notably David Maraniss, *When Pride Still Mattered: A Life of Vince Lombardi* (New York: Simon & Schuster, 1999).

Physics of football hits: Player size analysis based on several sources. Most helpful were two studies that used large databases of NFL players—"Heavy Pressure: NFL Players Struggle with Weight Game," *Palm Beach Post*, October 29, 2006, and "Supersized in the NFL: Many Ex-Players Dying Young," Scripps Howard News Service, January 31, 2006. Statistics on force of hits came from Brian Vestag, "Football Brain Injuries Draw Increased Scrutiny," *Journal of the American Medical Association* 287:437–39, 2002, and Tim Layden, "The Big Hit," *Sports Illustrated*, July 30, 2007. Statistics on force of concussive hits in NFL study came from Elliot J. Pellman et al., "Concussion in Professional Football: Reconstruction of Game Impacts and Injuries," *Neurosurgery* 53:799–814, 2003.

Steinberg's advocacy: Interviews with Leigh Steinberg provided the details on his awakening in the wake of Aikman's rookie concussion and his subsequent crusade for safety reforms.

NFL concussion data: The widely used per-game average was based on the league's released statistics for number of reported concussions per season.

Wayne Chrebet's story: Narrative of concussion controversy based on multiple news stories in *The New York Times* and the New York *Daily News*. Quotes came from "Jets' Chrebet Sustains Another Concussion," *New York Times*, November 6, 2003, and "Concussion and Its Aftereffects End Season for Jets' Chrebet," *New York Times*, November 13, 2003.

Elliot Pellman controversy: Background on the formation of the NFL's MTBI Committee came from Elliot J. Pellman, "Background on the National Football League's Research on Concussion in the National Football League," *Neurosurgery* 53:797–98, 2003. Background on Pellman's chairmanship came from Peter Keating, "Doctor Yes," *ESPN The Magazine*, October 28, 2006.

NFL concussion studies: Details on the NFL MTBI Committee's conclusion that multiple concussions did not lead to long-term consequences came from Elliot J. Pellman et al., "Concussion in Professional Football: Neuropsychological Testing—Part 6," *Neurosurgery* 55:1290–1305, 2004. Details on the committee's conclusion that it was safe to return certain players to the same game in which they were concussed and that that might extend beyond the pros to college and high school players came from Elliot J. Pellman et al., "Concussion in Professional Football: Players Returning to the Same Game—Part 7," *Neurosurgery* 56:79–92, 2005.

Fallout from NFL studies: Gerard Malanga's quote came from "N.F.L. Study Authors Dispute Concussion Finding," *New York Times*, June 10, 2007.

Football participation statistics: Figures for colleges and secondary schools came from the National Center for Catastrophic Sports Injury Research's 2010 report titled "Annual Survey of Football Injury Research: 1931–2009." Figure for youth leagues came from USA Football's "2007 Youth Football Participation Index Study."

Lack of concussion knowledge in college football: Data came from a 2003 study led by JoEllen Sefton at Central Connecticut State University for her master's thesis titled "An Examination of Factors That Influence Knowledge of and Reporting of Head Injuries in College Football."

Incidence of concussion in high school football: Disparity statistics based on comparison of numerous epidemiological studies. In player surveys, the low rate of 15 percent came from Michael McCrea et al., "Unreported Concussion in High School Football Players: Implications for Prevention," *Clinical Journal of Sports Medicine* 14:13–17, 2004, while the high rate of 47 percent came from Wayne Langburt et al., "Incidence of Concussion in High School Football Players of Ohio and Pennsylvania," *Journal of Child Neurology* 16:83–85, 2001. In trainer surveys, the low rate of 4 percent came from M. McCrea et al., "Standardized Assessment of Concussion in Football Players," *Neurology* 48:586–88, 1997, and John W. Powell and Kim D. Barber-Foss, "Traumatic Brain Injury in High School Athletes," *Journal of the American Medical Association* 282:958–63, 1999. The reasons players gave for not reporting came from McCrea's *Clinical Journal of Sports Medicine* article and Sefton's thesis.

Early college football: Analysis pieced together from multiple sources. Background and some details came from John Sayle Watterson, *College Football: History, Spectacle, Controversy* (Baltimore: Johns Hopkins University Press, 2000). Description of playing style, John L. Sullivan's quote, and Theodore Roosevelt's ultimatum came from Bruce K. Stewart, "American Football," *American History*, November 1995. Description of Harvard's flying wedge came from several sources, including Scott A. McQuilkin and Ronald A. Smith, "The Rise and Fall of the Flying Wedge: Football's Most Controversial Play," *Journal of Sport History* 20:57–64, 1993.

Theodore Roosevelt's intervention: History based on multiple sources, notably John Sayle Watterson, *College Football: History, Spectacle, Controversy* (Baltimore: Johns Hopkins University Press, 2000). Roosevelt's quote on football as a metaphor came from Theodore Roosevelt, *The Strenuous Life: Essays and Addresses* (New York: Century, 1899). His letter to Ted Jr. came from Joseph Bucklin Bishop, ed., *Theodore Roosevelt's Letters to His Children* (New York: Charles Scribner's Sons, 1923).

Hockey head injuries: Details on Eddie Shore, Ace Bailey, and Gordie Howe came from

Arthur Pincus, David Rosner, Len Hochberg, and Chris Malcolm, *The Official Illustrated NHL History* (London: Carlton Books, 1999). Details on Bill Masterton's death and its impact came from Richard Beddoes, Stan Fischler, and Ira Gitler, *Hockey! The Story of the World's Fastest Sport* (New York: Macmillan, 1969).

Physics of hockey hits: Data on the force of peewee hockey hits and its comparison to college football came from J. P. Mihalik et al., "Characteristics of Head Impacts Sustained by Youth Ice Hockey Players," *Journal of Sports Engineering and Technology* 222:45–52, 2008.

Pat LaFontaine's story: Narrative based on multiple sources. A first-person account, including the dialogue with the first neurologist he consulted, came from Pat LaFontaine, *Companions in Courage: Triumphant Tales of Heroic Athletes* (New York: Warner Books, 2001). The most helpful magazine articles included Leigh Montville, "Can't Quit Now," *Sports Illustrated*, August 24, 1997, and Mark Herrmann, "An American in Transition," *Rinkside*, January 1999. The account of the events leading to his retirement was pieced together from numerous news stories from all four New York City dailies.

Eric Lindros concussion controversy: Details came from multiple newspaper and magazine articles.

Incidence of hockey concussions: The statistic comparing NHL to NFL players came from newspaper research in "NHL Watches as Concussions Rise," *Orange County Register*, September 23, 2007. Data comparing concussions rates for U.S. college men's and women's hockey to each other and to football came from Jennifer M. Hootman et al., "Epidemiology of Collegiate Injury for 15 Sports: Summary and Recommendations for Injury Prevention Initiatives," *Journal of Athletic Training* 42:311–19, 2007.

Lack of concussion reporting in youth hockey: Data came from I. J. S. Williamson and D. Goodman, "Converging Evidence for the Under-Reporting of Concussions in Youth Ice Hockey," *British Journal of Sports Medicine* 40:128–32, 2006.

J. Scott Delaney's research: Narrative based on his studies and on quotes and information in Christopher Nowinski, *Head Games: Football's Concussion Crisis* (East Bridgewater, Mass.: Drummond, 2007). Details on Delaney's pro football research came from J. Scott Delaney et al., "Concussions during the 1997 Canadian Football League Season," *Clinical Journal of Sport Medicine* 10:9–14, 2000. Details on his college research came from J. Scott Delaney et al., "Concussions among University Football and Soccer Players," *Clinical Journal of Sport Medicine* 12:331–38, 2002.

Prevalence of problem in all sports: College data came from Kevin P. Kaut et al., "Reports of Head Injury and Symptom Knowledge among College Athletes: Implications for Assessment and Educational Intervention," *Clinical Journal of Sport Medicine* 13:213–21, 2003. High school data came from Ellen E. Yard and R. Dawn Comstock, "Compliance with Return to Play Guidelines Following Concussion in U.S. High School Athletes, 2005–2008," *Brain Injury* 23:888–98, 2009.

Incidence of soccer concussions: Comparisons based on data from Luke M. Gessell et al.,

"Concussions among United States High School and Collegiate Athletes," *Journal of Athletic Training* 42:495–503, 2007.

Melissa Inzitari's story: Narrative based on interviews with Melissa Inzitari, Katrina Majewski, and Jill Brooks, Ph.D. Additional details came from Peter Keating, "Heading for Trouble," *ESPN The Magazine*, March 23, 2009, and "Soccer: Head Start on Safety," Newark *Star-Ledger*, November 20, 2002. Brooks's research was described in the chapter titled "Concussion Management Programs for School-Age Children," which she contributed to Ruben J. Echemendía, ed., *Sports Neuropsychology: Assessment and Management of Traumatic Brain Injury* (New York: Guilford Press, 2006).

Chapter 4: Sudden Impact

Part I—Brian Radke's story: Narrative based on interviews with Brian and Nova Radke. Background information came from interviews with Jovita Bollig, Nova's mother, and Mike Bloomer, a friend who served with Brian in Iraq and remained close after they both returned to the Phoenix area. The quote from Brian's Walter Reed neurologist came from Jim Naughton, "Saving Sergeant Radke," *Neurology Now*, September/October 2006.

Part II—Chari Abb's story: Narrative based on interviews with Chari Abb; her mother, Chari Stoesser; Mark Sementilli, Ph.D.; and Tom Thompson. Background information came from an interview with Chris Abb and from Theodore Tsaousides and Wayne A. Gordon, "Cognitive Rehabilitation following Traumatic Brain Injury: Assessment to Treatment," *Mount Sinai Journal of Medicine* 76:173–81, 2009.

Chapter 5: Through the Cracks

Anne Forrest's story: Narrative based on interviews with Anne Forrest. Background information came from Sherri Dalphonse, " 'I Wanted My Brain Back,'" *Washingtonian*, March 2007.

Hidden TBIs: Discussion based on interviews with Wayne Gordon, Ph.D., and Tamar Martin, Ph.D. Some details came from Wayne A. Gordon et al., "The Enigma of 'Hidden' Traumatic Brain Injury," *Journal of Trauma Rehabilitation* 13:39–56, 1998, and Wayne A. Gordon, "Mild Traumatic Brain Injury: Identification, the Key to Preventing Social Failure," *Brain Injury Professional* 5:8–11, 2008. Background information came from "Studies Cite Head Injuries as Factor in Some Social Ills," *Wall Street Journal*, January 29, 2008.

Michael Zacchea's story: Narrative based on interviews with Michael Zacchea.

TBI in the military: Information was drawn from a variety of sources, including interviews with Charles Hoge, M.D.; Wayne Gordon, Ph.D.; and Warren Lux, M.D. Also helpful was the ABC television special *To Iraq and Back—Bob Woodruff Reports,* which aired on February 27, 2007. Details were also drawn from several studies, including Charles W. Hoge et al., "Mild Traumatic Brain Injury in U.S. Soldiers Returning from Iraq," *New England Journal of Medicine* 358:453–63, 2008; Charles W. Hoge et al., "Care of War Veterans with Mild Traumatic Brain Injury—Flawed Perspectives," *New England Journal of Medicine* 360:1588–91, 2009; Susan Connors et al., "Care of War Veterans with Mild Traumatic Brain Injury," *New England Journal of Medicine* 361:536–37, 2009; and Timothy Walilko et al., "Head Injury as a PTSD Predictor among Oklahoma City Bombing Survivors," *Journal of Trauma* 67:1311–19, 2009.

Chapter 6: Playing Defense

Mark Lenkiewicz's story: Narrative based on interviews with Mark and Diane Lenkiewicz and with Mark Lovell, Ph.D.

Development of neuropsychological testing: History based on interviews with Mark Lovell, Ph.D., and Joseph Maroon, M.D. Additional background came from several newspaper and magazine stories, including Michael Farber, "The Worst Case," *Sports Illustrated,* December 19, 1994. Details of the college study came from a chapter by Jeffrey T. Barth and colleagues titled "Mild Head Injury in Sports: Neuropsychological Sequelae and Recovery of Function," which was published in Harvey S. Levin et al., eds., *Mild Head Injury* (New York: Oxford University Press, 1989).

University of Pittsburgh Medical Center concussion program: Mark Lovell's background and his clinic's development based on interviews with Lovell, director of the UPMC Sports Medicine Concussion Program. Background information on the clinic came from interviews with Michael Collins, Ph.D., assistant director of the concussion program, and Freddie Fu, M.D., director of the UPMC Center for Sports Medicine.

Ben Roethlisberger's concussions: Details on the motorcycle crash and concussion came from multiple newspaper and magazine accounts. Details on the management of his football concussions came from an interview with Joseph Maroon as well as multiple newspaper stories in the *Pittsburgh Post-Gazette* and *New York Times,* including "Roethlisberger Case Stirs Debate Even after He Passes Concussion Tests," *New York Times,* November 5, 2006.

Angelica Kruth's story: Narrative based on interviews with Angelica and Doreen Kruth and with Mark Lovell, Ph.D.

Chapter 7: Anatomy of a Brain Injury

Part I—Phineas Gage's story: Narrative based on the original medical papers published by the treating physician. Chief among those were John M. Harlow, "Passage of an

Iron Rod through the Head," *Boston Medical and Surgical Journal* 39:389–93, 1848, and John M. Harlow, "Recovery from the Passage of an Iron Bar through the Head," *Publications of the American Medical Society* 2:327–47, 1868. Also referenced was Henry J. Bigelow, "Dr. Harlow's Case of Recovery from the Passage of an Iron Bar through the Head," *American Journal of the Medical Sciences* 20:13–22, 1850. A debt is owed to the world's leading authority on the case for reprinting those medical papers and providing comprehensive details in Malcolm Macmillan, *An Odd Kind of Fame: Stories of Phineas Gage* (Cambridge, Mass.: MIT Press, 2000). Details on the modern neuroimaging of the skull came from Hanna Damasio et al., "The Return of Phineas Gage: Clues about the Brain from the Skull of a Famous Patient," *Science* 264:1102–5, 1994. Perspective and background was provided in Antonio R. Damasio, *Descartes' Error: Emotion, Reason, and the Human Brain* (New York: Grosset/Putnam, 1994), and John Fleischman, *Phineas Gage: A Gruesome but True Story about Brain Science* (Boston: Houghton Mifflin, 2002).

Part II—Broca's brains: Details on Broca's patients and his discovery came from Francis Schiller, *Paul Broca: Founder of French Anthropology, Explorer of the Brain* (Berkeley: University of California Press, 1979), and J. M. S. Pearce, "Broca's Aphasiacs," *European Neurology* 61:183–89, 2009. MRI scans of Broca's brains described in N. F. Dronkers et al., "Paul Broca's Historic Cases: High Resolution MR Imaging of the Brains of Leborgne and Lelong," *Brain* 130:1432–41, 2007.

Part III—H.M.'s story: Details on Henry Molaison's life, surgery, and impact on memory research came from William Beecher Scoville and Brenda Milner, "Loss of Recent Memory after Bilateral Hippocampal Lesions," *Journal of Neurology, Neurosurgery & Psychiatry* 20:11–21, 1957; Philip J. Hilts, *Memory's Ghost: The Strange Tale of Mr. M and the Nature of Memory* (New York: Simon & Schuster, 1995); and "H.M., an Unforgettable Amnesiac, Dies at 82," *New York Times*, December 5, 2008.

Chapter 8: Deciphering the Damage

Discovery of diffuse axonal injury: Details came from an interview with John Polvishock, Ph.D., and from John Povlishock et al., "Axonal Change in Minor Head Injury," *Journal of Neuropathology & Experimental Neurology* 42:225–42, 1983; J. Hume Adams et al., "Diffuse Brian Damage of Immediate Impact Type: Its Relationship to Primary Brain Stem Damage in Head Injury," *Brain* 100:489–502, 1977; and Thomas A. Gennarelli et al., "Diffuse Axonal Injury: An Important Form of Traumatic Brain Damage," *Neuroscientist* 4:202–15, 1998.

Smith research on axon stretching: Discussion based on interviews with Douglas Smith, M.D., and on Douglas H. Smith and David F. Meany, "Axonal Damage in Traumatic Brain Injury," *Neuroscientist* 6:483–94, 2000; Min D. Tang-Schomer et al., "Mechanical Breaking of Microtubules in Axons during Dynamic Stretch Injury Underlies Delayed Elasticity, Microtubule Disassembly, and Axon Degeneration," *FASEB Journal* 24:1401–10, 2009; and Tracey J. Yuen et al., "Sodium Channelopathy Induced by Mild Axonal Trauma Worsens Outcome after a Repeat Injury," *Journal of Neuroscience Research* 87:3620–25, 2009.

Axonal injury in mild TBI: Information came from P. C. Blumbergs et al., "Staining of Amyloid Precursor Protein to Study Axonal Damage in Mild Head Injury," *Lancet* 344:1055–56, 1994.

Research on duration of concussion effects: Information came from interviews with David Hovda, Ph.D., and from Atsuo Yoshino et al., "Dynamic Changes in Local Glucose Utilization following Cerebral Concussion in Rats: Evidence of a Hyper- and Subsequent Hypometabolic State," *Brain Research* 561:106–19, 1991; and David A. Hovda et al., "Diffuse Prolonged Depression of Cerebral Oxidative Metabolism following Concussive Brain Injury in the Rat: A Cytochrome Oxidase Histochemistry Study," *Brain Research* 567:1–10, 1991.

Research on loss of plasticity: Discussion based on interviews with David Hovda, Ph.D., and on Christopher C. Giza et al., "Experience Dependent Behavioral Plasticity Is Disturbed following Traumatic Brain Injury in the Immature Brain," *Behavioral Brain Research* 157:11–22, 2005; Christopher C. Giza et al., "N-Methyl-D-Aspartate Receptor Subunit Changes after Traumatic Injury to the Developing Brain," *Journal of Neurotrauma* 23:950–61, 2006; Igor Fineman et al., "Inhibition of Neocortical Plasticity during Development by a Moderate Concussive Brain Injury," *Journal of Neurotrauma* 17:739–49, 2000; and Daniel J. Olesniewicz et al., "Repeated Measures of Cognitive Processing Efficiency in Adolescent Athletes: Implications for Monitoring Recovery from Concussion," *Neuropsychiatry, Neuropsychology, & Behavioral Neurology* 12:167–69, 1999.

Metabolic cascade: Discussion based on interviews with David Hovda, Ph.D.; Edward Hall, Ph.D., director of the University of Kentucky Spinal Cord and Brain Injury Research Center; and Jonathan Lifshitz, Ph.D., also with the University of Kentucky Spinal Cord and Brain Injury Research Center. Some details came from Christopher C. Giza and David A. Hovda, "The Neurometabolic Cascade of Concussion," *Journal of Athletic Training* 36:228–35, 2001.

Imaging: Discussion based on interviews with David Hovda, Ph.D.; Mark Lovell, Ph.D.; and Michael Lipton, M.D., Ph.D. Some details came from Marvin Bergsneider et al., "Dissociation of Cerebral Glucose and Level of Consciousness during the Period of Metabolic Depression following Human Traumatic Brain Injury," *Journal of Neurotrauma* 17:389–401, 2000, and Michael L. Lipton et al., "Diffusion-Tensor Imaging Implicates Prefrontal Axonal Injury in Executive Function Impairment following Very Mild Traumatic Brain Injury," *Radiology* 252:816–24, 2009.

Link between Alzheimer's and TBI: Narrative constructed from interviews with Douglas Smith, M.D., and from Kunihiro Uryu et al., "Multiple Proteins Implicated in Neurodegenerative Diseases Accumulate in Axons after Brain Trauma in Humans," *Experimental Neurology* 208:185–92, 2007; Victoria E. Johnson et al., "A Neprilysin Polymorphism and Amyloid-beta Plaques following Traumatic Brain Injury," *Journal of Neurotrauma* [epub 2009, ahead of print]; Xaio-Han Chen et al., "A Lack of Amyloid Beta Plaques Despite Persistent Accumulation of Amyloid Beta in Axons of Long-Term Survivors of Traumatic Brain Injury," *Brain Pathology* 19:214–23, 2009; and Victoria E. Johnson et al., "Traumatic Brain Injury and Amyloid-Beta Pathology: A Link to Alzheimer's Disease?" *Nature Reviews Neuroscience* [epub 2010, ahead of print].

Chapter 9: A Pocketful of Mumbles

Jerry Quarry's story: Narrative based on numerous newspaper and magazine articles chronicling his background, career, and decline. A special debt is owed to Steve Wilstein for his October 24, 1995, Associated Press feature providing the most comprehensive firsthand account of Quarry's descent into dementia. Another indispensable account came from William Plummer, "A Life on the Ropes," *People*, February 19, 1996. Additional details and quotes came from Pete Hamill, "Blood on Their Hands," *Esquire*, June 1996; "Damaging Blows for Boxing," *Newsday*, July 10, 1996; "Jerry Quarry," *Cyber Boxing Zone*, September 1998; obituaries in *The New York Times*, *Newsday*, and *Washington Times*; and information from the Jerry Quarry Foundation for Dementia Pugilistica.

Sports Illustrated neurological testing: Details came from the magazine's special report— Robert H. Boyle and Wilmer Ames, "Too Many Punches, Too Little Concern," *Sports Illustrated*, April 11, 1983, and Jeff Wheelwright, "A Conversation with The Greatest," *Sports Illustrated*, April 11, 1983. Other *Sports Illustrated* news and feature articles from 1965 to 1999 also informed accounts of heavyweight fights and of Quarry's upbringing, career, and dementia pugilistica.

Martland's landmark punch-drunk paper: Narrative based on the article as read before the New York Pathological Society at the New York Academy of Medicine—Harrison S. Martland, "Punch Drunk," *Journal of the American Medical Association* 91:1103–7, 1928. A debt is owed to the protégé who authored the definitive biography—Samuel Berg, *Harrison Stanford Martland, M.D.: The Story of a Physician, a Hospital, an Era* (New York: Vantage Press, 1978). Background information came from Lois R. Densky-Wolff, "Harrison S. Martland, MD," *Medical History Society of New Jersey*, 26:5, 2006, and Deborah Blum, "Will Science Take the Field?" *New York Times*, February 5, 2010. Nathan Ehrlich's identification as the parkinsonian patient in the "Punch Drunk" paper came from cross-referencing details in Martland's 1928 *Journal of the*

American Medical Association article with information contained in boxing references including *The Ring Boxing Encyclopedia and Record Book.*

Critchley's chronic traumatic encephalopathy study: Details came from Macdonald Critchley, "Medical Aspects of Boxing, Particularly from a Neurological Standpoint," *British Medical Journal* 5015:357–62, 1957.

Roberts's landmark epidemiological study: Narrative based on the original book-length report, A. H. Roberts, *Brain Damage in Boxers: A Study of the Prevalence of Traumatic Encephalopathy among Ex-Professional Boxers* (London: Pitman Medical and Scientific Publishing, 1969). Background on genesis of study came from "Medical Notes in Parliament," *British Medical Journal* 1:1423–24, 1962, and "Medical News," *British Medical Journal* 1:1099, 1963. Perspective on the study's significance provided by Barry D. Jordan's chapter titled "Boxing," which was published in Barry D. Jordan, ed., *Sports Neurology* (Philadelphia: Lippincott–Raven, 1998); and from Robert H. Boyle and Wilmer Ames, "Too Many Punches, Too Little Concern," *Sports Illustrated*, April 11, 1983.

Corsellis's landmark pathological study: Some details came from J. A. N. Corsellis, "Boxing and the Brain," *British Medical Journal* 298:105–9, 1989; T. J. Crow, "Obituary: J. A. N. Corsellis," *Psychiatric Bulletin* 20:508–9, 1996; and Robert H. Boyle and Wilmer Ames, "Too Many Punches, Too Little Concern," *Sports Illustrated*, April 11, 1983.

Slapsie Maxie Rosenbloom: Details came from several sources, notably Jeff Wheelwright, "How Punchy Was Slapsie Maxie?" *Sports Illustrated*, April 11, 1983, and "Damaging Blows for Boxing," *Newsday*, July 10, 1996.

Early CAT scan studies: Discussion based on Ira R. Casson et al., "Neurological and CT Evaluation of Knocked-out Boxers," *Journal of Neurology, Neurosurgery, and Psychiatry* 45:170–74, 1982; M. Kaste et al., "Is Chronic Brain Damage in Boxing a Hazard of the Past?" *Lancet* 320:1186–88, 1982; and Ronald J. Ross et al., "Boxers—Computed Tomography, EEG, and Neurological Evaluation," *Journal of the American Medical Association* 249:211–13, 1983.

Sugar Ray Robinson: Narrative based on multiple sources. Details and background came from Sugar Ray Robinson with Dave Anderson, *Sugar Ray* (New York: Viking Press, 1969); Herb Boyd with Ray Robinson II, *Pound for Pound: A Biography of Sugar Ray Robinson* (New York: Amistad, 2005); Kenneth Shropshire, *Being Sugar Ray: The Life of Sugar Ray Robinson, America's Greatest Boxer and the First Celebrity Athlete* (New York: Basic Civitas, 2007); and Wil Haygood, *Sweet Thunder: The Life and Times of Sugar Ray Robinson* (New York: Knopf, 2009).

Head injury's link to Alzheimer's: Statistic from Paul Dash and Nicole Villemarette-Pittman, *Alzheimer's Disease* (New York: Demos Medical Publishing, 2005).

Champions with dementia pugilistica: Background on Willie Pep and Sandy Saddler from "The Lonely Fight," *Newsday*, July 3, 1994. Details on Wilfred Benítez from "Taking Care of a Favorite Son," *New York Times*, May 5, 1996, and "Too Many Beatings," *New York Times*, November 12, 1997.

Physics of boxing: Data on force of heavyweight punches came from J. Atha et al., "The Damaging Punch," *British Medical Journal* 291:1756–57, 1985, and Peter Stoler, "Medicine: Ali Fights a New Round," *Time*, October 1, 1985.

Muhammad Ali's story: A special debt is owed to the definitive authorized biography, Thomas Hauser, *Muhammad Ali: His Life and Times* (New York: Simon & Schuster, 1991). Also indispensable were books authored by Ali's ringside physician—Ferdie Pacheco, *Fight Doctor* (New York: Simon & Schuster, 1976); Ferdie Pacheco, *Muhammad Ali: A View from the Corner* (New York: Birch Lane Press, 1992); and Ferdie Pacheco, *Blood in My Coffee: The Life of The Fight Doctor* (Champaign, Ill.: Sports Publishing, 2005). Additional details and background came from multiple sources, including David Remnick, *King of the World: Muhammad Ali and the Rise of an American Hero* (New York: Random House, 1998); Mark Kram, *Ghosts of Manila: The Fateful Blood Feud between Muhammad Ali and Joe Frazier* (New York: HarperCollins, 2001); "Fans, Friends Worried, But Ali Says 'I'm Fine,'" *Jet*, October 8, 1984; Rick Telander, "Facing Facts about Ali," *Sports Illustrated*, July 1, 1991; and Wallace Matthews, "Fighting Spirit," *Neurology Now*, March/April 2006.

Quarry brothers: Details of careers and family legacy based on multiple sources, notably Steve Wilstein's October 24, 1995, Associated Press feature on Jerry Quarry. Other helpful sources included William Plummer, "A Life on the Ropes," *People*, February 19, 1996; "Mike Quarry, 55; Had Boxing-Induced Dementia," *New York Times*, June 14, 2006; Jonathan Mahler, "Staying in the Ring," *New York Times Magazine*, December 31, 2006; and the Jerry Quarry Foundation for Dementia Pugilistica.

Genetic research: Discussion based on an interview with Barry Jordan, M.D. Details of his seminal apoE ε4 study came from Barry D. Jordan et al., "Apolipoprotein E E4 Associated with Chronic Traumatic Brain Injury in Boxing," *Journal of the American Medical Association* 278:136–40, 1997. Information on TBI raising risk for Alzheimer's in people with apoE ε4 came from R. Mayeux, "Synergistic Effects of Traumatic Head Injury and Apolipoprotein-ε4 in Patients with Alzheimer's Disease," *Neurology* 45:555–57, 1995. Background on Jordan's study came from "Research Hints at a Gene Link to Brain Afflictions of Boxers," *New York Times*, July 9, 1997. Background information on Jordan came from "Rebel Neurologists Say Boxing Can Be Safe," *New York Times*, May 22, 1990, and James Thornton, "A Genetic Link to Boxing Impairment?" *Physician and Sports Medicine*, September 1997.

Medical opposition to boxing: AMA editorial position came from George D. Lundberg, "Boxing Should Be Banned in Civilized Countries," *Journal of the American Medical Association* 249:250, 1983, and background information came from Maurice W. Van Allen, "The Deadly Degrading Sport," *Journal of the American Medical Association* 249:250–51, 1983. Details of smoking gun study came from Ira R. Casson et al., "Brain Damage in Modern Boxers," *Journal of the American Medical Association* 251:2663–67, 1984. Details on international crusade to ban boxing came from the British Medical Association's 1993 report titled "The Boxing Debate." AAN position came from multiple sources, notably an October 6, 1984, Associated Press story published in numerous newspapers. Fatality statistics came from multiple sources based on figures published annually in *The Ring Boxing Encyclopedia and Record Book*.

Safety reforms: Based on an interview with Barry Jordan, M.D. Additional information came from Arthur Allen, "Cruel Blows," *Salon*, April 30, 1999, and "Rebel Neurologists Say Boxing Can Be Safe," *New York Times*, May 22, 1990.

Floyd Patterson's story: Narrative based on multiple sources, notably Thomas Hauser, *Muhammad Ali: His Life and Times* (New York: Simon & Schuster, 1991); David Remnick, *King of the World: Muhammad Ali and the Rise of an American Hero* (New York: Random House, 1998); "No More Excuses: It's Time to Ban Boxing," *Holland Sentinel*, April 11, 1998.

Chapter 10: Ticking Time Bombs

Bennet Omalu's story: Narrative based on an interview with Bennet Omalu, M.D. Discussion of his seminal CTE case studies based on Bennet I. Omalu et al., "Chronic Traumatic Encephalopathy in a National Football League Player," *Neurosurgery* 57:128–34, 2005; Bennet I. Omalu et al., "Chronic Traumatic Encephalopathy in a National Football League Player: Part II," *Neurosurgery* 59:1086–93, 2006; Casson et al., "Correspondence: Chronic Traumatic Encephalopathy in a National Football League Player," *Neurosurgery* 58:E1003, 2006. Some details came from Bennet Omalu, *Play Hard, Die Young: Football Dementia, Depression, and Death* (Lodi, Calif.: Neo-Forenxis Books, 2008); " 'Brain Chaser' Tackles Effects of NFL Hits," *Washington Post*, April 25, 2007; and Jeanne Marie Laskas, "This Is Your Brain on Football," *GQ*, October 2009.

Mike Webster's story: Details came from multiple sources, notably Greg Garber's five-part series on *ESPN.com* ("A Tormented Soul," January 24, 2005; "Blood and Guts," January 25, 2005; "Man on the Moon," January 26, 2005; "Wandering through the Fog," January 27, 2005; "Sifting the Ashes," January 28, 2005), "Former Steeler's Family Wins Disability Ruling," *New York Times*, December 14, 2006; Jeanne Marie Laskas, "This Is Your Brain on Football," *GQ*, October 2009; "Research Finds Football Hits May Lead to Brain Injury," *ABCNews.com*, October 16, 2009; Bennet Omalu, *Play Hard, Die Young: Football Dementia, Depression, and Death* (Lodi, Calif.: Neo-Forenxis Books, 2008); and congressional testimony on June 26, 2007, by Cyril V. Smith, a partner in Zuckerman Spaeder, the law firm representing Webster.

Terry Long controversy: Details came from "Wecht: Long Died from Brain Injury," *Pittsburgh Post-Gazette*, September 14, 2005; "Surgeon Disagrees with Wecht That Football Killed Long," *Pittsburgh Post-Gazette*, September 15, 2005; "Steelers Doctor Says Concluding Football Led to Long's Demise Is Bad Science," *Pittsburgh Post-Gazette*,

September 16, 2005; "Document Says Former Steeler Drank Antifreeze in Suicide," *New York Times*, January 27, 2006; and Bennet Omalu, *Play Hard, Die Young: Football Dementia, Depression, and Death* (Lodi, Calif.: Neo-Forenxis Books, 2008).

Chris Nowinski's story: Narrative based on interviews with Chris Nowinski. Some details came from Christopher Nowinski, *Head Games: Football's Concussion Crisis* (East Bridgewater, Mass.: Drummond, 2007).

Andre Waters's story: Details came from "Expert Ties Ex-Player's Suicide to Brain Damage from Football," *New York Times*, January 18, 2007; "Brain Chasers," ESPN's *Outside the Lines*, August 12, 2007; and Bennet Omalu, *Play Hard, Die Young: Football Dementia, Depression, and Death* (Lodi, Calif.: Neo-Forenxis Books, 2008).

Justin Strzelczyk's story: Details came from multiple news sources, notably "Lineman, Dead at 36, Sheds Light on Brain Injuries," *New York Times*, June 15, 2007, and "Brain Chasers," ESPN's *Outside the Lines*, August 12, 2007. Background information came from interviews with Bennet Omalu, M.D., and Julian Bailes, M.D.

Chris Benoit's story: Details came from interviews with Nowinski and Omalu as well as from newspaper accounts.

Sports Legacy Institute and Center for the Study of Traumatic Encephalopathy: Details came from interviews with Nowinski, Cantu, and Robert Stern, Ph.D.

Ann McKee's research: Discussion based on interviews with Ann McKee, M.D., and on Ann C. McKee et al., "Chronic Traumatic Encephalopathy in Athletes: Progressive Tauopathy after Repetitive Head Injury," *Journal of Neuropathology & Experimental Neurology* 68:709–35, 2009. Additional background came from "What Football Did for Us and . . . What Football Did to Us," *Chicago Sun-Times*, June 25, 2010, and Caleb Daniloff, "Game Changers," *Bostonia*, Fall 2010.

Paul Pender's story: Details on announced cause of death came from an Associated Press obituary published in numerous newspapers on January 14, 2003. His identification as CTE patient came from cross-referencing details in Ann C. McKee's 2009 *Journal of Neuropathology & Experimental Neurology* article with information contained in numerous boxing books including *The Ring Boxing Encyclopedia and Record Book*.

John Grimsley's story: Details came from "Deadly Aftershocks," *Philadelphia Daily News*, May 28, 2009.

Rival labs: Details on the West Virginia University lab came from interviews with Brain Injury Research Center co-founders Julian Bailes, M.D., and Bennet Omalu, M.D. Details on the scientific rivalry came from Jeanne Marie Laskas, "This Is Your Brain on Football," *GQ*, October 2009, and Peter Keating, "Coming to a Head," *ESPN The Magazine*, January 10, 2011.

Sylvia Mackey's and Eleanor Perfetto's stories: Narrative based on an interview with Eleanor Perfetto. Details came from numerous newspaper and magazine articles. A debt is owed to Alan Schwarz for a series of articles on long-term consequences of concussions, notably "Wives United by Husbands' Post-N.F.L. Trauma," *New York Times*,

March 14, 2007; "N.F.L. Meeting Irks Wives of Ill Retirees," *New York Times*, December 13, 2008; "Worker Safety Case on Dementia Tests N.F.L.," *New York Times*, April 6, 2010; "In N.F.L., Women Lead the Way," *New York Times*, April 11, 2010. Also helpful were a host of newspaper stories, notably "A Trailblazer's New Path," *Baltimore Sun*, November 23, 2003; "NFL Neglect of Mackey Belongs in Hall of Shame," *Baltimore Sun*, December 27, 2005; and " '88 Plan': Honor for a Declining NFL Warrior," Associated Press, March 23, 2007. Some details came from radio and television broadcasts, including "John Mackey: From the NFL to Dementia," *CBSNews.com*, April 28, 2007; "Head On," HBO's *Real Sports*, May 14, 2007; "Concussions and the NFL," NPR's *On Point*, December 19, 2008; Frank Deford, "The Cautionary Tale of John Mackey, NFL Star," NPR's *Morning Edition*, January 6, 2009; and "A Blow to the Brain," CBS's *60 Minutes*, October 11, 2009.

Chapter 11: Seeds of Change

NFL concussion summit conference: Based on multiple news accounts, including "Compromise Reigns at Summit on Concussions," *Washington Post*, June 20, 2007; "Player Silence on Concussions May Block N.F.L. Guidelines," *New York Times*, June 20, 2007; and Jeanne Marie Laskas, "This Is Your Brain on Football," *GQ*, October 2009. Background information came from an interview with Julian Bailes, M.D., and from multiple news stories, including "Concussion Panel Has Shakeup As Data Is Questioned," *New York Times*, March 1, 2007; "Concussions Tied to Depression in Ex-N.F.L. Players," *New York Times*, May 21, 2007; "Update on Concussions and the NFL: Medicine Fast Framing Theories with Hard Data," *Pittsburgh Post-Gazette*, June 17, 2007.

Dementia research: Details came from interviews with Kevin Guskiewicz, Ph.D., and from the following studies—Kevin M. Guskiewicz, "Recurrent Concussion and Risk of Depression in Retired Professional Football Players," *Medicine & Science in Sports & Exercise* 39:903–9, 2007, and Kevin M. Guskiewicz, "Association between Recurrent Concussion and Late-Life Cognitive Impairment in Retired Professional Football Players," *Neurosurgery* 57:719–26, 2005.

Ira Casson controversy: Details came from multiple print and broadcast sources, notably "Head On," HBO's *Real Sports*, May 14, 2007.

Ted Johnson controversy: Details came from "Dark Days Follow Hard-Hitting Career in N.F.L.," *New York Times*, February 2, 2007; " 'I Don't Want Anyone to End up Like Me,' " *Boston Globe*, February 2, 2007; and "N.F.L. Culture Makes Issue of Head Injuries Even Murkier," *New York Times*, February 3, 2007.

Roger Goodell's concussion challenge: Characterization of the exploding epidemic from column by Michael Wilbon, "NFL Facing the Truth about Head Injuries," *Washington Post*, August 8, 2010.

NFL's 2007 policy changes: Announcement of policies and quotes from informational pamphlet came from the NFL's August 14, 2007, press release titled "NFL Outlines for Players Steps Taken to Address Concussions."

Super Bowl press conference: Narrative based on multiple news stories. Ann McKee's reaction to finding CTE in an eighteen-year-old brain came from "Parents, Doctors Prod NFL on Brain Injuries," *Boston Globe*, February 2, 2010.

NFL MTBI Committee meeting: Details came from an interview with Chris Nowinski and from Caleb Daniloff, "Game Changers," *Bostonia*, Fall 2010.

NFL dementia survey study: Details came from a report titled "Study of Retired NFL Players," which was prepared by David R. Weir and colleagues at the University of Michigan's Institute for Social Research and submitted to the NFL Player Care Foundation on September 10, 2009. Background information came from "Dementia Risk Seen in Players in N.F.L. Study," *New York Times*, September 30, 2009.

NFL's 2009 policy changes: Details came from the NFL's December 2, 2009, press release announcing stricter concussion guidelines.

Ben Roethlisberger concussion controversy: Details came from multiple news stories, including "With Roethlisberger's Injury, Team Goals and Player Safety Collide," *New York Times*, December 1, 2009.

NFL's change of direction: Details on overhaul of concussion committee came from "Leaders of N.F.L. Head Injury Study Resign," *New York Times*, November 25, 2009, and "N.F.L. Suspends Its Study of the Effect of Concussions on Retired Players," *New York Times*, December 20, 2009.

NFL's funding of outside research: Details on the NFL underwriting the Center for the Study of Traumatic Encephalopathy's research came from "N.F.L. Gives $1 Million to Brain Researchers," *New York Times*, April 21, 2010. Establishment reaction to Chris Nowinski's advocacy came from an interview with Nowinski and from "What Football Did for Us and . . . What Football Did to Us," *Chicago Sun-Times*, June 25, 2010. Reaction to Ann McKee's CTE discoveries came from Caleb Daniloff, "Game Changers," *Bostonia*, Fall 2010.

Roger Goodell's youth advocacy: Details of legislative campaign came from a May 23, 2010, Associated Press story titled "Goodell Sends Letter to 44 Governors." Details of meeting with Robert Cantu came from Caleb Daniloff, "Game Changers," *Bostonia*, Fall 2010, and Peter Keating, "Coming to a Head," *ESPN The Magazine*, January 10, 2011.

CTE cases involving younger brains: Details of Chris Henry's story came from multiple news accounts, including "Ex-Bengal Is First in N.F.L. Known to Play with Brain Trauma," *New York Times*, June 29, 2010. Details of Owen Thomas's story came from multiple news accounts, including "In College Player's Suicide, Signs of Disease That Haunts N.F.L.," *New York Times*, September 14, 2010.

Hit-impact research: Background on studies of head impacts in college football players came from an interview with Kevin Guskiewicz, Ph.D. Details on his own research came from various articles and published studies conducted by his Department of Exercise and Sport Science at the University of North Carolina–Chapel Hill. Additional information came from various articles, including Malcolm Gladwell, "Offensive Play," *New Yorker*, October 19, 2009, and "Safer Football, Taught from Inside the Helmet," *New York Times*, November 6, 2010. Details of the 2010 study involving three NCAA football teams came from "For Head Injuries, a Problem in Practice," *New York Times*, September 17, 2010. Details of the high school impact study came from Thomas M. Talavage et al., "Functionally-Detected Cognitive Impairment in High School Football Players without Clinically-Diagnosed Concussion," *Journal of Neurotrauma*, published early online in October 2010, and David Epstein, "The Damage Done," *Sports Illustrated*, November 1, 2010. Details on Virginia Tech's pioneering use of helmet-sensor technology came from the September 17, 2010, *Times* article and various other stories, including "Concussion Worries Renew Focus on Football Safety," NPR, September 25, 2010.

Certified athletic trainers: Statistic came from the National Athletic Trainers' Association.

Neuropsychological testing: Details on how trainers use neuropsych tests came from Tracey Covassin et al., "Immediate Post-Concussion Assessment and Cognitive Testing (ImPACT) Practices of Sports Medicine Professionals," *Journal of Athletic Training* 44:639–44, 2009. Details on the Washington state school district that rejected use of ImPACT came from "Despite Law, Town Finds Concussion Dangers Lurk," *New York Times*, September 23, 2010. Kevin Guskiewicz's quote came from Michael Popke, "Hit Hard," *Athletic Business*, December 2009.

College football controversy: Details came from "Put Me In, Doc: When Doctors Must Say No to Athletes," *American Medical News*, October 25, 2010.

Mayo Clinic concussion conference: Details came from multiple news stories, including "With Focus on Youth Safety, a Sport Considers Changes," *New York Times*, October 17, 2010; "Panel Urges Hockey to Ban Blows to Head at All Levels," *New York Times*, October 21, 2010; and "N.H.L. Declines to Modify Head-Checking Rule," *New York Times*, October 22, 2010.

Canadian youth hockey study: Concussion data in peewee leagues came from Carolyn A. Emery et al., "Risk of Injury Associated with Body Checking among Youth Ice Hockey Players," *Journal of the American Medical Association* 303:2265–72, 2010.

Philadelphia Eagles concussion controversy: Coverage of Stewart Bradley's missed concussion came from multiple news stories, including "Return of a Stumbling Eagle Raises Concerns," *New York Times*, September 14, 2010; "Too Little Time to Assess Injury," *Philadelphia Inquirer*, September 15, 2010; "Televised Collapse Delivers Warning on Unseen Injuries," *New York Times*, September 16, 2010; and "Silence Follows Announcers' Concern," *New York Times*, September 17, 2010.

Epilogue

Dave Showalter's story: Narrative based on interviews with Dave Showalter.

NFL crackdown: Details of the head hits that led to the tipping point and the NFL's response to them came from multiple news stories. James Harrison's quote came from "Defenders Criticize N.F.L. for Helmet-to-Helmet Fines," *New York Times*, October 21, 2010. Description of player pushback and relevant quotes came from Peter King, "Concussions: The Hits That Are Changing Football," *Sports Illustrated*, November 1, 2010, and "Urlacher Upset with NFL Flagrant Hits Policy," *Chicago Tribune*, October 19, 2010. The newspaper columns cited were by William Rhoden, "To Lower Violence, Escalate the Penalty," *New York Times*, October 18, 2010, and Brad Wilson, "Philadelphia Eagles' Head Coach Andy Reid Knows Preventing Head Injuries Is Worth Causing a Period of Uncertainty in the NFL," Easton *Express-Times*, November 9, 2010.

Madden NFL: Details on the video game's redesign came from "Madden Puts Concussions in New Light in His Game," *New York Times*, April 3, 2011. Background on the video game's history came from Tim Layden, "The Big Hits," *Sports Illustrated*, July 30, 2007.

Dave Duerson's story: Details came from the BU Center for the Study of Traumatic Encephalopathy's press conference on May 1, 2011; from several *New York Times* news stories; and from Paul Solotaroff with Rick Telander, "The Ferocious Life and Tragic Death of a Super Bowl Star," *Men's Journal*, May 2011.

Sidney Crosby's story: Details of his head injuries and their aftermath came from *Pittsburgh Post-Gazette* news stories of January 8, 2011; January 9, 2011; January 25, 2011; and April 30, 2011. Background on his concussion's impact on the NHL came from *New York Times* stories of January 21, 2011, and March 14, 2011. Pat LaFontaine's quotes came from Craig Custance, "LaFontaine: A Cautionary Tale," *Sporting News*, March 14, 2011.

Troy Aikman: Quotes came from Troy Aikman, "The NFL Should Proceed with Caution on Head Injuries," *Sporting News*, December 21, 2009.

Harry Carson's story: Details came from John Solomon, "Retirement Plan #2," *Sports Illustrated*, June 1, 1998; William Nack, "The Wrecking Yard," *Sports Illustrated*, May 7, 2001; Bob Drury, "This Is Your Brain on Multiple Concussions," *Men's Health*, July/August 2006; Greg Garber, "Concussions Still Carson's Concern," *ESPN.com*, February 2, 2010; and Victoria Schlesinger, "Heads Up," *Discover Presents The Brain*, Spring 2010.

Index

Page numbers in *italics* refer to illustrations.

About the Authors

Linda Carroll is a nationally respected health writer with an expertise in brain science. Over the past two decades she has covered a wide range of health topics for prominent publications, including *msnbc.com*, *Newsday*, and *The New York Times*. As a contract writer for *msnbc* for the past fifteen years, she has written investigative stories, news features, and the women's health column. She has also written investigative pieces for *Health* and *SmartMoney*.

David Rosner is a longtime journalist with extensive experience covering sports and health. While on staff at *Newsday*, he won national awards for sports writing and investigative reporting. In addition to writing for national magazines, he has co-authored a hockey history book and helped create an award-winning website serving athletes with disabilities. He developed brain injury expertise as managing editor of *Neurology Now*, the official patients' magazine of the American Academy of Neurology.